BIOLOGICAL HAZARDS

BIOLOGICAL HAZARDS

AN ORYX SOURCEBOOK

Joan R. Callahan

Oryx Sourcebooks on Hazards and Disasters

ORYX Press
Westport, Connecticut • London

The rare Arabian Oryx is believed to have inspired the myth of the unicorn. This desert antelope became virtually extinct in the early 1960s. At that time, several groups of international conservationists arranged to have nine animals sent to the Phoenix Zoo to be the nucleus of a captive breeding herd. Today, the Oryx population is over 1,000, and over 500 have been returned to the Middle East.

Library of Congress Cataloging-in-Publication Data

Callahan, Joan R.
    Biological hazards : an Oryx sourcebook / Joan R. Callahan.
       p.   cm.—(Oryx sourcebooks on hazards and disasters)
    Includes bibliographical references and index.
    ISBN 1–57356–385–4 (alk. paper)
       1. Environmentally induced diseases—Handbooks, manuals, etc.   2. Environmental toxicology—Handbooks, manuals, etc.   I. Title.   II. Series.
    RB152.5.C354   2002
    615.9′02—dc21   2001055184

British Library Cataloguing in Publication Data is available.

Library of Congress Catalog Card Number: 2001055184
ISBN: 1–57356–385–4

First published in 2002

Oryx Press, 88 Post Road West, Westport, CT 06881
An imprint of Greenwood Publishing Group, Inc.
www.oryxpress.com

Printed in the United States of America

∞™

The paper used in this book complies with the Permanent Paper Standard issued by the National Information Standards Organization (Z39.48–1984).

10 9 8 7 6 5 4 3 2 1

For Daniel

Contents

Preface

> What's true of all the evils in the world is true of plague as well.
> It helps men to rise above themselves.
> —Albert Camus, *The Plague* (1948)

The oldest known story, recorded on cave walls across Europe in the late Pleistocene, tells of a hunter who was killed by a bison. The oldest surviving book, the *Epic of Gilgamesh* (2700 B.C.), is about a hero who went out from the city to slay the great bull of heaven. Gilgamesh was less successful as a physician than as a cowpuncher; a snake foiled his quest for a medicinal plant, and he lost his best friend to a disease, sent by the gods as punishment for cutting a forest.

Of all the world's dangers, the living ones are the most reliable, both as literary themes and as hard fact. Biological hazards—poisons and pathogens, monsters and serpents—have packed theaters and grave-yards from antiquity. The purpose of this book is to acquaint readers with these hazards and with their associated risks and rewards. In the Oryx tradition, we have presented this material in the form of a compact reference handbook for library, personal, or classroom use.

As the book will serve a general readership with a wide range of backgrounds, the titles of the disease chapters reflect the modes of transmission (in other words, how people catch the disease) rather than a more technical classification. Later chapters deal with larger, more photogenic hazards, particularly those with teeth. As many diseases and other biological hazards propagate themselves in more than one way, each chapter also contains a cross-reference table of related references in other chapters. The book does not attempt to describe all known biological hazards, or to present all known facts regarding any hazard, but it provides reference lists to steer the interested reader in the right direction.

Within each chapter and section, the material appears in the sequence dictated by taxonomy, risk, the alphabet, or other criteria as applicable. For each biological hazard category, the book presents current scientific knowledge on causes, preventive measures, costs, outlook, and other topics of interest, with older examples to provide historical context. The source for most of this information is the published literature of science and history; in addition, each chapter ends with an anecdote that illustrates some of its major themes.

Chapter 1 discusses the nature of hazards and their influence on human history and behavior. It also defines some key terms and concepts that appear later in the book.

Chapters 2, 3, and 4 present examples of waterborne, foodborne, and airborne diseases, respectively. The focus is on topics in the news—disease outbreaks in North America caused by polluted wells, tainted hamburgers, and the like—but not at the expense of more exotic pathogens that threaten developing nations, and may one day reach our own shores.

Chapter 5 is about diseases that are transmitted by physical contact with a source or intermediary, such as a sex partner, a mosquito, or a cat's claws. The chapter contains three main sections: sexually transmitted diseases, vectorborne diseases, and diseases transmitted by other forms of contact.

Chapter 6 presents examples of diseases and pests that threaten agricultural crops and domestic animals that are important to our well-being. They are biological hazards in the sense that the loss of these resources can cause major economic hardship and famine, particularly in developing nations.

Chapter 7 begins the material that many readers may regard as the good stuff: venomous snakes, spiders, and scorpions, killer bees, poisonous plants and fungi, life-threatening allergic reactions, and addictive chemicals of biological origin, such as cocaine and nicotine.

Chapter 8 continues this trend with a discussion of animals that attack human beings for a variety of reasons, plus others that represent passive or mechanical biohazards, such as flocks of geese that fly in the vicinity of airplanes.

Chapter 9 discusses a range of popular controversies associated with biological hazards, such as the risks of immunization, the allegedly suspicious origins of certain disease epidemics, and the proper role of government in regulating addictive substances and herbal medicines.

The last four chapters present reference material: copies of relevant documents, print and nonprint resources, lists of organizations, and a glossary, respectively.

Despite its subject matter, this book is no dry catalog of sickness and despair. Although it is true that biological hazards are alive and well in the twenty-first century, it is equally true that, for the first time, our species has both the tools to fight these ancient enemies and, paradoxically, the leisure to enjoy them.

CHAPTER 1

Overview:
The Nature of Hazards

Where have all the good men gone
And where are all the gods?
Where's the street-wise Hercules
To fight the rising odds?
— Dean Pitchford and Jim Steinman, "Holding Out for a Hero"
© 1984 Ensign Music Corporation (BMI)
Lyrics Reprinted by Permission

It was a perfect summer's day in the beachfront community of Torbay, Devonshire, in the south of England—until the children started screaming.

By the time the authorities took charge, more than 130 injured people had staggered from the surf with blood streaming from their legs and feet. Amid general hysteria, the British Coast Guard and police evacuated the beach, posted warning signs, summoned air ambulances to transport the victims, and set out grimly in search of a would-be killer. The date was August 9, 1998.

And then came the letdown. The officers quickly discovered that the dangerous animals were nothing more than ordinary razor clams buried in the sand. Despite the name, razor clams are not particularly sharp-edged; perhaps some of the shells were broken. In any case, the combination of a low tide and a hot day had prompted bathers to wade out farther than usual, and they had simply stepped on clams. It was a milestone in the animal attack literature.

Legal and ethical issues notwithstanding, does anyone really want a beach so safe that no one can stub a toe? This chapter will briefly explore the importance of biohazards in human experience, and will present key terms and concepts.

HAZARD, RISK, AND DISASTER

Although the media tend to use these three terms interchangeably, their meanings are quite different. A **hazard** is an agent or event that can harm human beings (or, in some cases, their goods or environment). **Risk**, by contrast, is a measure of the expected loss resulting from a given hazard, based on how severe the harm might be and how likely it is to occur. A **disaster**—literally, an evil star—is something very bad that happens suddenly and affects a large number of people. It results from a hazard, but not necessarily one that its victims recognized in advance.

We speak of a hazardous material, for example, but not a risky material. Hazard is an intrinsic quality of the material itself, but risk is an attribute of a situation. If a thing is very bad but unlikely to happen, the risk is low; and if a thing is likely to happen, but not very bad, the risk is also low. The science of risk management, then, focuses on major hazards that people are likely to encounter.

There are many different types of hazards, each with its associated risks. Volcanoes and earthquakes are familiar examples of geological hazards. There are also meteorological hazards, such as hurricanes and floods; technological hazards, such as airplane crashes and nuclear power plant accidents; and biological hazards.

As defined in this book, a biological hazard is anything of a biological nature that can harm human beings.[1] More than half the text deals with infectious diseases, which, taken as a group, have caused more death and suffering than any other single biological hazard in human history (see Tables 1.1 and 1.2). The remaining chapters deal with crop pests, venomous animals, predators that attack humans, and related topics.

Some hazards are borderline. Fire, depending on its source, may belong to any of several hazard categories. By our definition it is not a biological hazard, even though a forest fire represents the combustion of biomass. Warfare and criminal behavior also might appear to be biological hazards, as they are the work of living human beings, but their complexity sets them apart as sociological or psychological hazards, instead.

Not every biological hazard, regardless of definition, qualifies as a significant risk. Few readers in North America will contract the Ebola virus, for example, despite all the publicity it has received. Few will be devoured by a Komodo dragon, either, or poisoned by a meal of polar bear liver. All these hazards have claimed human lives, but the risk is low except in specific circumstances. For some biological hazards, the reverse is true: we encounter them every day, usually without harmful effects. The flesh-eating *Streptococcus* (see Chapter 5) nearly killed one man after he scratched his arm on a suitcase, but his experience need not frighten the majority into wearing armor. Similarly, most people eat hamburgers, drink tap water, shake hands with strangers, and get bitten by mosquitoes without ever contracting a serious disease. Luck and the immune system both play important roles.

Disasters do not figure prominently in the biohazard literature. The most familiar disasters, such as hurricanes and floods, are not of biological origin (although they kill many people). True biological disasters are rare and often ambiguous. The available examples include large-scale epidemics of human disease; major crop failures from pathogens or pests; and various unusual

---

[1]There are at least three other definitions of biological hazards: (1) *anything*, living or nonliving, that can harm humans; (2) biomedical waste; or (3) long-term environmental changes, such as global warming.

Table 1.1
Leading Causes of Death (in Percentages), 1985–1997

	Year		
Cause of Death	1985	1990	1997
Developed World:			
Infectious and Parasitic Diseases	5	4	1
Perinatal and Maternal Causes	1	1	1
Cancers	21	21	21
Diseases of the Circulatory System	51	48	46
Diseases of the Respiratory System	4	3	8
Other and Unknown Causes	18	23	23
Developing World:			
Infectious and Parasitic Diseases	45	44	43
Perinatal and Maternal Causes	10	9	10
Cancers	6	7	9
Diseases of the Circulatory System	16	17	24
Diseases of the Respiratory System	6	7	5
Other and Unknown Causes	17	16	9

Source: World Health Organization.

Table 1.2
Deaths from Selected Causes, 1999

Tuberculosis is the *single* infectious disease that claims the most lives each year. In this table, each of the first four categories represents more than one pathogen. (HIV causes AIDS, but the actual cause of death may be any of several opportunistic infections.)

Cause	Estimated Deaths (Worldwide)
Respiratory Infections	4,039,000
Tobacco Use	4,023,000
HIV/AIDS	2,673,000
Perinatal Conditions	2,356,000
Diarrheal Diseases	2,213,000
Tuberculosis	1,669,000
Malaria	1,086,000
Measles	875,000
Venomous Animal Bites and Stings	3,000
Other Animal Attacks	2,000

Source: World Health Organization.

events, such as a 1945 incident in which crocodiles allegedly ate more than 900 soldiers (see Chapter 8). The popular press describes some long-term environmental trends (such as biodiversity loss) as biological "disasters," but these processes are too gradual to qualify as disasters by the usual definition.

TYPES OF BIOLOGICAL HAZARDS

A biological hazard affects people either directly or indirectly. Depending on its nature, it may lie in wait at the salad bar, in a pristine mountain lake, or in a lover's bed; it may crawl inside its host and lay eggs; it may bite, sting, maul, or eat its victims; it may defecate in the attic, kill the sheep, rot the potatoes, or clog the jet engine. Exposure may be voluntary or involuntary, or something in between.

Biological hazards include a wide range of agents and outcomes:

- Bacteria, fungi, viruses, protozoans, or nonliving infectious agents (such as prions) that can cause acute or chronic disease in humans. Such organisms are **pathogens**.
- Larger multicellular parasites that live in or on the human body.
- Toxic chemicals, or **toxins**, produced by many living organisms.
- Chemicals of biological origin that produce allergic reactions in some people.
- Any material (such as medical waste, untreated sewage, rodent feces, or spoiled food) that is likely to contain pathogens or biological toxins. The universal biohazard symbol (see Figure 1.1) usually represents this type of biological hazard.
- Animals that kill or injure humans for any reason.

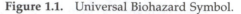

Figure 1.1. Universal Biohazard Symbol.

- Animals whose behavior causes hazards of a mechanical nature, such as deer that cross highways at night.
- Organisms (pathogens, parasites, or predators) or their products that cause famine or economic harm, by damaging resources such as livestock or crop plants.

Note that some organisms represent more than one type of hazard. Ticks, for example, are widely disliked for many reasons. They can transmit pathogens and cause disease epidemics; in this case, the pathogen is the real hazard, and the tick is only the vehicle or **vector**. But certain ticks also produce toxins that can cause paralysis or death, particularly in children. A third hazard is the irritating presence of the tick itself, which may frustrate the host's efforts at removal until nothing remains but the dismembered parasite's head and mouthparts embedded in an infected wound. Thus, the tick is a disease vector, a venomous organism, and an ectoparasite (a parasite that lives on the exterior of its host). All these effects might be called primary biological hazards, as they cause direct physical harm to humans. Ticks also produce secondary biological hazards: by transmitting disease to livestock, they can cause economic harm, food shortages, or even mass starvation.

Ticks even contribute to hazards of a non-biological nature. When people use pesticides to control tick populations, they may inadvertently create a technological hazard that is worse than the original problem. The recent publicity over Lyme disease has demonized ticks (see Chapter 5), creating what amounts to a sociological hazard. In some rural areas, it is traditional to control ticks by burning brush; but such fires may run out of control, thus producing a fire hazard. Finally, the link between tickborne diseases and deer population growth has added fuel to an old argument about wildlife management and predator control; this is an example of a political hazard.

MORE TERMINOLOGY

It is easy to describe how a hippopotamus injures a human being ("It bit him in half"), but harder to explain in everyday words how a bacterium does the same job ("It releases an enterotoxin"). Thus, this book contains many specialized terms and a large glossary. For the reader's convenience, here are a few terms that will appear often:

When public health officials see more cases of a given disease than usual, they declare an **epidemic**. An **outbreak** usually is a more localized, short-term rise in the number of cases, but in practice, the terms outbreak and epidemic often are used interchangeably. If an epidemic is more or less worldwide, it is a **pandemic**.

These terms are relative; the 1993 hantavirus epidemic in the American Southwest, for example, consisted of about 30 cases and 20 deaths. These numbers do not diminish the tragedy, but would scarcely impress the inhabitants of developing nations, where thousands of children die of malaria and other infectious diseases every day. Malaria itself, by contrast, does not represent an epidemic at present, because its "normal" background death rate has always been high. We refer to HIV as an epidemic because the number of cases per year has risen steadily since 1982, and society is still reeling. Before that, the number was zero, because HIV either did not exist or doctors did not recognize it. Once the incidence of this disease levels off, the epidemic will be over, even if HIV remains a major cause of death.

An **infection** occurs when a harmful bacterium or some other pathogen takes up residence in the body. When a parasite does the same thing, the result is an **infestation**. An **intoxication** or **toxicosis** occurs when a person ingests or otherwise encounters a toxic chemical, or **toxin**, that some other organism has produced. An **infectious disease** is one caused by infection or infestation. If a disease can spread from one person to another, it is said to be **contagious**. Inhalation anthrax, for example, is infectious because a bacterium causes it, but it is not usually contagious, because the infective dose—the number of bacterial cells required to start an infection —is too large.

A **virus** is an extremely small entity that can reproduce only inside a living cell. The virus itself is quite unlike a cell, and some biologists regard viruses as nonliving. **Prions** are not even remotely alive; they are proteins that seem to induce other proteins to change shape and cause disease. A **bacterium** (plural, bacteria) is a small, one-celled organism that is definitely alive, but it has no nucleus and differs in other ways from the cells of animals and plants. Rickettsiae and chlamydiae are specific types of bacteria.

Next on the way up the scale are **protozoa**, which are not exactly single-celled animals, as their name might suggest, but close to it. The protozoa, together with some possibly unrelated algae, are known as **protista**. Finally, a lot of unrelated small animals are lumped together as **multicellular parasites**, a group that includes everything from microscopic nematode worms to things like parasitic fish and vampire bats.

The easiest creatures in the previous paragraph to kill (usually) are the bacteria, because certain other bacteria and fungi figured out how to do it a long time ago, and we can borrow their chemical weapons, called **antibiotics**. The hardest things to kill, at least when they are living in our bodies, are the organisms that are most like humans. A medicine used against a protozoan disease such as malaria, for example, generally makes us feel a great deal sicker than taking an antibiotic for a sinus infection. To kill the parasite, we must partly kill the patient.

There are many different ways to classify diseases—for example, by the type of organism that causes them, by the part of the world where they occur, or by their level of severity. In this book, we have chosen to sort diseases into groups according to the way they spread from one person to another. For most diseases, however, there is more than one mode of transmission. Rabies, for example, appears in Chapter 5 with diseases transmitted by animal bites or other contact, but it is also possible to catch it by inhalation. There are even a few diseases, such as leprosy, for which the principal mode of transmission is not yet known. Such diseases appear in the most likely chapter, with an explanatory note.

HAZARDS AND HEROES

As we said, modern readers (including emergency response agencies) tend to focus their attention on hazards and disasters of a nonbiological nature. In developed nations, large-scale biological plagues are largely a thing of the past; at the time this book went to press, even the recently awakened fear of anthrax was already fading. And yet the memory of these hazards cannot lurk very far beneath the surface of memory. As every science-fiction writer knows, the most successful monsters closely resemble bugs, worms, and venomous serpents, and the most dreaded weapons are those that disfigure their victims rather than killing them cleanly.

Thus, to understand the subject matter of this book, the reader should first consider the world from the viewpoint of a man or woman living several thousand years ago. This hypothetical person (a man, for purposes of the example) is standing on an eastern European hillside, tending his goats, breathing the unpolluted air (if the nearby volcano has not recently erupted), and dreaming of a better life. Take the world as it is, and subtract the world of this man's dreams, and the items left over will consist largely of biological hazards.

He has fathered 11 children, of whom seven have already died. Six succumbed to common childhood diseases, one with fearful convulsions, said to be carried on the night air; one never returned from a trip to the well, and he suspects wolves, despite his neighbor's blathering about the evil eye. His present wife is his third, thanks to childbed fever, and each pregnancy is a new occasion for fear as well as joy. The man himself is limping, for a black scorpion stung him recently on the foot. He cannot file Worker's Compensation or drive to the emergency room; instead, he must endure the pain and continue working. If he dies, neighbors or predators will take the goats, and his family may starve. The stored grain seemed like a fine safeguard against such emergencies, but now it is moldy, and people who eat it seem to go crazy. All these problems demand action, if only someone knew what to do.

On the subject of goats, it would also be helpful to rid the pasture of poisonous plants. One man cannot pick them all, and goats never seem to learn. But worst of all is the shaking sickness that claimed half the herd last year. He felt uneasy about serving that meat to his family, fearing that the same malady might strike them. But the village elders insist that food has nothing to do with disease—although there are rumors of another tribe that has laws against eating certain animals, such as pigs, and their people seem to stay healthier. Yes, the man did everything possible to prevent the loss, even burned two of his last healthy goats as a sacrifice, but all in vain.

The people, in short, need a hero—but not every hero is a warrior. To the farmers, in fact, warriors have usually meant bad luck. The last time an army camped nearby, they drank all the wine, bothered the women, and generally made a mess. By the time they left, many people had developed strange rashes. No, the hero this village needs is more like a public health officer.

In the classic Greek myths, the hero Heracles (or Hercules) had to complete 12 tasks, known today as the Labors of Hercules. Scholars have interpreted the Labors as symbols of the obstacles that people must overcome in order to reach their full potential. And what were these tasks? No fewer than eight involved capturing or killing large animals that were a menace to public safety. Two of Hercules' targets—a marsh-dwelling serpent called the Hydra, and a flock of evil marsh birds—appear to symbolize malaria or other diseases associated with swamps. Another of his tasks was to cleanse a king's stables, where large amounts of unsanitary manure had accumulated over the years.

Finally, Hercules had to steal a jeweled belt; a sacred deer that destroyed its pursuers, by eluding them until the hunt became an obsession; and three magic apples that prevented sickness and death. Indeed, of all the 12 Labors, only the jeweled belt finds no obvious counterpart in the biological hazards literature. Hercules even dabbled briefly in biological warfare. After killing the Hydra, he saved some of its toxic blood to use against his enemies; but, as so often happens, one of those enemies eventually turned the tables, by killing Hercules with his own poison.

It is noteworthy that, after completing his 12 Labors—plus side trips, including a visit to a tribe whose crops were being destroyed by birds—Hercules crowned his achievements by creating the Olympic Games. In a civilized society, heroes simply cannot go around stealing treasures and killing everything in sight. Organized sports (and, unfortunately, psychoactive drugs) mimic some of the feelings associated with fighting and surviving a real-life hazard. Some of these surrogate hazards can even be deadly in their own right. We conclude that, without hazards, there are no heroes.

HAZARDS AND SOCIETIES

A sign bearing the words "Everything is dangerous if you're stupid" was once a familiar sight in military and industrial facilities in the United States (and, for all we know, throughout the world). The point is that, except in the case of unavoidable disasters, we are all responsible to some extent for our own safety. Children are unlikely to catch diphtheria if their parents have them immunized; hardly anyone dies of mushroom poisoning without eating unidentified wild mushrooms. But most of us apparently need some danger, and every society fulfills that need by defining acceptable hazards and surrogates. Sociobiologist E.O. Wilson put it this way: "We're not just afraid of predators, we're transfixed by them, prone to weave stories and fables and chatter endlessly about them, because fascination creates preparedness, and preparedness, survival. In a deeply tribal sense, we love our monsters."[2] A generation earlier, author John Steinbeck wrote: "Men really do need sea-monsters in their personal oceans. . . . An ocean without its unnamed monsters would be like a completely dreamless sleep."[3]

Take predators, for example. The majority of people in the developed world can easily avoid predators and other dangerous animals—and so we seek them out, instead.

The news media report that a woman was mauled by a bear that she insisted on feeding at Yellowstone, or that an anaconda nearly choked a man who was showing off for a TV camera. For those who cannot travel, there are imaginary predators (see Surrogate Hazards, Chapter 9). Every human culture has created an unseen world filled with animals more terrible than the real ones: great hairy manlike beasts that tear limbs from unwary travelers, giant birds that carry off children, and snakes hundreds of feet long. And yet this unseen world always contains a hero who goes out from the safety of the village and slays the beast. If a world with danger is bad, apparently a world without heroes is worse.

Real, unavoidable monsters are not nearly so appealing as exotic ones. In some parts of Africa, a woman will stand in a river to wash her laundry, invariably facing the riverbank. She knows a crocodile could take her—thousands of people in Africa and Asia reportedly suffer this fate every year—but the crocodile is a part of life, and so she turns her back on the river and enjoys the day. Later, safe at home, she and her family indulge in monster lore (or, nowadays, a violent American video game). In the United States, we apply the same logic to such necessary activities as commuting on the freeway. Given familiarity and consent, even the most terrible hazards lose their punch. And if danger retreats too far, sometimes we pursue it (see Figure 1.2).

In developed nations, the removal of necessary monsters from our lives created a vacuum that was quickly filled with seem-

---

[2]Quoted in Richard Ellis, *Monsters of the Sea* (New York: Knopf, 1994).
[3]John Steinbeck, *The Log from the Sea of Cortez* (New York: Viking Press, 1951).

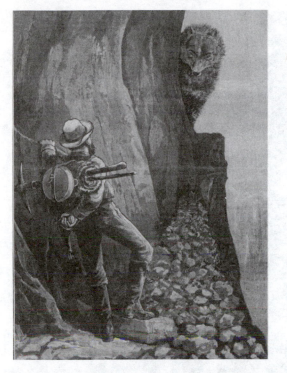 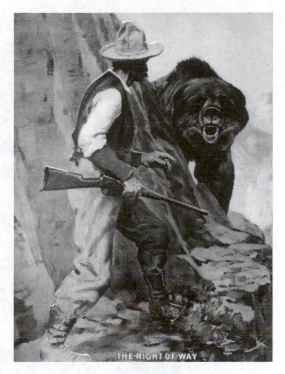

THE RIGHT OF WAY

Figure 1.2. Dealing with a biological hazard.

(left) "The Dangers of Prospecting—A Scene in the Rocky Mountains," by nineteenth-century artist Paul Frenzeny. The terrified man has picked up a rock, although the bear probably could not attack him from its present position. (Reproduced from *The American West* by L. Beebe and C. Clegg [E.P. Dutton, 1955], with permission of Ann Clegg Holloway.)

(right) Remington Arms Company's famous advertisement "The Right of Way." The man from the older painting has left his pack somewhere, but has acquired a rifle and a new air of confidence. Apparently he intends to shoot the bear, which will then fall into the canyon. (Reproduced with permission from Remington Arms Company, Inc.)

ingly pointless ones. "Splat" movies and soccer matches are examples that come to mind, but other forms of voluntary risk-taking behavior turn up in the oddest places. Many U.S. residents, for example, have begun to reject pasteurized milk, cooked fish, and childhood vaccinations in favor of the alternatives. Painful foods have enjoyed a renaissance (see Figure 1.3). Even "safe sex," the buzzword of a generation, has recently fallen out of favor (see Chapter 5).

Now contrast this love of monsters and danger with the prevalent modern belief that nothing in nature has either the inclination or the right to harm us, unless we accept the risk voluntarily. By this view,

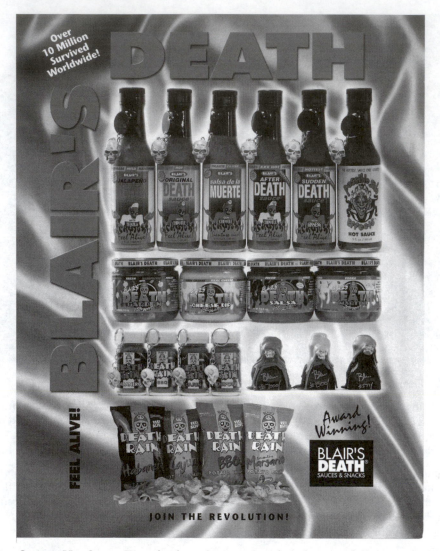

Figure 1.3. Serious Hot Sauce. Even food products are marketed successfully using product labels that emphasize pain and risk rather than enjoyment. (Courtesy of Gardner Resources, Inc.)

predation and disease are unnatural new elements in a world out of balance. A wolf or a disease is not supposed to harm us unless we somehow earn its wrath. And if it breaks the rules that we have invented, it must be a bad wolf or a man-made disease. It is the beast within, whom we must tame or else banish. "Problem" bears, cougars, and even turkeys (see Chapter 8) are routinely executed; in 2001, California authorities arrested and imprisoned a sea otter for allegedly raping seals.

The underlying premise (and bias) of this book, by contrast, is that bears act like bears and prions act like prions. When a bear attacks a pet dog or an unprotected child in a national park, that bear is simply hungry. It is acting on knowledge that we have largely forgotten—that people are food and have always been food. And if we insist on feeding and tolerating predators in residential areas, we teach those predators that people are harmless and safe to eat, if nothing better is available. Accepting the predator's role in our fantasy lives, in other words, also means accepting its place in the food chain.

THE ENEMY WITHIN

So there are real monsters, and imaginary ones, and surrogate ones that will do in a pinch. But there are also monsters tiny enough, and elusive enough, to haunt the dreams of every culture that has invented soap.

Scenario: An ambulance arrives at a trauma center with an unconscious man in critical condition. Doctors find that his skin is covered with fungi and other microorganisms, including the potentially deadly bacteria that cause toxic shock syndrome and necrotizing fasciitis. His sputum is positive for several species of viruses and bacteria that cause meningitis, pneumonia, and scarlet fever. And his mouth defies description; there are more bacteria here than in his rectum.

A microscopic examination of his face reveals parasitic mites wiggling in every eyelash follicle, and thriving communities of tiny worm-like animals just beneath the surface of his skin. Farther inside, the man is even more disgusting. His colon is filled with masses of dead bacteria and undigested food, and there is mucus in his lungs.

Finally, using an electron microscope, we find that every cell in his body has been invaded by what appear to be primitive bacteria. What is wrong with this man?

Answer: He fell off the roof and fractured his skull. That explains his unconsciousness. Otherwise, he is perfectly healthy and normal.

Just as we sometimes feel that nothing has the right to kill us or make us sick, so we may be shocked to discover that we are not alone. And yet each of us is a walking menagerie and fungus garden. Reasonable hygiene and laundry habits are beneficial to health, but excessive bathing and purging can destroy protective skin oils and helpful bacteria. Products that allegedly stimulate our glands, energize our immune systems, cleanse our guts, and empty our wallets are the basis of a thriving and largely unregulated industry. People are afraid that they are not clean, and therein may lie the greatest biological hazard of all (see Chapter 9).

HAZARDS AS CAREERS

Medicine and allied fields offer a wide range of career opportunities for students with an interest in biological hazards. At present, only a small percentage of people in Western nations officially die of diseases that doctors now recognize as infectious (see Table 1.1); but this situation may change with the next "emerging" pathogen, and some of our assumptions about non-communicable diseases are already wavering.

In the United States, heart disease, cancer, and Alzheimer's disease are major killers. Many other people suffer from multiple sclerosis, Lou Gehrig's disease, arthritis, schizophrenia, and Gulf War syndrome. Until recently, doctors believed that all these conditions resulted from genetic or environmental factors or from "stress." In the past decade, however, studies have shown that most, if not all, may have an infectious component:

- At least two common bacteria, *Chlamydia pneumoniae* and *Porphyromonas gingivalis,* appear to be associated with heart disease. The influenza virus also may play a role, as flu shots offer some protection from second heart attacks in cardiac patients.

- Scientists now believe that some (possibly most) cancers may result from viral infections. Examples are breast cancer, which is associated with the Epstein-Barr virus, plus a second virus similar to one that causes mammary tumors in mice; and mesothelioma, which may be linked to the SV-40 virus (see Chapter 9).

- At least 13 percent of Alzheimer's patients may actually be suffering from an infectious prion disease similar to Creutzfeldt-Jakob syndrome (see Chapter 3).

- Multiple sclerosis has been linked to so many different pathogens that one of them, at least, seems likely to be causative. Three promising candidates are human herpesvirus-6, *Chlamydia*, and the Epstein-Barr virus.

- A 2000 study has tentatively linked Lou Gehrig's disease (amyotrophic lateral sclerosis) to a virus similar to echovirus-7 (see Chapter 5).

- Some forms of arthritis result from treatable bacterial infections, such as ehrlichiosis and Lyme disease (see Chapters 5 and 6).

- In 1996, University of Texas researchers reported that many veterans with Gulf War syndrome were infected with a little-known bacterium called *Mycoplasma fermentans*, and that antibiotic treatment appeared to relieve their symptoms. (Later studies, however, failed to confirm this finding.)

- Perhaps most surprising of all, researchers have found a strong association between the Borna disease virus of horses (see Chapter 6) and schizophrenia in humans.

Thus, there is evidence that some of the most important diseases of our time may ultimately yield to vaccination or to improved pharmaceutical treatment. Ironically, however, when a 1999 survey in England showed that 50 percent of men and 30 percent of women thought cancer might be contagious, the press derided these people as "ignorant." In fact, they had simply read the latest health bulletins about viruses causing cancer.

In many countries, these issues have a lower priority, as fewer people survive long enough to worry about the causes of Alzheimer's disease or cancer. Well-known infectious diseases and parasites are commonplace, and the need for health care in the developing world has never been greater. Health professionals seeking new challenges might consider the U.S. Centers for Disease Control and Prevention's Epidemic Intelligence Service (CDC EIS), a two-year program of disease investigation and public service at various locations around the world. The logo of this program, a shoe with a hole in the sole (Figure 1.4), suggests the level of commitment and adventure that such a tour of duty may entail.

But medicine and allied professions are not the only occupations that deal with biological hazards (Table 1.3). Every year, biochemists and ethnobotanists discover new uses for animal and plant toxins. Biological

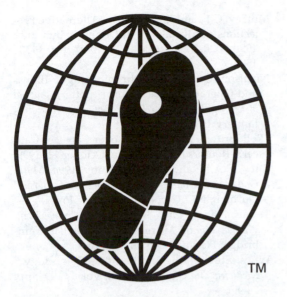

Figure 1.4. Logo of the Epidemic Intelligence Service, U.S. Public Health Service, Centers for Disease Control and Prevention (CDC). (Reproduced with permission of the U.S. Centers for Disease Control and Prevention.)

warfare and terrorism are important challenges facing military officers, city planners, public health managers, and medical technicians. Even food service workers and parents who wash their hands make a great contribution to public health. Farmers may face the greatest challenge of all, safeguarding their own health while also feeding the world and combating every imaginable hazard, from economic circumstances and bad weather to imported crop pests and possible agroterrorism.

Although this book does not mince words, its purpose is not to shock the reader, but rather to impart a real appreciation for its subject matter: heroes who died fighting disease, and heroes who lived to protect and feed their communities, and creatures of unsurpassed beauty and complexity—yes, we mean the parasites, too— and opportunities enough to challenge any student in search of a career.

Table 1.3
Some Careers Related to Biological Hazards

Professional	Technical	Other
Agrogeneticist	Agricultural Inspector	Animal Control Officer
Biochemist	Agricultural Technician	Child Care Worker
Entomologist	Animal Breeder	Crop Duster
Epidemiologist	Animal Care Technician	Farm Worker
Microbiologist	Farmer	Food Service Worker
Parasitologist	Forest Ranger	Home Care Aide
Pharmacologist	Food Science Technician	Law Enforcement Officer
Physician	Medical Technologist	Lifeguard
Toxicologist	Nurse	Military, Special Forces
Urban and Regional Planner	Nutritionist	Parent
Virologist	Paramedic	Pest Control Operator
Wildlife Biologist	Pharmacist	
Wildlife Manager		

REFERENCES AND RECOMMENDED READING

Aronowitz, Robert A. 1999. *Making Sense of Illness: Science, Society, and Disease*. Cambridge University Press.

Beck, David L. "Sexually Predatory Sea Otter Captured." *San Jose Mercury News*, April 17, 2001.

Ewald, Paul W. 2000. *Plague Time: How Stealth Infections Cause Cancers, Heart Disease, and Other Deadly Ailments*. New York: Free Press.

Gold, Stephen. "The Rise of Markets and the Fall of Infectious Disease." *The Freeman*, November 1992.

Kennedy, Dominic. "Bathers Injured by Plague of Razor-Sharp Molluscs." *The Times* (UK), August 10, 1998.

Kumate, J. "Infectious Diseases in the 21st Century." *Archives of Medical Research*, Summer 1997, pp. 155–161.

Murray, C.J., and Lopez, A.D. "Alternative Projections of Mortality and Disability by Cause 1990-2020." *Lancet*, May 24, 1997, pp. 1498–1504.

Nicolson, G.L., et al. "Chronic Fatigue Illness and Operation Desert Storm" [letter]. *Journal of Occupational and Environmental Medicine*, January 1996, pp. 14–16.

"Poll: Britons in Dark Ages over Cause of Cancer." Reuters News Service, October 11, 1999.

Ruck, C.A.P., and Staples, Danny. 1994. *Myth: Gods and Goddesses, Heroines and Heroes*. Durham, NC: Carolina Academic Press.

Tomes, Nancy. 1998. *The Gospel of Germs: Men, Women, and the Microbe in American Life*. Cambridge: Harvard University Press.

Wing, Steve. "The Limits of Epidemiology." *Medicine and Global Survival*, Vol. 1, 1994, pp. 74–86.

CHAPTER 2

Human Pathogens in Water

How many ova have I swallowed? Who knows what will be hatched within me? . . . The man must not drink of the running streams, the living waters, who is not prepared to have all nature reborn in him,—to suckle monsters.

— Henry David Thoreau, *Journal*, 1851

Improved access to clean drinking water is a major goal of public health programs throughout the developing world. Countries such as Mexico have made outstanding progress in modernizing their water and sanitation systems; at the close of the millennium, however, tap water in most Mexican cities remained undrinkable, and Mexico was the world's largest market for bottled water. In less prosperous nations, clean water often is a luxury beyond reach.

Most waterborne pathogens and parasites begin their work when a person swallows them, but others infect wounds, chew through the skin, or enter the brain through the nose. Water also promotes disease indirectly by providing a breeding ground for insects and other animals that act as disease vectors (see Chapter 5). Thus, water projects intended to solve one public health problem may inadvertently create another.

A small human population in an arid area, far from any major river or lake, may find its growth severely limited by a lack of water; but as long as the demand for water does not exceed the supply, the people may be reasonably healthy. They dig for underground springs, eat fruit, and take advantage of seasonal rains. But if a new factor (such as colonialism) breaks down traditional social structures and allows population growth to outstrip the local carrying capacity, the people begin to die. Next, a health agency arrives on the scene and builds a dam. The people now have plenty of water for their farms. But even if they have enough surplus fuel to boil their new drinking water, parasitic diseases such as schistosomiasis are likely to increase, replacing famine as the primary health concern. Mosquitoes breed in the new ecosystem, causing epidemics of malaria and other vectorborne diseases. The water project may also bring immigrants and their diseases to the area.

To literal-minded Westerners, the African proverb "Filthy water cannot be washed" speaks volumes. In fact, it means something along the lines of *quis custodiet custodes*; but it sounds more like a description of the developing world's dilemma. We think of water as a place to get clean, but in many countries, it is probably safer to stay dirty.

CROSS REFERENCE

The titles of Chapters 2–5 reflect the principal modes of disease transmission. Most pathogens, however, can be transmitted in more than one way. Waterborne microorganisms, for example, can also contaminate food during irrigation and washing. For the reader's convenience, Table 2.1 lists some potentially waterborne pathogens that are covered in other chapters. Note that certain waterborne pathogens disperse in aerosol droplets and are defined as airborne (see Chapter 4).

THE IMPORTANCE OF DIARRHEA

Most of the diseases in the next two chapters are variations on a single disconcerting theme: diarrhea. Although Western readers

Table 2.1
Cross-Reference: Other Waterborne Diseases

Disease	Chapter	Notes
Botulism	3	Food or water
Campylobacteriosis	3	Food or water
Crohn's disease/MAP	3	Food or water
E. coli	3	Food or water
Echinococcosis	3	Food or water
Fasciolopsiasis	3	Food or water
Hepatitis A	3	Food, contact, or water
Norwalk Virus	3	Food or water
Paratyphoid Fever	3	Food or water
Pork Tapeworm	3	Food, water, or contact
Beef Tapeworm	3	Food or water
Typhoid Fever	3	Food or water
Salmonellosis	3	Food or water
Toxoplasmosis	3	Transplacental infection, food, or water
Viral gastroenteritis	3	Contact, food, or water
Yersiniosis	3	Food or water
Astrovirus	5	Contact, food, or water
Poliomyelitis	5	Contact, milk, or possibly water
Rotavirus	5	Contact, food, water, or airborne
Tularemia	5	Contact, food, water, or (rarely) airborne
Biting Aquatic Insects	7	May also act as disease vectors

may dismiss diarrhea as a minor inconvenience, waterborne diarrheal diseases kill over two million people each year worldwide, many of them children. This is the number of reported deaths; according to the National Center for Infectious Diseases, the annual toll is more like five million. The total incidence is estimated at three to five billion cases per year—one case for every one or two people on earth. About 80 percent of these cases result from drinking polluted water.

It is likely that, for thousands of years, diarrhea has ranked alongside tuberculosis and malaria as one of the most important biological hazards. When any hazard exists long enough, evolution tends to produce countermeasures; Chapter 5 explains how sickle-cell anemia and thalassemia, seemingly undesirable genetic traits, protect their carriers from malaria. Similarly, researchers now believe that another deleterious gene—the one that causes cystic fibrosis—may confer some protection against diarrhea.

Like many genetic traits, the CF gene is recessive—that is, a person needs to inherit it from both parents in order to have the disease. About 5 percent of all Caucasians have one copy of the CF gene; based on its prevalence in various populations, and the number of variations that have appeared, geneticists estimate that the CF mutation occurred over 50,000 years ago. The fact that it has lasted this long suggests that it must provide some benefit. Apparently, the answer lies in the unusually salty sweat of children with CF. The mutation reduces the number of chloride channels that normally funnel salt out of a cell and recycle it back into the body. When salt leaves a cell, water goes with it; in severe diarrhea, this normal process runs amok and the body becomes dehydrated.

Studies have shown that one copy of the CF gene reduces the number of chloride channels by one-half, thus reducing fluid loss without causing illness. This trait could enable its carriers to survive in a diarrhea epidemic. Children born with two copies of the gene, however, do not secrete enough fluid inside their lungs or intestines for these organs to function normally. At some time in prehistory, the gene apparently saved more lives than it destroyed, and natural selection favored its spread.

EXAMPLES OF WATERBORNE BACTERIAL DISEASES

As many of the bacteria that cause human illness occur both in water and in food, some diseases that the reader might expect to find in this section are in Chapter 3 instead.

Buruli Ulcer. Most Americans have never heard of Buruli ulcer—a severe infectious disease associated with shallow, stagnant water, primarily in West Africa. The mode of transmission is not yet understood, but the agent is waterborne and may enter the body through a small break in the skin. Some recent studies suggest that certain biting aquatic insects also serve as vectors, and that freshwater fish may be the reservoir; others have proposed airborne dispersal in droplet form.

First described in Uganda in 1897, this disease was later found in several other West African countries, and has recently turned up in parts of Asia, Australia, and the New World tropics. At present, the only known hosts are human beings and (in

Australia) koalas, but researchers have successfully inoculated armadillos and rodents with the disease. The agent, *Mycobacterium ulcerans*, is one of several related bacteria collectively known as saprophytic mycobacteria. A related species, *Mycobacterium marinum*, causes a less serious skin disease in North America known as swimming pool granuloma. Both these pathogens are related to the bacteria that cause tuberculosis and leprosy, but the agent of Buruli ulcer is unique in that it destroys tissue and bone and suppresses the immune system, apparently by releasing a lipid toxin, called mycolactone, that causes cells to self-destruct. Extensive necrosis may result, usually on the leg, foot, or hand (Figure 2.1). Most cases occur in children under 15 years of age.

Buruli ulcer has recently become the focus of a World Health Organization (WHO) global initiative. At present, there is no reliable method of early diagnosis and no vaccine. Heat treatment has proven useful in some cases; when the ulcers become extensive, skin grafting may be required, but the cost of such treatment is beyond the means of most patients.

The world's sudden interest in this tragic disease, after more than 100 years, may reflect the perception of risk in developed nations. In 1999, a Canadian man who visited Africa contracted Buruli ulcer. Some doctors now believe that this and other diseases caused by environmental mycobacteria represent a serious health threat that merits further study.

Cholera. This disease, caused by the bacterium *Vibrio cholerae*, is the first one that comes to mind when most people think of a waterborne disease epidemic. Today, chol-

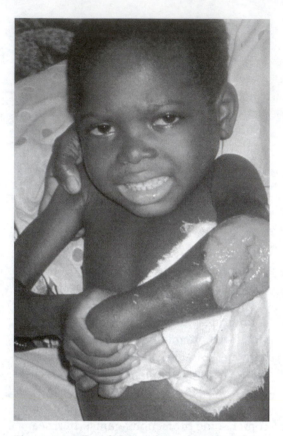

Figure 2.1. Buruli Ulcer. (Reproduced with permission from the World Health Organization.)

era occurs mainly in developing nations, where over two billion people are considered to be at risk. Cholera epidemics tend to follow natural disasters, such as hurricanes and floods; they can also happen when a region stops chlorinating its drinking water supply, as happened in Peru in 1991. That nation's first cholera epidemic in nearly a century quickly spread to the rest of South America, where a total of one million people contracted cholera and some 11,000 died.

The cholera bacterium is a natural occupant of warm estuaries and coastal waters.

Two of its less famous relatives that share the same habitat are *Vibrio parahaemolyticus*, which contaminates seafood (see Chapter 3), and *Vibrio alginolyticus*, which can cause wound infections in swimmers. In 2000, a related marine bacterium called *Photobacterium damsela* infected a wound on a Florida man's leg and caused a severe case of necrotizing fasciitis—the media's favorite "flesh-eating bacteria disease," but actually an infection caused by any of several bacteria.

It is not entirely clear how a cholera epidemic starts, but apparently people ingest the vibrios in seafood or in contaminated drinking water from a source near an estuary. As human populations are concentrated near coastlines, the highly contagious disease then spreads from person to person. Fecal contamination of other water sources is likely to occur in areas that lack modern sanitation. Some sources claim that the 1991 cholera epidemic in Peru resulted from an El Niño plankton bloom; as noted above, however, the epidemic closely followed the Peruvian government's decision to stop chlorinating its water. Ironically, the government made that decision in the interest of public health, after years of reports suggesting that chlorine might cause cancer. In 1992, the influential U.S. Environmental Protection Agency finally decided that chlorine (below a concentration of 100 parts per billion[1]) was safe after all, but many Peruvians were dead by then.

The earliest available records indicate that cholera originated in India and spread to Europe and North America in the nineteenth century. Europe had its first documented cholera epidemic in 1817, and North America had a series of cholera outbreaks in the mid-1800s. Today, thanks to improved water quality, there are only about 50 reported cases of cholera in the United States each year, most of them foodborne.

In 1831, cholera reached England, where it claimed thousands of lives in repeated epidemics until it met its match in Dr. John Snow. In 1849, he published a famous pamphlet entitled "On the Mode of Communication of Cholera," which proposed that cholera resulted from drinking water that was contaminated with sewage from the houses of cholera victims. This might sound obvious today, but apparently it had not occurred to anyone else, although the River Thames was so polluted that its odor interfered with the work of Parliament. Sewage was deposited in open cesspools that were often located near water wells. The available water was so vile that many people turned to alcohol as an alternative, thus compounding the problem.

When the next cholera outbreak occurred in 1854, Dr. Snow tested his theory by determining where the victims had obtained their drinking water. Nearly all had drunk from the same contaminated well. Once the authorities removed its pump handle, forcing people to use other sources, the number of new cases decreased and the epidemic stopped. These findings led to better sewage systems and other public health reforms. In 1883, Robert Koch confirmed the existence of the cholera bacterium.

This radical new idea was not without its detractors. One of them, Dr. Max von

---

[1]EPA reduced the safe limit to 80 parts per billion in 2002.

Pettenkofer, had a strong personal belief that airborne poisons in soil transmitted cholera and that the bacterium was at most a minor player. After obstructing the acceptance of Dr. Snow's contagion theory for many years, Dr. von Pettenkofer and his colleagues tested the theory by drinking a culture of cholera bacteria. All of them promptly developed diarrhea, but none of them died, and this outcome somehow reinforced their belief. Fortunately for the world, most scientists eventually figured it out.

Cholera's mode of action appears very simple: victims have such profuse watery diarrhea that some die of dehydration within a few days or hours. The fatality rate in modern epidemics usually is below 1 percent, because most people survive cholera if fluids and electrolytes can be replaced quickly enough. (Some of these survivors become carriers who can start new epidemics.) Before doctors understood how to treat cholera, however, up to 50 percent died in some epidemics. Rehydration is still a problem in many developing nations, where clean water is hard to obtain for everyday use, much less for treating cholera. Researchers in India have developed a starch-based rehydration fluid that yields superior results; antibiotics also are helpful in some cases. A cholera vaccine also is available, but at present it offers only 50 percent protection for a period of two to six months.

Despite the apparent simplicity of cholera, recent discoveries have shown that the infection is a highly complex process. Its agent, like many pathogenic bacteria, contains a cluster of disease-causing genes called a virulence factor or pathogenicity island. The once-harmless cholera bacterium acquired these genes by infection with a virus called VPIF. The VPIF genes, in turn, act as a receptor for a second virus called CTXF, which produces the cholera toxin. When this second virus attaches to the bacterial cell, it also injects its own genes. Thus, the VPIF virus has effectively commandeered a bacterium and is using it to control a second virus. Studies have shown that bacteria may acquire their virulence factors while inside the human intestine, rather than in polluted coastal waters or sewage systems.

One observer has compared the VPIF virus to an armed terrorist who hijacks a tank (the bacterium) and forces an innocent bystander (the CTXF virus) to drive it on a mission of destruction. But the metaphor need not end there. The team's mission is not over until its tank climbs the ramp of a colossal landing craft—the human body—and enlists the body's resources for its own manufacture, finally to emerge by the billion on a foreign shore. Without technology, a simple marine virus has managed to invade the land, circle the globe, and change history.

Leptospirosis. Often called swine fever, this disease actually occurs in many domestic and wild animals. Swine, cattle, horses, dogs, rodents, deer, raccoons, and even reptiles and amphibians may serve as reservoir hosts. The possible modes of transmission also are numerous. The disease often is waterborne or foodborne, but it can also spread by contact with infected animals or objects contaminated with their urine.

The agents of leptospirosis include over 150 different pathogenic serotypes of spirochetes in the genus *Leptospira*. The disease occurs in two forms: anicteric leptospirosis, a mild flu-like illness, and Weil's disease, which may involve kidney and liver damage, internal bleeding, and loss of consciousness. Antibiotic treatment is effective if started by the second day of the illness.

In 1995, at least 16 people in Nicaragua died from an unusual form of leptospirosis that affected the lungs rather than the liver or kidneys, causing severe respiratory hemorrhaging. For a more typical case of leptospirosis, see Chapter 10 (Naval Facilities Engineering Command, Abstract of an Accident). In 2000, several U.S. athletes contracted leptospirosis while participating in the Eco-Challenge Race in Malaysian Borneo. A similar incident occurred in 1998 in Illinois, when 110 triathlon participants caught this disease and 23 were hospitalized.

Melioidosis. This disease can spread by various routes but is often waterborne. It is an uncommon infection that usually turns up in agricultural workers who have been in contact with contaminated water or soil. Cases have occurred in Southeast Asia, the Middle East, Australia, Papua New Guinea, and South America. For unknown reasons, excessive consumption of alcohol and kava (a traditional root beverage) are risk factors.

The agent, *Pseudomonas* (or *Burkholderia*) *pseudomallei*, is closely related to the bacterium that causes glanders in horses (see Chapter 6). The disease ranges in severity from clinically inapparent cases to severe pulmonary infection with rapidly fatal septicemia. Abscesses of the spleen, prostate, brain, and other organs may occur. Treatment usually involves a combination of antibiotics, such as chloramphenicol, doxycycline, and trimethoprim-sulfamethoxazole, and/or ceftazidime.

Shigellosis. The agents of this disease are *Shigella dysenteriae* and related bacteria. Typical sources include water contaminated by fecal matter, vegetables that have been washed or irrigated with such water, or vegetables fertilized with raw sewage. Like many waterborne pathogens, *Shigella* is also foodborne; in 2000, an outbreak in the western United States was traced to a chip dip. Large outbreaks of shigellosis often occur in crowded situations with inadequate sanitation, such as jails, camps, and ships. In 1954, an epidemic occurred among residents of a trailer park in Los Angeles. In male homosexuals, shigellosis can also be a sexually transmitted disease.

The incidence of this disease may be declining, as the CDC reported a 44 percent decrease between 1996 and 2000. A 1999 study reported an average of 448,240 cases per year in the United States, 80 percent of them waterborne. Symptoms often include bloody diarrhea (dysentery) with a fever and abdominal cramps. To avoid contracting this disease, people who work with young children should wash their hands carefully after changing diapers.

Like the agents of cholera, diphtheria, and several other diseases, the shigellosis bacterium is virulent only because of blocks of genetic material that may have come from a virus. In *Shigella*, these genes code for the shiga toxin, which produces the disease symptoms by inhibiting protein synthesis and causing cell death.

Typhoid Fever. Although many books describe typhoid as a waterborne disease, today it is primarily foodborne; thus, the main account is in Chapter 3. The near-elimination of typhoid from the United

21

States in the last century often is attributed to the construction of water and sewage treatment systems, but the connection may be an indirect one. For example, vegetables and fruits are unsafe to eat when irrigated with contaminated water, and shellfish that live in polluted coastal waters are known to concentrate typhoid and other pathogens.

Ulcer Disease. This name, for lack of a better one, is often applied to upper gastrointestinal ulcers caused by the bacterium *Helicobacter* (formerly *Campylobacter*) *pylori*. Recent studies have shown that this bacterium can survive for up to three years in river water, and in 1999 a microbiologist in Pennsylvania confirmed a direct link between contaminated drinking water and stomach ulcers. Thus, stomach ulcers are actually a waterborne disease that at least 10 percent of U.S. residents contract at some point in their lives.

Until the early 1980s, physicians believed that such ulcers resulted from stress, rich food, or other vague lifestyle factors. Treatments ranged from years of bland diets and antacid drugs to freezing or removal of the stomach. Then two Australian physicians, Drs. Barry Marshall and Robin Warren, discovered the agent. When other doctors ridiculed their theory, one of the researchers infected himself with the bacterium and quickly developed ulcer symptoms. Although this experiment did not impress everyone, later studies of patients with ulcers showed that most had *Helicobacter pylori* infections and that antibiotic treatment usually healed the ulcer. In 1994, the NIH issued a consensus statement acknowledging that about 90 percent of ulcers result from a treatable bacterial infection. If untreated, these ulcers may increase the risk for cancer of the stomach or pancreas.

EXAMPLES OF WATERBORNE VIRAL DISEASES

Some human viral diseases can be waterborne, but for most of them it is not the primary mode of transmission. The polio virus, for example, is an important indicator of human fecal contamination in coastal waters—because recently vaccinated children excrete it—but polio has never been primarily a waterborne disease (see Chapter 5). Other human enteric viruses commonly found in water include echovirus and Coxsackie virus, both associated with the common cold (see Chapter 5). Hepatitis A and Norwalk viruses can be waterborne, but are more often spread through contaminated food (see Chapter 3).

Hepatitis E. This form of hepatitis, called HEV, is the world's most common form of hepatitis transmitted by ingestion. Most cases are in Africa, southern Asia, India, Mexico, and Central America. Large outbreaks often result from drinking water contaminated with feces, but in endemic areas, HEV also accounts for more than half of all sporadic cases of hepatitis. Unlike hepatitis A (see Chapter 3), HEV is rarely transmitted from person to person. It is foodborne at times, but most often waterborne.

The illness typically lasts several weeks, with symptoms similar to those of other forms of viral hepatitis: abdominal pain, loss of appetite, dark urine, fever, swelling of the liver, jaundice, nausea, and vomiting. There may also be a rash, joint pain, and other symptoms. Victims tend to be young adults; children may get the disease in a milder form. At present, there is no evidence of chronic infection or long-term liver damage.

EXAMPLES OF WATERBORNE PROTOZOAL DISEASES

Amebic Dysentery or *Amebiasis*. Several different microorganisms can cause dysentery (severe bloody diarrhea). Bacillary dysentery is another name for shigellosis, a bacterial disease described earlier in this chapter. The usual agent of protozoal dysentery is an ameba called *Entamoeba histolytica*, which exists in two stages: an active stage in the intestine of the human host, and a dormant form (called a cyst) that can survive outside the body in water, soil, or food. Unlike some other amebas, this species is not free-living.

People contract amebiasis by drinking or swimming in contaminated water, or by eating food that has become contaminated by the fecal-oral route or by flies or irrigation water. It is particularly common among residents of institutions for the developmentally disabled. In male homosexuals, it is also a sexually transmitted disease (see Chapter 5). At present, an estimated 40 million people worldwide suffer from amebiasis. Compared to shigellosis, amebic dysentery is less likely to occur in large epidemics, but more likely to cause permanent damage to the intestine, liver, or other organs.

The symptoms of amebic dysentery include abdominal and rectal pain with frequent watery stools containing blood and mucus. The amebae invade the walls of the colon, sometimes causing ulceration; they may also spread to the liver and cause ab-

scesses there. If the ulcer or abscess ruptures, peritonitis may result. Several thousand cases of amebiasis occur in the United States each year, but the fatality rate is low. Metronidazole and other amebicides are effective as treatment.

Amebic Meningitis. This disease is extremely rare but uniformly fatal. Florida health officials estimate that there is about one case for every 2.5 million hours people spend in that state's lakes and streams. The agent (*Naegleria fowleri*) is a free-living ameba that probably occurs in every nonchlorinated body of fresh water in North America, and the only way to avoid it for certain is to wear nose clips when diving. Nationwide, at least eight people died from amebic meningitis in 1998, including a 14-year-old boy in Florida and a three-year-old girl in Oklahoma. Some cases have been attributed to heat and drought, which can lower the water levels in lakes, thus concentrating pathogens and making transmission more likely.

Most of the publicized cases are especially tragic because they involve young people, who are more likely than senior citizens to jump repeatedly into a lake or stream. When they hit the surface, water is forced into the nasal cavity, along with any amebae it may contain. In rare cases, the amebae then travel up the nasal passages to the brain, where their life cycle interferes with that of the host. Swelling of the brain results, and death occurs after five or six days.

The free-living soil ameba *Balamuthia mandrillaris* also can invade the human brain, possibly through a skin lesion, causing a lethal form of encephalitis. Only about 100 known cases have occurred, and only one of those survived.

A freshwater ameba called *Acanthamoeba* sometimes causes a mild form of meningitis, but it is more famous as the organism that can damage the cornea of contact lens wearers. The condition is called acanthamoeba keratitis. On the bright side, this ameba produces a blood clot-dissolving enzyme that may have important medical uses.

Cryptosporidiosis. This worldwide disease results from an infestation by *Cryptosporidium parvum*, (Figure 2.2) one of a large group of parasitic protozoans called Sporozoa. Waterborne or foodborne members of this group, called coccidians, usually take up residence in the host's intestine, where they can cause severe diarrhea or dysentery.

Briefly, the host swallows a cell called an oocyst, out of which swim a large number of immature forms called sporozoites. These enter epithelial cells in the lining of the intestine, where they go through a series of developmental stages, finally resulting in the production of more oocysts. Some of these oocysts pass out of the body in feces, which may contaminate water or food; the

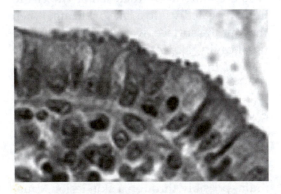

Figure 2.2. Although we cannot show you the effects of cryptosporidiosis, here is the bug itself, attached to the lining of the intestine. (*Source*: Armed Forces Institute of Pathology.)

oocyst has a hard shell and can even survive in chlorinated water. Other oocysts remain in the intestine, starting a new cycle. Cryptosporidiosis apparently is not transmitted directly from person to person, as the oocyte needs to spend some time in water before it develops to an infective stage.

Most domestic and wild animals have their own coccidian parasites, but similar infestations in humans received little publicity until the 1970s. In 1976, *Cryptosporidium* turned up in a man who was being treated with immune suppressants for another disease. In the 1980s and 1990s, outbreaks of diarrhea caused by the same organism occurred in healthy children and adults. One such outbreak in Wisconsin involved over 400,000 people (Table 2.2), apparently after cattle waste contaminated a public water supply. Public health investigators have traced outbreaks to contaminated swimming pools, fountains, drinking water, and foods. The illness rarely lasts more than two weeks, but patients have commented that it seems longer. There are about 300,000 cases each year in the United States, 90 percent of them waterborne.

At the time this book was written, there was no standard treatment for cryptosporidiosis other than antidiarrheal medications and replacement of lost fluid and electrolyte. Some sources recommend the drug paromomycin, but other drugs are being evaluated.

Cyclosporiasis. This is another coccidial disease of human beings. Its life cycle, mode of transmission, and symptoms are similar to those of cryptosporidiosis, except that cyclosporiasis often involves a series of remissions and relapses over a period of several weeks, sometimes with substantial

Table 2.2
Examples of Waterborne Disease Outbreaks

Disease	Date	Location	Estimated Cases	Estimated Deaths
Cholera	1849	Chicago, IL	NR	678
Cholera	1849	Canada	NR	6000
Cholera	1854	Chicago, IL	NR	1424
Cholera	1991–99	South America	1 million	11,000
Cryptosporidiosis	1993	Milwaukee, WI	403,000	104
Cyclosporiasis	1990	Chicago, IL	21	0
Giardiasis	1995	New York	1449	0
Giardiasis	1997	Oregon	100	0
E. coli O157	1999	Albany, NY	1000+	2
Norwalk-like Virus	1987	PA, DE, NJ	5000	NR
Salmonellosis	1965	Riverside, CA	15,000	NR
Shigellosis	1997	Lubbock, TX	480	0
Shigellosis	1998	Minnesota	83	0

Sources: Anderson (1991); Huang et al. (1995); Mead et al. (1999); *Morbidity and Mortality Weekly Reports*, various.

weight loss. The first known human outbreak in the United States was in Chicago in 1990, when 21 healthy adults became ill from a hospital water supply that was contaminated with *Cyclospora cayetanensis* of domestic origin. Ducks and various wild mammals may serve as reservoir hosts.

In 1996, cyclosporiasis received a great deal of publicity when health officials traced a large outbreak to imported raspberries from Guatemala. Texas authorities had first blamed the California strawberry industry, and the ensuing panic prompted an intensive search for other sources. Test methods available in 1996 found no *Cyclospora* on any berries, Guatemalan or otherwise, and the conclusions relied on epidemiological data. Two 1997 outbreaks in Florida were traced by similar means to lettuce grown in the United States. New test methods reported in 2000 may help verify the sources of future outbreaks.

By the latest estimates, about 16,000 Americans contract cyclosporiasis each year. Few people with moderate diarrhea contact their physicians, however, and the true incidence probably is much higher. Most recently reported cases have been foodborne, possibly due to media coverage of the raspberry issue. As discussed in Chapter 3, this is primarily a waterborne disease, but raw raspberries and lettuce have surfaces that may trap contaminated irrigation water.

A clinical trial in 1995 showed that trimethoprim/sulfamethoxazole (TMP/SMX) is effective in treatment of cyclosporiasis. Ciprofloxacin was slightly less effective in a 2000 study.

Giardiasis. Many people claim to remember the days when it was safe to drink directly from a flowing mountain stream, without resorting to an arsenal of water filters and chlorine tablets. In reality, even the most delicious untreated water has never been entirely "safe" to drink, and many a backpacker has learned that the fiercest creatures in the woods are not the bears.

The agent of giardiasis is a protozoan (*Giardia lamblia*), but it is not closely related to the ones that cause cryptosporidiosis and cyclosporiasis. It is less likely to occur in tap water than those organisms, as it is sensitive to chlorine. The symptoms it produces are similar, but arguably worse; the diarrhea can last for six weeks without relief, and tends to be accompanied by nausea, cramps, fatigue, and weight loss. In rare cases, severe giardiasis can damage the small intestine.

Boiling water for five minutes will kill *Giardia*, but iodine tablets will not. Backpackers sometimes carry special filters for removing *Giardia*; these generally work, but the resulting clean water may become recontaminated if the container is rinsed with untreated water or allowed to come in contact with the used filter. An estimated two million people in the United States contract giardiasis every year, and about 90 percent of cases are waterborne. Some cases are foodborne, and in male homosexuals this can be a sexually transmitted disease (see Chapter 5). Wild beavers and some domestic animals may serve as a reservoir. The same antibiotics used to treat other protozoan diseases usually are effective against giardiasis.

EXAMPLES OF WATERBORNE MULTICELLULAR PARASITES

The 1979 motion picture *Alien* was largely an exaggeration of what real parasites do to their hosts. The important differences are that real-life parasites are not intelligent and do not grow to enormous size. A person's body can contain a guinea worm a meter long, or a family of tapeworms with a total length of 50 meters, but these are narrow, soggy creatures that cannot pursue us on dry land.

Candirú Catfish (**Vandellia cirrhosa** *and related species*). This fish appears to be the only vertebrate animal that can live as a parasite inside the human body, and the only one that habitually enters by swimming up the urethra.

Humans are not the candirú's normal host; there are not enough of us in its habitat. Its usual strategy is to enter the gill chamber of a larger fish, which it finds by following the emerging stream of flavored water. Once inside, it uses its rasp-like mouth to feed on the host's blood. But a human will do in a pinch—and we have no gills. If a person urinates while swimming or wading, the candirú follows the stream of urine up the concentration gradient to its source, and then swims inside (it is a very small fish). Contrary to urban legend, the person cannot be standing beside the stream urinating into the water, nor can the candirú leap through the air to its victim like a tiny salmon climbing a waterfall. The victim must be *in* the water.

A doctor must remove the candirú quickly, before it locks itself in place with its spines and starts making a mess. Otherwise, the victim will die. The best way to avoid the problem is to wear tight clothing while swimming, or possibly take up tennis instead. This little darling is a native of Central and South America, but has recently taken up residence in at least two Florida counties.

*Guinea Worm Disease (**Dracunculiasis, Dracontiasis**).* Of all the parasites that afflict humans, guinea worm is one of the most devastating. The process begins when a tiny shrimp-like animal called a copepod swallows a guinea worm larva. Inside the copepod, the larva develops to the infective stage. Then a person, let us say a man, drinks water contaminated with copepods. The guinea worm larvae released in his stomach are now free to migrate through his body and pursue their own interests, including reproduction.

By the time the gravid female worm reaches the subcutaneous tissues of the man's foot, it is a meter long. A blister appears on his foot, accompanied by pain, fever, and diarrhea. Finally, the blister ruptures. Every time the man steps in water, the female worm discharges larvae to start the cycle again. The female worm may dangle from the open sore (Figure 2.3), and an old method of treatment was to wind the worm carefully onto a stick.

Until recently, Guinea worm disease was particularly common in India. In 1984, the country had 40,000 reported cases. It was a joyous day when, in 1999, WHO declared India free of guinea worm disease after a successful program of health education and improved water quality. Several African nations have also eradicated or greatly reduced the incidence of this disease. Former U.S. president Jimmy Carter has led a campaign to eradicate Guinea worm disease worldwide.

Leeches. Although leeches often attach to humans, and are known to serve as disease vectors in some animals (mainly fish), they do not transmit any major human disease. During the Vietnam War, many U.S. soldiers had streptococcal infections from leech

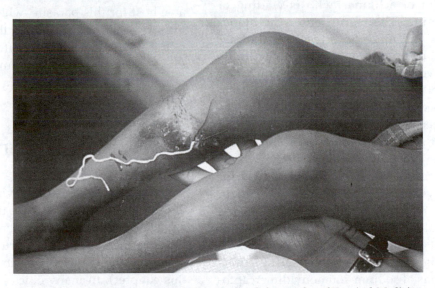

Figure 2.3. Emerging Guinea Worm. (Reprinted from the *Colour Atlas of Tropical Medicine and Parasitology*, 4th ed., edited by W. Peters and H. M. Gilles, p. 159, copyright 1995, by permission of the publisher Mosby.)

bites, but any dirty skin puncture can become infected. Mainly, these familiar freshwater worms are annoying, and people seem to find them repulsive. They have a sucker at each end, which is confusing the first time you see one.

For centuries, doctors have used leeches to remove excess blood from tissue, but public acceptance remains low. In 2001, researchers at the University of Wisconsin announced that they had invented a mechanical leech.

Schistosomiasis or *Bilharziasis*. This parasitic infestation kills an estimated 14,000 people each year worldwide and causes severe illness in millions more. Worldwide, at least 200 million people have schistosomiasis. The agents include several species of blood flukes or trematodes in the genus *Schistosoma*. After their larvae (called cercariae) mature in freshwater snails, they emerge into the water, where they penetrate the skin of a human who is wading or swimming. The worms enter the bloodstream and migrate to the liver, kidney, spleen, or other organs. They mate in the blood vessels that feed the intestines, and some of the resulting eggs find their way to the intestinal lumen or urinary bladder. The host then sheds them into the environment to start another cycle in water. But that is not the end of the infestation; the worms may continue living in the same host for many years, even adjusting their growth rate in response to changes in the host's physical condition.

Until about 1970, doctors treated schistosomiasis with dangerous intravenous injections of sodium antimony dimercaptosuccinate and sodium antimony tartrate. Safer, more effective drugs such as praziqantel, oxamniquine, and metrifonate

are now available in pill form. In the 1920s, before the pills were available, Egypt started a mass injection program to control schistosomiasis. Despite good intentions, the use of inadequately sterilized equipment resulted in an epidemic of hepatitis C (see Chapter 5), which now infects an estimated 20 percent of the Egyptian population.

Swimmer's Itch. It may be stretching a point to call this parasite a "hazard," but we include it because of its close relationship to the agent of schistosomiasis, one of the most devastating diseases in the developing world.

The agent of swimmer's itch is a fluke called *Trichobilharzia*. It is most common in the Great Lakes area of North America, but outbreaks have occurred in all 50 states, and the incidence seems to be increasing. Just as in schistosomiasis, the larvae mature inside a snail and then penetrate the skin of a person who is swimming or wading in the water—but human beings are not an acceptable host for this parasite, which normally lives in a duck or goose. Thus, the larvae die in the skin, and the body's efforts to expel the dead bugs create itchy pimples or blisters that last two or three days. No treatment usually is required.

OUTLOOK FOR THE TWENTY-FIRST CENTURY

Water treatment is improving in many developing nations, and those that have not already done so are likely to embrace chlorine treatment, in light of Peru's recent experience with cholera (described earlier in this chapter). In many cities in the developed world, however, existing water treatment and delivery systems have far exceeded their shelf life. They will continue to deteriorate unless repaired; at the same time, population growth will increase the demand for clean water. Some newly discovered human pathogens may require more effective water filtration and monitoring systems. *Cryptosporidium*, for example, can survive chlorine treatment.

The subject of global warming has been done to death elsewhere, including its potential effects on waterborne and vector-borne disease distribution. Not all experts agree, however, that the present warming trend will even continue, much less that it will restore malaria to Los Angeles. Local management of wetlands, discarded tire repositories, and other mosquito breeding grounds will most likely make a bigger difference in vector management in the foreseeable future.

Global programs to eradicate specific waterborne diseases, such as Guinea worm disease, cholera, and Buruli ulcer, are expected to yield dramatic results if funding continues.

THE GOOD OLD DAYS

In its 1996 *World Health Report*, WHO reported that "Almost half the world's population suffers from diseases associated with insufficient or contaminated water." For the most colorful and uncompromising descriptions of the human consequences of water pollution, however, we turn to the medical literature of the nineteenth century, when this problem was nearly universal:

I introduced a polypus forceps into the lower part of the pharynx and toward the esophagus, where a body, distinctly moving, was felt. This body I seized with the forceps, and with considerable force managed to remove it. It was a leech between 2½ and three inches in length. . . . This man had drunk the pea-soup-like water of a tank dug in the side of the hill, rather than go a few hundred yards to a spring where the water is perfectly clear and pure.

There is a somewhat similar case of a military pharmacist, a member of the French army in Spain, who drank some water from a pitcher and exhibited, about a half hour afterward, a persistent hemorrhage from the nose. Emaciation progressively continued, although his appetite was normal. . . . Three weeks afterward he carried in his nostril a tampon of lint, wet with an astringent solution, and, on the next day, on blowing his nose, there fell from the right nostril a body which he recognized as a leech.[2]

Cholera, now restricted largely to developing nations with inadequate water treatment and sewage facilities, was once a serious problem throughout North America (see Table 2.2). In a letter dated June 29, 1849, a Mr. Chambers of Mount Pleasant, Tennessee describes the ravages of one such epidemic (original spelling preserved):

I have not heard from there [Memphis, Tennessee] now for several days—at the last account the Cholera was raging to a fearful extent, upwards of Nine Thousand have left and died together. . . . Such times were never seen. None are exempt. Young Men and Ladies in the very bloom of health perhapse in on hour are no more. Business is almost entirely suspended. Nor can you see a face that looks bright, nor an Eye looks drye—As yet we have had no case of true Cholera in the Country only those who contract it in Memphis or some where on the river.[3]

---

[2]G.M. Gould and W.L. Pyle, *Anomalies and Curiosities of Medicine* (New York: Bell Publishing Co., 1896). (This is not a tall tale; the Israeli journal *Harefuah* reported several similar cases in September 1989.)
[3]Source: Collection of Frederick Smoot (published on the Internet in 1997).

FROM THE AUTHOR'S FILE CABINET

In May 1997, a 13-year-old boy in a small southern California town contracted a severe watery diarrhea that caused him to miss four days of school. As he had only a slight fever and no abdominal pain, his parents did not take him to a doctor, and by the fifth day he had apparently recovered. Soon afterward, his father developed similar but more severe diarrhea, losing 15 pounds in five days. As the father wanted to lose weight anyway, and had no pain, he did not see a doctor either. The family concluded that some minor gastrointestinal virus was at work. The mother expected to be next, having mopped up after both patients, but neither she nor her 15-year-old daughter became ill.

About four weeks later, the young man had a relapse, this time with severe vomiting and bloating as well as watery diarrhea. But he recovered after a day or two, and did not want to see a doctor. His father, who had not regained the lost weight, had a second bout of diarrhea at about the same time—and yet the mother and daughter remained healthy. As all four family members were in close contact and ate the same foods, it seemed unlikely that the cause was either a food prepared at home or a pathogen that was transmissible from person to person.

Two weeks later, the young man was sick again, this time with a moderate fever and headache in addition to nausea and abdominal cramping. As he had rarely been sick before in his life, his mother began to worry, particularly after her still-slim husband reported a third bout. The recurring illness seemed to resemble cyclosporiasis, the subject of media coverage that year. Pos-

sible sources were the tap water, which only the male household members drank, and a fast-food meal that the father and son had shared eight days before the first symptoms appeared. A teacher remarked that several local children were absent from school with a similar illness during the same week in May.

For many years, the town's rural water company had failed to meet federal water quality standards (which is why the mother and daughter refused to drink it), but there were no reports of protozoa in the water. A quick literature search revealed, however, that *Cyclospora* had been detected in water samples from nearby drainages, and that the organism had contaminated other public water supplies.

When the young man became ill for the fourth time in late June, the mother called a doctor's office assigned by the family's insurance plan. She did not get past the nurse, who said the doctor was booked up for eight weeks and that the illness was probably either a virus or "nerves." Without seeing the patient, the nurse advised the mother to try an over-the-counter diarrhea medicine and an herbal tea. The mother hung up. (The father also had a fourth recurrence, but liked his new waistline and was not sure he wanted to recover.)

Finally, the mother called a doctor at the CDC in Atlanta, who told her that cyclosporiasis had been linked only to imported raspberries; thus, if no family member had eaten raspberries, the illness could not be cyclosporiasis. The mother pointed out that *Cyclospora* had also been found in water and lettuce, but the doctor said this was unlikely. The mother offered to pay for testing to rule out cyclosporiasis; the doctor referred her to another doctor at the California State Health Department, who, in turn, referred her to the local County Health Department.

The County Health Department said they could indeed provide testing, and told the mother to bring her son to a certain address—which turned out to be a dilapidated clinic for low-income people. Sitting in that waiting room for five hours, surrounded by rash-covered children and coughing adults, may have raised the political consciousness of this upper-middle-class family, but did little to solve the young man's immediate problem. The doctor who eventually saw him was not familiar with cyclosporiasis or other coccidioses, and said he was not sure what tests to order. The mother thanked him, paid at the desk, drove her son home with his sample container, and bought a water filter. But as the illness did not return for a fifth round, reliable testing for coccidia was no longer possible, and the cause never was identified. There were no long-term sequelae except that the father kept the weight off for two years.

In 2000, one of the doctors mentioned in this story coauthored an article about the 1997 California cyclosporiasis outbreaks.[4] The article concluded that "media reports and enhanced laboratory surveillance improved detection of these outbreaks" by alerting the public. Several cases were cited in which people became ill after eating raspberries and asked their physicians to test them for *Cyclospora*. Another interpretation of the same data, however, is that this self-selected sample was biased by the media focus on the risks of "foreign" raspberries.

Although cyclosporiasis is known to be waterborne as well as foodborne, the investigation was limited to food-related clusters. If other potential sources are not tested, none can be found.

REFERENCES AND RECOMMENDED READING

"After Smallpox, Guinea Worm Disease Eradicated from India." Associated Press, December 24, 1999.

American Water Works Association. 1997. *Cryptosporidium and Water: A Public Health Handbook*. Denver, CO: AWWA Working Group on Waterborne Cryptosporidiosis.

Anderson, Christopher. "Cholera Epidemic Traced to Risk Miscalculation." *Nature*, November 28, 1991, p. 255.

Berkman, Alan, and Bakalar, Nicholas. 2000. *Hepatitis A to G: The Facts You Need to Know about All Forms of this Dangerous Disease*. New York: Warner Books.

Bilson, Geoffrey. 1980. *Darkened House: Cholera in Nineteenth-Century Canada, 1832–1871* (Social History of Canada, No. 31). Toronto: University of Toronto Press.

"Bottled Water in Mexico." *Beverage World*, April 15, 1997.

Bovsun, Mara. "Man Attacked by Saltwater Flesh-Eating Bug." United Press International, March 15, 2000.

Collins, Andrew E. 1998. *Environment, Health, and Population Displacement: Development and Change in Mozambique's Diarrhoeal Disease Ecology*. Brookfield, MA: Ashgate.

Craun, Gunther F. (Editor). 1986. *Waterborne Diseases in the United States*. CRC Press.

Davies, S.J., et al. "Modulation of Blood Fluke Development in the Liver by Hepatic CD4+ Lymphocytes." *Science*, November 9, 2001, pp. 1358–1361.

"Defeat of a Superbug? An Experimental Virus May Have Cured a Deadly Infection." ABCNews.com, September 16, 1999.

[4] J.C. Mohle-Boetani, et al., "The Impact of Health Communication and Enhanced Laboratory-based Surveillance on Detection of Cyclosporiasis Outbreaks in California" (*Emerging Infectious Diseases*, March–April 2000, pp. 200–203).

Environmental Working Group. 1996. *Just Add Water: Violations of Federal Health Standards in Tap Water, 1994–1995*. Washington, DC: Environmental Working Group.

"Eye Researchers Make Serendipitous Lab Discovery of Blood-Clot Buster that May Help Heart Attack Patients." News Release, University of Texas Southwestern Medical Center at Dallas, March 5, 1996.

Fayer, Ronald (Editor). 1997. *Cryptosporidium and Cryptosporidiosis*. Boca Raton, FL: CRC Press.

"Federal Government: Chip Dip Sickens At Least 30." Reuters News Service, January 27, 2000.

Gleeson, Cara, and Gray, N.F. 1997. *Coliform Index and Waterborne Disease: Problems of Microbial Drinking Water Assessment*. London: E. & F.N. Spoon.

Gorbach, Sherwood L. (Editor) 1986. *Infectious Diarrhea*. St. Louis, MO: Blackwell Mosby Book Distributors.

Gudger, Eugene W. 1930. *The Candirú: The Only Vertebrate Parasite of Man*. New York: P.B. Hoeber, Inc.

"*Helicobacter pylori* in Peptic Ulcer Disease." NIH Consensus Statement, January 7–9, 1994.

Herman, J.R. "Candirú: Urinophilic Catfish, Its Gift to Urology." *Urology*, March 1973, pp. 265–267.

Holman, Robert E. 1993. *Cryptosporidium: A Drinking Water Supply Concern*. Raleigh, NC: Water Resources Research Institute, University of North Carolina.

Huang, P., et al. "The First Reported Outbreak of Diarrheal Illness Associated with Cyclospora in the United States." *Annals of Internal Medicine*, Vol. 123, 1995, pp. 409–414.

Hunter, Paul R. 1997. *Waterborne Disease: Epidemiology and Ecology*. New York: John Wiley.

Huq, M.I. 1979. *Isolation, Purification, and Characterization of a Shigella Plague*. Bangladesh: International Centre for Diarrhoeal Disease Research.

Jordan, Peter, et al. 1993. *Human Schistosomiasis*. New York: CABI Publishing.

Keutsch, Gerald T. (Editor). 1991. Workshop on Invasive Diarrheas, Shigellosis, and Dysentery: Bangkok, Thailand, 7–9 December 1988.

Reviews of Infectious Diseases, Vol. 13, Suppl. 4. University of Chicago Press.

Klemm, Donald J. 1982. *Freshwater Leeches (Annelida: Hirudinea) of North America*. Washington, DC: U.S. Government Printing Office.

Kretschmer, R.R. (Editor). 1990. *Amebiasis: Infection and Disease by* Entamoeba histolytica. Boca Raton, FL: CRC Press.

Kumate, J. "Infectious Diseases in the 21st Century." *Archives of Medical Research*, Vol. 28 No. 2, 1997, pp. 155–161.

"Lake Users Warned of Health Hazards." Associated Press, August 16, 1998.

Logsdon, Gary S. (Editor) 1988. *Controlling Waterborne Giardiasis: A State of the Art Review*. Reston, VA: American Society of Civil Engineers.

Long, Peter L. (Editor). 1982. *The Biology of the Coccidia*. Baltimore, MD: University Park Press.

Los Angeles County Health Department. 1954. *Report on Epidemic of Shigellosis in a Trailer Village*. Los Angeles, CA: Los Angeles County Health Department.

"Many Bacterial Epidemics Stem from Virus Conspiracy." News Release, University of Maryland, May 27, 1999.

Marshall, B.J., and Warren, J.R. "Unidentified Curved Bacilli in the Stomach of Patients with Gastritis and Peptic Ulceration." *Lancet*, June 16, 1984, pp. 1311–1315.

Martinez-Palomo, A. (Editor). 1986. *Amebiasis*. Human Parasitic Diseases Series, Vol. 2. New York: Elsevier Science Publishers.

Mead, Paul S., et al. "Food-Related Illness and Death in the United States." *Emerging Infectious Diseases*, September–October 1999, pp. 607–625.

"Mechanical Leech Does Icky Job Better." Reuters News Service, December 15, 2001.

Meisel, J.L., et al. "Overwhelming Watery Diarrhea Associated with a *Cryptosporidium* in an Immunosuppressed Patient." *Gastroenterology*, June 1976, pp. 1156–1160.

National Research Council. 1999. *From Monsoons to Microbes: Understanding the Ocean's Role in Human Health*. Washington, DC: National Academy Press.

Olson, Betty H. 1999. *Geographical and Seasonal Occurrence of* Cyclospora cayetanensis *in Southern California Waters*. Davis, CA: University of California Water Resources Center.

Olson, Erik. 1995. *You Are What You Drink*: Cryptosporidium *and Other Contaminants Found in the Water Served to Millions of Americans*. New York: Natural Resources Defense Council.

Orlandi, P.A., and Lampel, K.A. "Extraction-free, Filter-based Template Preparation for Rapid and Sensitive PCR Detection of Pathogenic Parasitic Protozoa." *Journal of Clinical Microbiology*, June 2000, pp. 2271–2277.

"Outbreaks of *Cyclosporiasis* and Guatemalan Raspberries." News Release, U.S. Food and Drug Administration, June 10, 1997.

Panisset, Ulysses B. 2000. *International Health Statecraft: Foreign Policy and Public Health in Peru's Cholera Epidemic*. Lanham, MD: University Press of America.

Parent, G., et al. "Grands Barrages, Santé et Nutrition en Afrique: Au-delà de la Polémique." [Dams, Health and Nutrition in Africa: Beyond the Polemic.] *Sante*, November–December 1997, pp. 417–422.

Portaels, Françoise, et al. "Insects in the Transmission of *Mycobacterium ulcerans* Infection." *Lancet*, March 20, 1999, p. 986.

Ravdin, Jonathan I. 1999. *Amebiasis*. London: Imperial College Press.

Rosenberg, Charles E. 1987. *The Cholera Years: The United States in 1832, 1849, and 1866*. Chicago: University of Chicago Press.

Sansonetti, P.J. (Editor). 1992. *Pathogenesis of Shigellosis*. Berlin: Springer-Verlag.

Sawyer, Roy T. 1986. *Leech Biology and Behaviour*. New York: Oxford University Press.

Semret, M., et al. "*Mycobacterium ulcerans* infection (Buruli ulcer): First Reported Case in a Traveler." *American Journal of Tropical Medicine and Hygiene*, November 1999, pp. 689–693.

Snowden, Frank M. 1996. *Naples in the Time of Cholera, 1884–1911*. New York: Cambridge University Press.

"Special Starch May Help in Treatment of Cholera." Reuters News Service, February 2, 2000.

"Stomach Bacteria Linked to Pancreatic Cancer." Reuters News Service, July 10, 2001.

"Trouble in the Water." Earthwatch, University of Wisconsin, August 11, 1999.

Van Heyningen, W.E., and Seal, J.R. 1983. *Cholera: The American Scientific Experience, 1947–1980*. Boulder, CO: Westview Press.

Van Hogendorp, K. 1998. *Survival in the Land of Dysentery: The World War II Experiences of a Red Cross Worker in India*. Fredericksburg, VA: Sergeant Kirkland's.

Wang, Joseph. 2000. *Miniaturized DNA Biosensor Systems for Detecting Cryptosporidium in Water Samples*. Las Cruces, NM: New Mexico Water Resources Research Institute.

CHAPTER 3

Human Pathogens in Food

Diseased nature oftentimes breaks forth
In strange eruptions.
— William Shakespeare, *King Henry IV, Pt. I, III, i, 27*

Of all the topics that people commonly discuss, food may inspire the most heated controversy. Many religions have dietary laws or food-based rituals; the exchange of food has always been a sacred bond. Health-food dealers serve these needs by providing consumers with more natural-tasting and less processed foods. Meanwhile, the vectors of urban legends circulate variations on the "Kentucky Fried Rat" theme, and hundreds of books and tabloid articles explain how our food is killing us and how we can be saved.

The current epidemic of obesity suggests that most Americans do not really believe these claims. The fear of food is just another hazard to be enjoyed and overcome. But with so much emphasis on food, it is understandable that every new outbreak of foodborne illness elicits public outrage and often becomes headline news.

In the United States alone, foodborne illnesses kill some 5,000 people each year, send over 300,000 to the hospital, and cause severe discomfort in millions more.[1] In 1997, ground beef caused 130,000 such illnesses. The U.S. Centers for Disease Control and Prevention (CDC) announced in 1999 that each American now has one chance in 840 of being hospitalized for food poisoning at some point in his or her life, and one chance in 55,000 of dying from this cause.

It is not clear whether the frequency of foodborne disease is actually increasing, or health departments and the media are simply paying more attention to it. Some journalists have blamed the alleged epidemic on the usual suspects: women, for seeking professions instead of majoring in home economics; young people, for inexperience at food preparation; and foreigners, for no clear reason. Others have cited the fast-food

[1]Paul S. Mead, et al., "Food–Related Illness and Death in the United States" (*Emerging Infectious Diseases*, September–October 1999, pp. 607–625).

industry, whose meat-mixing practices can quickly spread contamination through a thousand hamburgers; lawyers, for encouraging litigation every time someone gets a stomachache; and health-food dealers, for promoting unpasteurized milk and juices, unprocessed soft cheeses, vegetables grown on fresh manure, and other marginally safe products. Raw milk, in particular, has been a vehicle for several diseases, including tuberculosis, Brainerd diarrhea, and severe diarrhea caused by *E. coli*, *Salmonella*, and *Campylobacter*.

CROSS-REFERENCE

The titles of Chapters 2–5 reflect the principal modes of disease transmission. Most pathogens, however, can be transmitted in more than one way. Many pathogens found in food also occur in water (see Chapter 2). Some of these same diseases are transmissible by contact (Chapter 5), or result from bacterial or fungal toxins (Chapter 7). Thus, for the reader's convenience, Table 3.1 lists potentially foodborne pathogens that appear in other chapters.

FECAL-ORAL TRANSMISSION

Transmission of foodborne illnesses often follows the fecal-oral route. This disagreeable term simply means that people often do not wash their hands adequately after using the toilet—or after various dirty jobs, such as changing the kitty litter or shoveling manure on the farm. Later, when preparing a meal, they may inadvertently transfer the remaining traces of fecal mate-

rial or other body fluids to the food. A person who handles a contaminated raw chicken in the kitchen, for example, and then touches the baby's spoon, may transmit a disease such as salmonellosis. Bacteria find their way from the intestine of the chicken (or the butcher) to the baby's mouth, even if no one in the household ever eats the chicken.

People must have figured out the connection between dirty hands and foodborne illness a long time ago, judging by the "clean hand" customs that exist in many cultures. In some countries where soap and water are not readily available, it is still considered proper to wipe with one hand and eat or shake hands with the other. These customs may partly explain why left-handed people were once subject to discrimination.

A recent study with hidden video cameras revealed that the most spotless home kitchen can be the setting for high-risk behavior, usually involving contact with raw meat.[2] Similar studies in restaurants have shown that many food service workers fail to wash their hands—or dry them adequately, which is equally important—after using the toilet; others scrub properly, but then touch a contaminated surface (such as the bathroom doorknob) on the way out. Still others rely on the new hand sanitizer gels, but a 1999 study showed that some of these products actually increase the bacterial count on hands. Such hygiene problems are unintentional; but sometimes the fecal-oral route takes a more literal form, particularly among very young children, disgruntled restaurant employees, and inmates of mental institutions. In January

[2]Paula Kurtzweil, "Keeping Food Safety Surveys Honest" (*FDA Consumer Magazine*, September–October 1999, p. 14).

Table 3.1
Cross–Reference: Other Foodborne Diseases

Disease	Chapter	Notes
Amebic Dysentery	2	Water or food
Cholera	2	Water or food
Cyclosporiasis	2	Water or food
Hepatitis E	2	Water or food
Leptospirosis	2	Water, food, or contact
Shigellosis	2	Water or food
Ulcer Disease	2	Water or food
Diphtheria	4	Airborne, contact, or milk
Q Fever	4	Airborne, contact, or milk
Tuberculosis	4	Airborne or from raw milk
Astrovirus	5	Contact, food, or water
Hepatitis A	5	Contact, food, or water
Listeriosis	5	Contact, food, or airborne
Poliomyelitis	5	Contact, milk, or possibly water
Rabies	5	Usually contact; occasionally milk
Rat–bite Fever	5	Contact, milk, or possibly airborne
Rotavirus	5	Contact, food, or airborne
Streptococcal Disease	5	Contact or food
Tularemia	5	Contact, food, water, or (rarely) airborne
Brucellosis	6	Foodborne or contact; mainly in livestock

2001, the U.S. Food and Drug Administration (FDA) issued new safety guidelines that include background checks on food service workers, to prevent possible terrorism as well as less organized mischief.

Now that the reader is thoroughly queasy, we must point out that colonies of bacteria and fungi thrive under everyone's fingernails. Life is dirty, and there is nothing we can do about it. Nevertheless, the solution to fecal-oral transmission is fairly simple: Don't touch the raw hamburger, cover your hands with plastic bags when you make a salad—reuse the bags, if you wish, but don't turn them inside out—and, in the words of everyone's mother, before putting anything

in your mouth, think twice about where it has been.

OTHER ROUTES OF FOOD CONTAMINATION

Some of the worst foodborne illnesses result when bacteria in the gut of a domestic animal come in contact with the meat during processing. Examples include *Salmonella* and *Campylobacter* in poultry and the infamous *E. coli* 0157:H7 in beef. Another source of contamination occurs when flies land on food after walking on feces or garbage. Studies have shown that a single housefly (*Musca domestica*) can carry as many as six million bacteria and assorted viruses on its feet. Depending on where the fly acquired them, these passengers may be harmless, or they may be agents of diseases such as cholera, typhoid, dysentery, poliomyelitis, and infectious hepatitis. The eggs of parasitic worms also may cling to a fly's feet.

Polluted water is a frequent source of food contamination. Such water may be used for irrigation before a crop is harvested, or it may be sprinkled on vegetables to keep them fresh at the produce stand, or used to wash a carcass to remove visible contamination. *Cyclospora* (see Chapter 2) is a waterborne protozoan that often contaminates food. Note that the foods most often responsible for its transmission, such as raspberries and lettuce, have rather complicated surfaces and are eaten raw. Polluted water is likely to run off the smooth surface of a tomato, for example, whereas a head of lettuce provides nooks and crannies where the water can collect.

It is important to understand that diseases with similar symptoms may have entirely different causes. A person who contracts acute viral gastroenteritis (see Chapter 5) from another person, for example, almost always attributes it to "something I ate." In such a situation, throwing out the potato salad will not help; everyone in the family is likely to come down with the same illness anyway. Some food allergies (see Chapter 7) also may have symptoms that resemble those of a foodborne bacterial disease.

For the benefit of any reader who may associate food contamination with backward societies or individuals, we will conclude this introduction with the results of a 1995 survey by the Center for Food Safety and Applied Nutrition. The survey showed that 53 percent of Americans consumed raw eggs (in various mixtures), 23 percent ate undercooked hamburgers, and 25 percent did not wash their cutting boards after preparing raw meat or other foods. Such behavior was most frequent among well-educated people and males.

EXAMPLES OF FOODBORNE BACTERIAL DISEASES

Bacteria growing in food cause illness in two different ways. If the bacteria produce toxins, and the toxins cause symptoms, the illness is called an **intoxication**, more specifically **food poisoning**. (Intoxication, in this sense, means getting poisoned rather than getting drunk.) If, however, the bacteria simply colonize some part of the body and begin multiplying there, whether they release a toxin or not, the illness is called an **infection**.

Table 3.2 lists some examples of foodborne disease outbreaks, and Table 3.3 provides estimates of annual incidence in the United States.

Foodborne Bacteria that Cause Intoxication

Bacillus cereus *Food Poisoning*. This intoxication strikes about 27,000 people each year in the United States. The agent, *Bacillus cereus*, is a spore-forming bacterium that occurs in soils worldwide under anaerobic conditions (without oxygen). The spores can survive boiling, and when a cooked rice or vegetable dish stands at room temperature for a long time, the spores can germinate, allowing the bacteria to multiply rapidly

Table 3.2
Examples of Outbreaks of Foodborne Disease

Disease or Pathogen	Date	Location	Est. Cases	Est. Deaths
Campylobacter	1989	Missouri	101	0
Clostridium perfringens	1991	Wisconsin	600	0
Clostridium perfringens	1994	Australia	230	0
Hepatitis A	1989	Washington State	192	0
Listeriosis	1985	United States	142	48
Listeriosis	1998	United States	75	15
Norwalk–like Virus	1982	Minnesota	3,000	NR
Norwalk–like Virus	1999	Alaska	100	0
Salmonellosis	1996	United States	224,000	NR
Salmonellosis	1994	Finland	210	NR
Salmonellosis	1994	Sweden	282	NR
Salmonellosis	1996	California	450	0
Shigellosis	1988	Michigan	3,175	0
Staphylococcus	1998	Texas	1,364	0
Toxigenic E. coli	1993	Washington State	500	4
Toxigenic E. coli	1996	Western U.S., Canada	70	1
Toxigenic E. coli	1996	Japan	12,000	10+
Typhoid	1891	Chicago, IL	NR	1,997
Vibriosis	1997	Pacific Coast	209	1

Sources: Hennessy et al. (1996); Chicago Public Library, Web site; *Morbidity and Mortality Weekly Reports*, various.

Table 3.3
Estimated Annual Incidence of Some Foodborne Diseases, United States

Disease or Pathogen	Cases	Percent Foodborne	Fatality Rate
Norwalk–Like Virus	23,000,000	40	low
Campylobacteriosis	2,443,926	80	0.0010
Salmonellosis	1,412,498	95	0.0078
E. coli (all serotypes)	269,060	variable	variable
Clostridium perfringens	248,520	100	0.0005
Toxoplasmosis	225,000	50	low
Staphylococcus	185,060	100	0.0002
Yersiniosis	96,368	90	0.0005
Streptococcus	50,920	100	0.0000
Listeriosis	2,518	99	0.2000
Typhoid Fever	824	80	0.0040
Botulism	58	100	0.0769
Trichinosis	52	100	0.003

Source: Mead et al. (1999).

and release toxins. The illness usually lasts no longer than 24 hours and is rarely fatal. Symptoms include abdominal pain, diarrhea, nausea, and vomiting.

Clostridium botulinum *Food Poisoning.* Botulism is perhaps the most feared of all food intoxications, partly because of its high lethality (at least one-third of untreated cases) and partly because of its association with canned food (Figure 3.1). If, for example, people decide to eat a potato salad that has stood in the sun for several hours, at least they can feel responsible for the outcome; but they expect canned food to be clean and wholesome, particularly home-canned food without preservatives.

The botulinum bacillus is associated with canned food because it grows and produces its toxin (called botulin, botulinum, or BTX) only under anaerobic conditions. Nearly all commercially canned foods nowadays are safe, and boiling the food before serving will destroy any botulin that may be present. Most people who can foods at home use a pressure cooker and read the directions. As a result, this dreaded intoxication strikes only about 60 people each year in the United States (see Table 3.3). Thanks to public awareness, most victims now receive prompt medical treatment, and over 90 percent survive.

Unfortunately, the bacterium can occasionally grow in situations other than canned foods. In 1984, several people in California contracted botulism from foods such as meat loaves and stews that had been cooked and then left overnight at room temperature. In all such cases, the problem could have been avoided by thoroughly reheating the food.

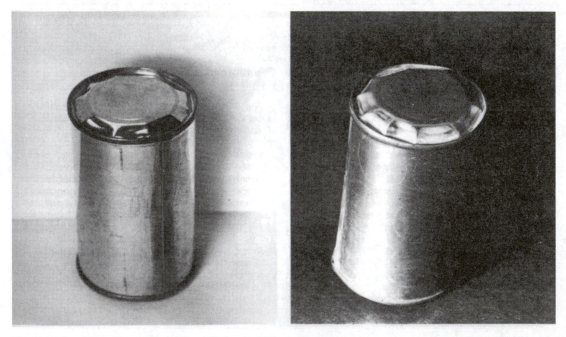

Figure 3.1. Cans to avoid. (*Source*: Biological Photo Service.)

Other forms of botulism affect infants, whose immature digestive systems allow them to contract the disease from "natural" raw honey; intravenous drug users, who sometimes contract wound botulism from dirty needles; and wildlife, such as ducks, which sometimes perish by the hundreds of thousands after feeding at polluted lakes with anaerobic waters. The toxin also has potential as an aerosolized or foodborne biological weapon.

This same bacterium provides an unexpected benefit to the youth industry: plastic surgeons routinely inject its neurotoxin (marketed as Botox®) under patients' skin to reduce wrinkles by relaxing the facial muscles. The same drug, properly administered, is useful in treating various neuromuscular disorders. When swallowed in food, however, the toxin relaxes other muscles, notably the ones that enable you to breathe. Symptoms of botulism poisoning include blurred vision, difficulty in speaking and swallowing, and paralysis. Doctors advise people to seek medical help at the first appearance of any of these symptoms. (Even if it is not botulism, it might be a stroke or other serious disorder.)

Never eat food from a bulging can (see Figure 3.1), and if you return such a can to the store, ask the clerk not to put it back on the shelf.

Clostridium perfringens *Food Poisoning*. This is another anaerobic, soil-dwelling, spore-forming bacterium that causes an estimated 248,520 foodborne illnesses per year in the United States (see Table 3.3). The most commonly encountered strain, known as Type A, causes a mild disease with a low case fatality rate. Certain other strains, however, can cause severe intestinal damage

and have caused deadly outbreaks in Germany and New Guinea. The usual sources are inadequately cooked or reheated meat dishes. The best way to prevent this and several other forms of food poisoning is to cook food thoroughly and then keep it at a temperature where bacteria are unlikely to multiply—in other words, either hot or cold.

When this same bacterium enters a wound through soil contamination, it can colonize poorly aerated tissues, causing a dreadful disease called gas gangrene. (This is one reason to avoid using a tourniquet for snakebite treatment, as discussed in Chapter 7.)

Escherichia coli *Food Poisoning*. The bacterium *Escherichia coli* (Figure 3.2), or E. coli for short, lives harmlessly in everyone's intestines, where it pursues its own interests and provides us with some vitamin K. In recent years, however, one unusual serotype

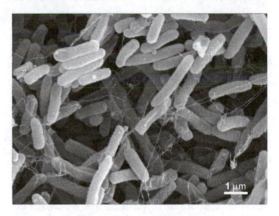

Figure 3.2. The Bacterium *Escherichia coli* (E. coli). This microbe is a normal occupant of the human intestine, but certain strains found in cattle cause severe illness in humans. The presence of any coliform bacteria in food or water is a good indicator of fecal contamination. (*Source*: Dr. Shirley Owens, Michigan State University.)

of E. coli (known as 0157:H7) has received a great deal of publicity because of the deadly toxin it produces. These diarrhea-causing E. coli live in cows, not in people, but they sometimes contaminate beef during the slaughtering process. Crops fertilized with untreated cow manure also may be contaminated, and the bacteria may enter water wells and lakes near dairy farms or feedlots.

Some scientists believe the 0157:H7 strain originated in Central America in the 1970s during a pandemic of shigellosis (see Chapter 2), when a bacterial virus transferred a toxin-producing gene from the *Shigella* bacteria to the intestinal bacteria of cattle. Others have implicated the cholera bacterium as the source of the gene; still others believe that the increased use of antibiotics in cattle has somehow produced this strain. Whatever its origin, 0157:H7 does not harm the cattle themselves, but in humans it causes food poisoning that is sometimes lethal, especially for children and elderly people. Nor is it clear how 0157:H7 has expanded its range so rapidly, but it now exists in as many as one-half of all cattle in the United States.

The largest recent E. coli outbreak occurred at a New York state fair in 1999, when more than 1000 people became ill and two died (Table 2.2, Chapter 2). Smaller outbreaks have occurred at various restaurants, such as the Sizzler chain in the Milwaukee area in 2000.[3]

The most frequent source of E. coli 0157:H7 is undercooked ground beef, but major outbreaks have also been associated with raw milk and unpasteurized apple juice (Table 3.2). Symptoms include cramps, nausea, and bloody diarrhea, sometimes leading to kidney failure—a condition known as hemolytic uremic syndrome, or HUS. The 0157:H7 strain alone causes about 73,480 cases and 250 deaths in the United States each year. Public health officials emphasize that doctors must *not* treat E. coli 0157:H7 patients with antibiotics or with antidiarrheal medications. Those who receive antibiotics are 14 times more likely than others to develop the deadly hemolytic uremic syndrome.

Although 98 percent of all fruit juice sold in the United States is pasteurized, between 16,000 and 48,000 Americans become ill each year from drinking unpasteurized fruit juice. One way to protect yourself is to add cinnamon to the juice; it will kill some of the bacteria, but it will not destroy any toxin that may already be present. Similarly, researchers report that adding finely ground prunes to hamburger meat (one tablespoon per pound) can kill more than 90 percent of any E. coli it contains. Alternatively, consumers can simply buy pasteurized fruit juice and cook their meat.

In 1998, the U.S. National Institute of Child Health and Human Development (NICHD) announced successful clinical trials for an experimental vaccine against E. coli 0157:H7. Although this vaccine is promising, its large-scale use seems unlikely in view of the low incidence of severe E. coli intoxication and the current widespread suspicion of new vaccines. A more effective strategy would be to eradicate the source, by vaccinating cattle rather than humans. Yet another promising (and controversial) strategy is to irradiate beef at processing plants.

---

[3]J. Warrick, "An Outbreak Waiting to Happen" (*Washington Post*, April 9, 2001).

Staphylococcal Food Poisoning. Staphylococcus aureus, a bacterium that causes various diseases ranging in severity from acne to toxic shock syndrome (see Chapter 5), also can contaminate food. Some strains release enterotoxins that cause nausea, vomiting, and diarrhea.

In a typical outbreak in Texas, 1364 children became ill with staphylococcal food poisoning, of a total of 5824 who had eaten lunch at 16 elementary schools. Investigators traced 95 percent of these cases to contaminated chicken salad. Other frequent vehicles are cream-filled pastries, sandwich fillings, and other foods that require handling during preparation and are stored at near-room temperatures. Canned mushrooms also have caused outbreaks.

Vibrio parahaemolyticus *Food Poisoning*. This bacterium is related to the one that causes cholera (see Chapter 2), but the disease, called vibriosis, is less severe and rarely causes death. Like the cholera bacterium, it lives in marine coastal areas and often contaminates fish and other seafood. Sushi lovers are prime candidates; cooking destroys the bacteria, but not the toxins they produce. Symptoms include watery diarrhea, cramps, chills, and frequently a headache. The largest known outbreak occurred in 1997, when 209 persons became ill and one died after eating raw oysters in the Pacific Northwest. Antibiotic treatment is usually unnecessary.

Foodborne Bacteria That Cause Infection

Anthrax. The bacterium *Bacillus anthracis* is the agent for this dreaded disease of cattle and other livestock. Modes of transmission include contact (Chapter 5), inhalation (Chapter 4), or ingestion of contaminated meat. The gastrointestinal form in humans tends to occur in large outbreaks when people eat undercooked meat of infected animals. Symptoms include abdominal distress and fever, often followed by septicemia and death.

The only reported outbreak of gastrointestinal anthrax in the United States occurred in 2000, after six members of a Minnesota family ate meat from a cow later found to be infected with anthrax. Two family members had relatively mild gastrointestinal distress with fever, but all recovered before the problem was identified. The report seems inconsistent with the reported high case fatality rate for gastrointestinal anthrax, but at the time this book went to press, no further information was available. For the main discussions of anthrax, see Chapters 4 and 5.

Campylobacteriosis. The bacterium *Campylobacter jejuni* may be the most common human foodborne bacterium, causing illness in more than two million people in the United States each year (Table 3.3). It is considerably less famous than *Salmonella* or *E. coli*, however, as *Campylobacter* tends not to occur in large, headline-grabbing epidemics. It is a normal occupant of the intestinal tract of many mammals and birds. A typical outbreak might involve a small number of people who all ate the same turkey or chicken at a social gathering. Larger outbreaks occur infrequently when *Campylobacter* contaminates water rather than food; in 1978, more than 2000 people in Vermont contracted the disease when their town switched temporarily to a nonchlorinated water source.

In a November 1999 study, the Center for Science in the Public Interest tested 50 supermarket turkeys and found that eight contained *Campylobacter* and none contained *Salmonella*. A similar study in 1998, before turkey processors adopted new safety standards, revealed *Campylobacter* in 90 percent of turkeys and *Salmonella* in 18 percent. In all fairness, consumers were not planning to eat those turkeys raw anyway, and thorough cooking destroys both types of bacteria; but the turkeys could easily have contaminated other foods in the kitchen, by way of unwashed hands or work surfaces. Thus, we repeat: Wear gloves, or wash, or both.

Besides poultry, sources of *Campylobacter* include red meat, eggs, raw milk, and contaminated water. The symptoms are similar to those of most foodborne bacterial infections: abdominal cramping, diarrhea, and nausea. In some cases, the disease causes a bloody diarrhea or dysentery that is severe enough to be lethal if untreated, and relapses may occur. Worse, researchers in 1996 reported that victims of a paralytic disease called Guillain-Barré syndrome showed a higher than expected frequency of antibodies for *Campylobacter*, suggesting that this foodborne infection is a major precursor.

Like most foodborne illnesses, campylobacteriosis is self-limiting and usually is allowed to (excuse the expression) run its course. Early treatment with an antibiotic such as erythromycin reduces the length of time that infected individuals shed the bacterium.

Crohn's Disease (**Mycobacterium avium** *subspecies* **paratuberculosis, or MAP).** The most likely agent of Crohn's disease is closely related to the pathogens that cause tuberculosis and leprosy. Before pasteurization became a common practice, people often caught a form of tuberculosis called scrofula by drinking raw milk contaminated with another related bacterium, *M. bovis*, as discussed in Chapter 4. The MAP bacterium causes, instead, a chronic inflammation of the intestine that has only recently gained recognition as an infectious disease.

Like stomach ulcer disease, Crohn's disease was formerly attributed to a personal idiosyncrasy, stress, or an autoimmune disorder. Although some studies have linked Crohn's unequivocally with MAP, others have yielded conflicting results, and the issue remains controversial. Genetic susceptibility to Crohn's disease also appears to be a factor.

Listeriosis. This relatively rare but potentially fatal disease is caused by the bacterium *Listeria monocytogenes*. About 2500 Americans contract listeriosis each year, and about 20 percent of them die. Most victims are infants, elderly persons, or those with weakened immune systems. The disease also is dangerous for pregnant women, because it can cause birth defects, miscarriage, or stillbirth.

The symptoms of listeriosis vary depending on the part of the body affected. When it causes meningoencephalitis, it may start with a sudden fever, intense headache, and nausea. More often, it is a less severe flu-like illness. The incubation period varies from three to 70 days, but is usually about a month. Ampicillin and other antibiotics usually are effective.

Perhaps the most famous outbreak of listeriosis in the United States occurred in 1985 when at least 142 people contracted listeriosis from a contaminated batch of soft cheese;

48 of those victims died. Smaller outbreaks in Europe, with similar fatality rates, also have been linked to soft cheeses. Other foods that have caused listeriosis include hot dogs, smoked fish products, and foie gras. In 2000, a major U.S. manufacturer recalled nearly 17 million pounds of turkey and chicken products with possible *Listeria* contamination.

Salmonellosis. Many readers probably are acquainted with this disease, either from news reports or from personal experience. Each year in the United States, about 1.4 million people contract salmonellosis. Usually it is foodborne, which is why we placed it in this chapter; but people also catch this disease by drinking contaminated water or by handling pets, particularly reptiles (see Chapter 5).

There are many different strains of salmonella, usually grouped into three species: *Salmonella typhi*, the agent of typhoid fever (below); *Salmonella cholerae-suis*, which causes a disease in swine (see Chapter 6); and *Salmonella enteriditis*, which causes the foodborne disease usually known as salmonellosis and also a typhoid-like disease called paratyphoid fever. Some authorities combine all these bacteria into one species with various serotypes.

The infective dose needed to contract salmonellosis may be fewer than 100 bacterial cells, depending on the strain and other variables. The bacteria then multiply in the small intestine and release an enterotoxin that causes severe diarrhea and vomiting. Usually the disease is self-limiting and lasts only two or three days, but a few people become chronic carriers. Salmonellosis may have long-term effects, including arthritis.

Salmonella bacteria occur naturally in mammals, birds, and reptiles. They can contaminate a wide range of foods, including raw or undercooked poultry, meat, or eggs; unpasteurized milk and juice; raw cheese; and produce such as alfalfa sprouts and cantaloupe. One of the largest recorded outbreaks of salmonellosis occurred in the United States in 1996 when some 224,000 people became ill from eating Schwan's ice cream (see Table 3.2). The problem resulted from the company's former practice of transporting unpasteurized raw eggs in the same trucks used to carry the ice cream mixes. Schwan's changed its procedures, and no similar outbreaks have occurred. Large *Salmonella* outbreaks and serious long-term consequences are rare, and the egg industry is concerned about what it regards as media exaggeration of the problem.

Typhoid Fever. Although typhoid fever outbreaks can result from floods and other natural disasters (see Chapter 2), about 80 percent of cases are foodborne. Until the twentieth century, typhoid caused large epidemics in the United States, but at present this disease affects only about 800 U.S. residents each year. The agent, *Salmonella typhi*, is closely related to the bacteria that cause salmonellosis and paratyphoid fever.

Typhoid fever was known in ancient times, and it is one of several candidates for the mysterious disease that killed Alexander the Great in 323 B.C. More than a century ago, Army surgeon Walter Reed investigated outbreaks of typhoid fever during the Spanish-American War. Reed found that, under the unsanitary and crowded conditions that prevailed in military camps, most cases were spread by interpersonal contact rather than by food or water. He also recognized the important role of asymptomatic carriers in spreading the disease.

The symptoms of typhoid fever vary so greatly that diagnosis may be difficult without a blood or stool test. It often starts with a fever, headache, and either constipation or (less often) diarrhea, followed by the appearance of pink spots on the body and enlargement of the spleen and liver. In severe cases, the intestine may hemorrhage or rupture. Typhoid usually responds well to antibiotic treatment, but the fatality rate for untreated cases is about 10 percent. Milder cases also occur, and about 3 percent of patients (like the famous Typhoid Mary) become lifelong carriers of the disease. A vaccine is available for persons traveling to developing nations where typhoid is endemic.

As discussed in Chapter 2, a recent study suggests that the human gene responsible for cystic fibrosis also protects its carriers against typhoid and other diseases affecting the gastrointestinal tract.

Yersiniosis. This foodborne infection has received little publicity, but it affects nearly 100,000 people each year in the United States alone. The agents, *Yersinia enterocolitica* and *Y. pseudotuberculosis*, are related to the agent of plague (see Chapter 5). Although yersiniosis usually is not serious, the symptoms can mimic appendicitis: abdominal pain (often in the right lower quadrant) with vomiting and diarrhea. Adults may also have joint pain, and in children the diarrhea may be bloody.

These same bacteria also infect dogs, cats, and other domestic animals, and food or water may become contaminated by feces. Like the typhoid bacillus and a few other foodborne pathogens, this one can persist in

the body in a chronic carrier state. *Yersinia* is often resistant to penicillin and other common antibiotics, but severe cases usually respond to third-generation cephalosporins in combination with aminoglycosides.

EXAMPLES OF FOODBORNE VIRAL DISEASES

Hepatitis A. This potentially serious liver disease can be spread by the fecal-oral route, by direct contact (including sex), or in contaminated water. There are about 83,000 reported cases each year in the United States; only 5 percent of individual cases are foodborne, but most of the major outbreaks are foodborne.

In Kentucky in 1994, health officials traced 91 cases to a single infected employee of a catering company. Several cases occurred in 1999 among members of a family that operated a North Carolina restaurant. In the latter case, because of the high risk of an outbreak, the local health department immunized over 1,800 potentially exposed diners as a precaution, but no one outside the affected family became ill. Similar cases occurred during 1999 in Seattle, San Diego, and other cities.

Although Americans tend to regard hepatitis A only as a risk for travelers to developing nations, the CDC now recommends hepatitis A vaccination for all children in areas where the incidence exceeds the national average, particularly in 11 states: Arizona, Alaska, California, Idaho, Nevada, New Mexico, Oklahoma, Oregon, South Dakota, Utah, and Washington.

Symptoms of hepatitis A include nausea, diarrhea, fatigue, and jaundice. Although the illness may last several weeks or longer, it is rarely fatal.

Norwalk and *Norwalk-like Viruses*. These viruses are responsible for an estimated 23 million cases of viral gastroenteritis each year in the United States, about 40 percent of them foodborne. (The accuracy of this estimate is uncertain, as most cases go unreported.) Thus, Norwalk-like viruses may be the most common foodborne pathogen.

Symptoms are the same as for most other organisms in this chapter: nausea, vomiting, diarrhea, and abdominal cramps, sometimes with a headache and low-grade fever. The illness usually lasts only two or three days, and long-term effects are rare. The most frequent known sources are raw oysters, which may be contaminated by infected food handlers, contaminated water or ice, or sewage dumped near oyster beds.

Other Viruses. Although rotavirus and astrovirus are recognized agents of foodborne illness, only about 1 percent of reported cases are food-related. Unknown viruses are most likely responsible for some foodborne illnesses, as the cause is not determined in over 80 percent of cases. Brainerd diarrhea, for example, is associated with untreated water or raw milk and has occurred in outbreaks since 1983, but researchers have not yet identified the infectious agent.

EXAMPLES OF FOODBORNE FUNGAL DISEASES

As all the entries in this section would be intoxications rather than infections per se, they appear in Chapter 7, along with poisonous mushrooms and similar topics.

EXAMPLES OF FOODBORNE PROTOZOAL DISEASES

The protozoa most often associated with food poisoning are the marine dinoflagellates, a major component of so-called "red tides." These organisms at times kill billions of fish, and many of the fish that survive contain traces of the dinoflagellate toxins, which can cause severe illness in humans. Oysters and other filter-feeders also accumulate these toxins. But dinoflagellates do not live or multiply in food per se, either at the fish market or in your refrigerator; the fish acquire the toxin in the ocean. Thus, it would not be correct to call these organisms foodborne pathogens. They appear in Chapter 7 instead.

The other protozoa that often cause food poisoning are the coccidians, such as cryptosporidium and cyclospora. These organisms are mainly associated with water, although they often contaminate fruits or vegetables during irrigation. Thus, they appear in Chapter 2.

Only one other protozoan commonly causes foodborne illness in humans in the United States, and that is a coccidian called *Toxoplasma gondii*. The resulting disease, called toxoplasmosis, may be familiar to some readers because of magazine articles about the hazards of cat litter boxes. Adults contract this disease by eating contaminated food (and also by direct and indirect contact with contaminated feces), but the real danger of toxoplasmosis is to the developing fetus. If a pregnant woman contracts this disease, her baby may have birth defects, even if the woman herself has no symptoms.

An estimated 225,000 Americans contract toxoplasmosis every year, and about half of these cases are foodborne.

EXAMPLES OF FOODBORNE MULTICELLULAR PARASITES

Most residents of the United States are at low risk for infestation with a foodborne multicellular parasite. Exceptions might include pig farmers who have not kept up on the U.S. Department of Agriculture (USDA) literature, bear hunters who like raw meat, and children whose play areas are heavily contaminated with feces. A few ethnic groups that consume raw pork also are at risk.

In 1999, doctors at the University of Iowa announced a surprising discovery: patients with inflammatory bowel disease—ulcerative colitis or Crohn's disease—showed great improvement after swallowing the eggs of a parasitic worm. (At latest word, the name of the worm was not available, but it was a small species that can live for only a few weeks in the human intestine.) We infer that these people were either very brave or in very great distress; in either case, apparently it worked. The investigators noted that human beings had intestinal parasites for millions of years before the present hygienic age, and that it might take a while for our bodies to adjust to their absence.

Ascariasis. The agent is a roundworm or helminth called *Ascaris lumbricoides*. After a person swallows the eggs (either by the fecal-oral route or on food such as a raw salad), they hatch in the intestine. The larvae penetrate the gut wall and travel through the lymphatic and circulatory systems until they reach the liver and lungs. From the lungs, they ascend the bronchi until the person coughs them up and swallows them again. Finally, they grow to maturity in the small intestine, where they mate and produce eggs, which the host discharges in feces to start a new cycle. The mature worms may be up to eight inches long. At present, an estimated 1.4 billion people are infested with roundworms, most of them in developing nations.

The usual symptoms are coughing, fever, abdominal pain, and, of course, worms moving in the stool or occasionally emerging from the mouth. If adult worms migrate into the liver, gallbladder, peritoneal cavity, or appendix, the host may die. Some readers may be startled to learn that ascariasis is fairly common in the southern United States, and very common in tropical regions of the world. (A well-known journalist recently suggested that roundworm infestation may be the cause of chronic fatigue syndrome—a buzzword that probably refers to several illnesses—but he assumed soldiers must have brought the worms back from Vietnam.)

Several effective worm medications are available. Prevention is better; children should be taught proper health habits, and should stay out of areas with fecal contamination.

Beef Tapeworm (Taeniasis), Pork Tapeworm (Cysticercosis), and Fish Tapeworm (Diphyllobothriasis). These are three different diseases, but they have enough in common that it is preferable to describe them only once. The agents are the tapeworms *Taenia saginata*, *Taenia solium*, and *Diphyllobothrium latum*, respectively. People usually contract the first two diseases by eating undercooked meat and the third by eating undercooked fish.

Beef tapeworm is not fatal; the adult worms simply grow in the intestine, becoming extremely long and causing symptoms such as loss of weight, indigestion, and insomnia. Segments of the worm that pass in the stool look like grains of rice.

Fish tapeworm usually is not fatal either. In 1980, four Los Angeles physicians contracted fish tapeworm by eating sushi made of raw tuna, red snapper, and salmon. Most outbreaks have occurred under similar circumstances. This tapeworm can grow to a length of 32 feet inside the human intestine. It deprives its victims of vitamin B_{12} and can cause severe anemia.

The pork tapeworm is a more serious matter. When its eggs hatch in the intestine, the larvae migrate through the body, often causing serious complications or death when they reach the ear, eye, central nervous system, or heart. In some developing nations, more than one-third of all adult-onset epilepsy cases result from pork tapeworm; even in the United States, there are more than 1000 such cases per year. The larvae of the pork tapeworm are transmissible not only in contaminated food and water, but also by direct interpersonal contact. In 2001, Arizona doctors successfully removed a large cyst and decayed tapeworm from the brain of a woman who had eaten an undercooked pork taco.

To avoid contracting these three diseases, cook all meat and fish thoroughly, and do not allow pigs and humans to use the same toilet. (We are serious; some people even train their pet pigs to flush.) Several cestocidal drugs are effective against these three diseases, but pork tapeworm infesta-tion may also require surgery. For a fourth tapeworm disease, see the next paragraph.

Echinococcosis (Hydatid Disease). The agent is a dog tapeworm (*Echinococcus granulosus*), but few people contract it by eating dog meat. The usual vehicle is food or water contaminated with dog feces, and it is most common in areas where people live in close contact with dogs used for hunting or herding. The dogs eat the raw viscera of herbivores and then transmit the tapeworm to their owners by the fecal-oral route. The eggs hatch in the intestine, and the larvae form fluid-filled cysts in the liver, lungs, heart, or other organs. As these cysts may exceed eight inches in diameter, they are often lethal; death also may result from anaphylaxis (Chapter 7). Symptoms may include pain, jaundice, bone fractures, coughing, or pericarditis, depending on the location. The only effective treatment is to remove the cysts surgically.

Fasciolopsiasis. The agent is a large trematode or fluke called *Fasciolopsis buski* that lives in the small intestine. Infected humans pass the eggs in their feces; in water, the eggs hatch into larvae that develop further in snails, then emerge to form cysts on aquatic plants, including some vegetables such as the water caltrop and water chestnut. People ingest the cysts by eating the plants raw, and the cycle starts over. Worldwide, an estimated 40 million people are infested with foodborne trematodes. Prevalence is extremely high in some parts of Asia, but effective drugs are available. This parasite does not occur in North America, but we have a related trematode that causes a similar disease in cattle and sheep.

Trichinosis. The agent of this disease is an intestinal roundworm called *Trichinella spiralis*. It occurs in many animals, including dogs, cats, rodents, and some marine mammals. The only hosts that most people are likely to encounter are pigs and possibly bears, but two recent outbreaks in Alaska were traced to walrus meat. In the United States today, there are only about 88 human cases of trichinosis per year, as compared with 300–400 cases per year in the 1940s. Nearly all commercially available pork is safe, and adequate cooking kills the parasite anyway.

Once swallowed, the worms do not stay in the intestine, but migrate through the body by way of the lymphatic system and form cysts in muscle tissue. Symptoms of trichinosis include muscle pain, swelling of the upper eyelids, a skin rash, diarrhea, and fever. Mebendazole and other drugs are effective, but without treatment, trichinosis may be fatal. A recent study suggests that composer Wolfgang Amadeus Mozart died of this disease after eating undercooked pork.

OTHER FOODBORNE PATHOGENS

Prions, formerly called nonconventional pathogens, are smaller than any known virus and are composed entirely of protein. They are not exactly foreign invaders, but abnormal versions of certain membrane-associated proteins found in the mammalian brain. A prion contains no genetic material and is not alive, but it can somehow "train" other proteins to assume its own abnormal shape. In 1997, Stanley Prusiner and Stephen DeArmond won the Nobel Prize in Medicine for discovering the nature of prions. These pathogens cause several diseases in humans, livestock, and wild mammals.

Creutzfeldt-Jakob Disease (CJD). This invariably fatal neurological disease, which kills about 250 Americans each year, starts with progressive mental deterioration and jerking movements. It is one of a group of diseases called transmissible spongiform encephalopathies, or TSEs. Until recently, doctors regarded CJD as a tragic but rare disease of older people, often those with a history of some unusual contact with brain tissue of humans or other species. There was a relatively high incidence among Libyans who ate sheep's eyes and brains; some neurosurgeons, their patients, and recipients of corneal transplants also contracted CJD. Several recent cases also have occurred in people who ate the brains of wild goats and squirrels. Because of the connection to sheep, researchers suspected a possible link to a well-known sheep disease called scrapie (see Chapter 6).

Except for the Libyan examples, no known cases of CJD have resulted from eating lamb, but an indirect link to scrapie now appears to be fairly well established. First, a bit of history:

Bovine spongiform encephalopathy (BSE), popularly called mad cow disease, first appeared in the United Kingdom in about 1985, and researchers officially recognized it as a spongiform encephalopathy in 1986. The BSE epidemic peaked in 1992–1993, with nearly 1000 new cases per week in England. The disease also turned up in several European countries (see Figure 3.3), but not in the United States. The discovery of 32 infected cows in Germany in 2000 caused beef sales to plummet in that coun-

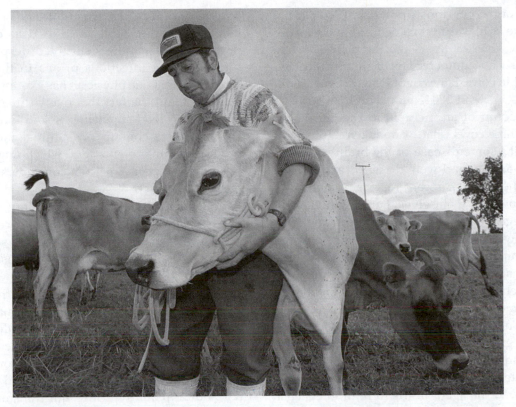

Figure 3.3. A Mad Cow. In this photograph, a Danish farmer hugs one of many cows that had to be destroyed during the BSE (bovine spongiform encephalopathy) epidemic in Europe. (*Source*: Reuters NewMedia Inc./Corbis.)

try; after much laboratory testing and humanitarian debate, part of the resulting beef surplus was sold to North Korea to help alleviate famine.

Most researchers now believe that BSE originated when a new rendering process in the 1980s made it possible for cattle feed to contain sheep remains that were potentially contaminated with the prion agent of scrapie. It was not until 1996, however, that scientists proposed a link between BSE and a recent outbreak of CJD in England. These cases were unusual in that most of the CJD victims were in their teens and twenties.

The most widely accepted explanation was that cattle caught scrapie from the sheep, and humans who ate beef from infected cows developed an atypical form of CJD, known as vCJD. In 1996, the cattle and rendering industries banned the use of all ruminant parts in animal feed. A 1999 study confirmed that the agent of BSE can travel from the mammalian digestive tract to the brain via the lymphatic system.

According to a minority viewpoint, however, a bovine disease similar to BSE has existed in the British Isles for a long time, and was somehow exacerbated by the use of organophosphate pesticides. Scrapie, unlike BSE, was first recognized in the British Isles over 250 years ago, but there were also early anecdotal reports of abnormal behavior in cows. Playwright John M. Synge, writing in about 1904, quoted an Irish farmer's account of an incident in the late 1800s: "Three cows I had were taken in the night with some disease of the brain, and they swam out and were drowned in the sea."[4] (There are no recent reports of mad cows drowning themselves, but BSE in its early stages causes disorientation, and few cows nowadays get close enough to the ocean to jump in.) Nor does everyone accept the conclusion that the vCJD outbreak resulted entirely from beef consumption. Apparently, some of its victims were vegetarians.

In 2001, Professor Chandra Wickramasinghe and Sir Fred Hoyle proposed that mad cow disease might have originated in outer space, when cows in England swallowed the agent in the form of interstellar dust that had fallen on their pasture. (A year earlier, the same two scientists proposed that influenza epidemics also originate in outer space.)

In short, the connection between BSE and CJD is not yet fully understood, and further research is vitally important. Autopsy results of Alzheimer's disease patients show that up to 13 percent actually had CJD that was wrongly diagnosed. Also, as some cases of "classic" CJD do not appear until decades after the causal event, there is some concern about a possible epidemic of future cases in people who were exposed to contaminated beef in Europe in the 1990s. A 2000 study suggests that prions alone may not cause

scrapie or other TSEs; when infected with hamster scrapie, some mice died as expected, whereas others survived despite high levels of infectious prions in their brains. At least one physician has expressed concern about the fact that many unregulated health-food supplements sold in the United States contain raw animal meat products of unknown origin, which might potentially expose American consumers to BSE.

Under conditions of such uncertainty, rumors spread like any epidemic. The recent resistance of many U.S. and Canadian soldiers to the anthrax vaccine was based partly on the belief that the vaccine was made using British bovine products that might be contaminated with BSE. To make matters worse, similar prion diseases affect many animals other than cows and sheep. A disease of dogs called canine spongiform encephalopathy (CSE) has been linked to BSE, but apparently CSE is not transmissible to humans by ordinary contact. BSE also has turned up in British zoo animals that received contaminated food. In the United States, a prion disease called chronic wasting disease (CWD) is common in wild deer and elk, affecting up to 15 percent in some herds; between 1998 and 2000, several young deer hunters exposed to this disease later died of CJD. At the time this book went to press, the FDA was considering a ban on blood donations from deer and elk hunters, although researchers had not proven a link between CWD and CJD.

Kuru. This disease occurs (or historically occurred) only among the Fore people of the New Guinea highlands, who practiced

---

[4]John M. Synge, *In Connemara* (Cork: Mercier Press, reprinted 1979).

ritual cannibalism and contracted the disease by eating human brains. Few readers are likely to encounter this situation, and we mention kuru mainly because a study of this disease led to Carleton Gajdusek's discovery of prions, for which he received a Nobel Prize in 1976.

OUTLOOK FOR THE TWENTY-FIRST CENTURY

Despite improved safeguards, the booming fast-food industry and its mass production of mixed ground beef will most likely continue to cause occasional outbreaks of foodborne illness. Shellfish poisoning incidents also may increase, as a result of dinoflagellate blooms associated with climate change and coastal pollution.

There is a widespread belief that global free trade will endanger residents of developed nations by allowing the import of contaminated foods. This belief appears to combine legitimate concerns about food safety standards with a less rational fear of anything foreign. The outcome may depend largely on the willingness of exporters to test their products, and on the objectivity of future studies of foodborne disease outbreaks.

A recent invention that may help in the detection of foodborne pathogens is a biosensor device (Figure 3.4) invented at the Georgia Institute of Technology. It can detect *Salmonella enteriditis*, *Listeria monocytogenes*, *Yersinia enterocolitica*, *Escherichia coli* (including 0157:H7), *Campylobacter jejuni*, and several other bacteria in food samples.

In 2000, the U.S. Food and Drug Administration released a major report on foodborne illness risk factors. It identifies the

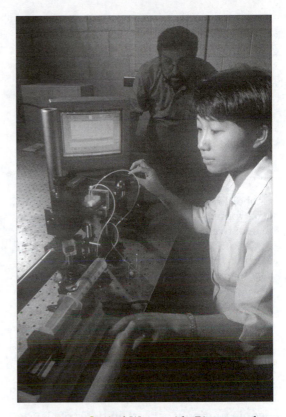

Figure 3.4. Optical Waveguide Biosensor for Detection of Foodborne Pathogens. This device, recently developed at Georgia Institute of Technology, can detect a dozen different micro-organisms including *Salmonella*, *E. coli*, and *Campylobacter*. (Photo by Gary Meek, Georgia Institute of Technology. Reproduced with permission.)

highest-priority risk factors as improper holding times and temperatures; contaminated equipment; cross-contamination; and poor personal hygiene.

THE GOOD OLD DAYS

With regard to the alleged goodness and purity of unprocessed food, untreated water, and natural remedies, we now offer two quotations from the medical literature of the nineteenth century, when all these products were as natural as anyone could wish.

In a famous 1896 work that rivals today's *Guinness Book of World Records* in matters of sheer astonishment, a physician of that era wrote:

Cobbold reports the case of four simultaneous tapeworms; and Aguiel describes the case of a man of twenty-four who expelled a mass weighing a kilogram, 34.5 meters long, consisting of several different worms. Garfinkel mentions a case which has been extensively quoted, of a peasant who voided 238 feet of tapeworms, 12 heads being found.[5]

Readers of the next example should not dismiss the clay-eating Irishwoman as an obvious lunatic. Even today, in many rural areas in the United States and elsewhere, people routinely eat certain types of clay as a "natural" source of dietary calcium and other minerals. The fact that this woman chose clay from a churchyard probably reflects her belief that the soil would be blessed, rather than some vile impulse to consume dead clergymen:

My favorite case report is that of an Irish woman who passed thousands of coprophagous beetles of the genus *Blaps* in her stools. She presumably ingested eggs or larvae inadvertently when she ate clay and chalk taken from the graves of priests.[6]

FROM THE AUTHOR'S FILE CABINET

A recent study of the life and death of Robert Louis Stevenson turned up the strange case of George Marshall, an Ohioan and Civil War veteran who was briefly famous in the last century for circuitous reasons (his wife's sister Fanny married the Scottish author). Like so many of his generation, George died in 1864 from a foodborne disease, or, more precisely, from the combined effects of two foodborne diseases—but that is not the way the family tells it in several published biographies of the Stevenson family.

By the official version, George and his best friend Sam Osbourne (Fanny's first husband) served in the Union Army until both received medical discharges in 1863. By that time, Sam's health was broken in some unspecified way, and George was allegedly dying of pulmonary tuberculosis (TB). TB was then considered a romantic malady, and a fashionable cure was to move to California. Sam wanted a silver or gold mine, and George's lungs wanted drier air; so the two friends left their wives in Indiana and boarded a ship bound for Panama in the winter of 1863–1864. (The biographies neglect to mention that George's wife was then in her seventh month of pregnancy.) But George coughed his last in Sam's company while crossing the Isthmus, never to see the promised land.

Several aspects of that story are untrue, but the only one that belongs here is George's cause of death, which his military

---

[5]G.M. Gould and W.L. Pyle, *Anomalies and Curiosities of Medicine* (New York: Bell Publishing Co., 1896).
[6]J.O. Westwood, *An Introduction to the Modern Classification of Insects* (London: Longman, 1839); cited by E.G. Matthews, "The Mediterranean beetle *Blaps polychresta* Forskal in South Australia" (*South Australian Naturalist* 49[3]: 35–39).

record clearly identifies as "camp diarrhea" contracted during the war. The record further states, however, that George suffered from "a vilent [sic] disease of the glands of the throat and neck of a scrofulous character." Although this was not the cause of death, it might have been scrofula—a nonfatal form of TB often contracted in that era by drinking raw milk, but not the consumption that claimed the lives of poets.

Contrary to most accounts, Robert Louis Stevenson himself most likely did not have pulmonary TB either. His famous hemorrhages, and the stroke that ended his life, may have resulted from a genetic bleeding disorder.[7] But he, too, suffered from at least one foodborne disease—tapeworm, possibly contracted from his favorite raw fish with miti sauce.

REFERENCES AND RECOMMENDED READING

"Anthrax in Minnesota: Family Receiving Treatment after Eating Diseased Meat." Associated Press, September 8, 2000.

Baker, Harry F., and Ridley, Rosalind M. (Editors). 1996. *Prion Diseases*. Totowa, NJ: Humana Press.

Bellenir, Karen, and Dresser, Peter D. 1995. *Food and Animal Borne Diseases Sourcebook*. Detroit, MI: Omnigraphics.

Berger, J.R., et al. "Creutzfeldt-Jakob Disease and Eating Squirrel Brains" [letter]. *Lancet*, August 30, 1997, p. 642.

Berkman, Alan, and Bakalar, Nicholas. 2000. *Hepatitis A to G: The Facts You Need to Know about All Forms of this Dangerous Disease*. New York: Warner Books.

"Botulism from Fresh Foods—California." *Morbidity and Mortality Weekly Report*, March 22, 1985.

Brasher, Philip. "Food Companies Seek Bacteria Killers." Associated Press, June 26, 2001.

Brink, Pamela J. "Clean Hand—Dirty Hand." *Western Journal of Nursing Research*, April 1996, pp. 118–119.

Bryan, Frank L. 1973. *Guide for Investigating Foodborne Disease Outbreaks and Analyzing Surveillance Data*. Atlanta, GA: U.S. Department of Health and Human Services, Public Health Service, Centers for Disease Control and Prevention (reprinted 1985).

Buzby, J.C., et al. 1996. *Bacterial Foodborne Disease Medical Costs and Productivity Losses*. Washington, DC: U.S. Department of Agriculture.

"*Campylobacter* Appears to be Major Cause of Guillain-Barré Syndrome." *Food Chemical News*, June 3, 1996.

Cerexhe, Peter, and Ashton, John. 1999. *Risky Food, Safer Choices: Avoiding Food Poisoning*. Kensington, NSW, Australia: New South Wales University Press.

Chase, Marilyn. "Vaccine Campaign Targets Outbreaks of Hepatitis A." *Wall Street Journal*, November 15, 1999.

Coghlan, Andy. "Wonderful Worms." *New Scientist*, August 7, 1999.

Collinge, John. "Variant Creutzfeldt-Jakob Disease." *Lancet*, July 24, 1999, pp. 317–323.

Donnelly, Christl A., and Ferguson, Neil M. 1999. *Statistical Aspects of BSE and vCJD: Models for Epidemics*. Boca Raton, FL: CRC Press.

Dyer, David L., et al. "Testing a New Alcohol-Free Hand Sanitizer to Combat Infection." *AORN Journal*, August 1998, pp. 239–251.

Eley, A.R. 1996. *Microbial Food Poisoning*. 2nd ed. New York: Aspen Publishers.

Evans, Carlton, et al. "Controversies in the Management of Cysticercosis." *Emerging Infectious Diseases*, Vol. 3, 1997, pp. 403–405.

Fox, Maggie. "Mad Cow Mystery Solved: Disease Travels from Food to Brain." Associated Press, March 29, 1999.

Fox, Nicols. 1998. *Spoiled: Why Our Food Is Making Us Sick and What We Can Do about It*. Bergenfield, NJ: Penguin USA.

Fox, Nicols. 1999. *It Was Probably Something You

---

[7]A.E. Guttmacher and J.R. Callahan, "Did Robert Louis Stevenson Have Hereditary Hemorrhagic Telangiectasia?" (*American Journal of Medical Genetics*, Vol. 91 [2000], pp. 62–65).

Ate: A Practical Guide to Avoiding and Surviving Foodborne Illness. Bergenfield, NJ: Penguin USA.

Gajdusek, D. Carleton. 1963. *Kuru Epidemiological Patrol from the New Guinea Highlands to Papua, August 21, 1957 to November 10, 1957*. Bethesda, MD: National Institute of Neurological Diseases and Blindness.

Greenburg, Bernard. 1973. *Flies and Disease, Volume 2: Biology and Disease Transmission*. Princeton, NJ: Princeton University Press.

Hartman, N., et al. "Rapid Response Biosensor for Detection and Identification of Common Foodborne Pathogens." *Proceedings of the Society of Photo-optical Instrumentation Engineers*, January 1995, pp. 128–137.

Hennessy, Thomas W., et al. "A National Outbreak of *Salmonella enteritidis* Infections from Ice Cream." *New England Journal of Medicine*, May 16, 1996, pp. 1281–1286.

Hermon-Taylor, J., et al. "Causation of Crohn's Disease by *Mycobacterium avium* subspecies *paratuberculosis*." *Canadian Journal of Gastroenterology*, June 2000, pp. 521–39.

Hirschmann, J.V. "What Killed Mozart?" *Archives of Internal Medicine*, June 11, 2001, pp. 1381–1389.

Hobbs, Betty C., and Roberts, Diane. 1993. *Food Poisoning and Food Hygiene*. London: Edward Arnold.

Hornsby, M. "Ministry in U-Turn on 'Crank' Farmer's Mad Cow Theory." April 13, 1998, *The Times*, London.

Hui, Y.H., et al. 1994. *Foodborne Disease Handbook*. New York: Marcel Dekker.

Kamin, M., and Patten, B. "Creutzfeldt-Jakob Disease: Possible Transmission to Humans by Consumption of Wild Animal Brains." *American Journal of Medicine*, January 1984, pp. 142–145.

Klitzman, Robert. 1998. *The Trembling Mountain: A Personal Account of Kuru, Cannibals, and Mad Cow Disease*. New York: Plenum Press.

Knight, Jonathan, and Day, Michael. "Killer in Hiding." *New Scientist*, September 2, 2000.

Latta, Sara L. 1999. *Food Poisoning and Foodborne Diseases*. Hillside, NJ: Enslow Publishers.

Lindenbaum, Shirley. 1979. *Kuru Sorcery: Disease and Danger in the New Guinea Highlands*. Mountain View, CA: Mayfield Publishing Company.

Massoudi, M.S., et al. "An Outbreak of Hepatitis A Associated with an Infected Foodhandler." *Public Health Reports*, Vol. 114, pp. 157–164.

Mead, Paul S., et al. "Food-Related Illness and Death in the United States." *Emerging Infectious Diseases*, September–October 1999, pp. 607–625.

"New E. Coli Beef Danger: Deadly Bug Could Affect Half of U.S. Cattle." Reuters News Service, November 10, 1999.

Norton, Scott A. "Raw Animal Tissues and Dietary Supplements." *New England Journal of Medicine*, July 27, 2000.

"Pesticide Tie to Britain's Mad Cow Epidemic." April 8, 1996, Reuters News Service.

Prusiner, Stanley B. (Editor). 1999. *Prion Biology and Diseases*. Cold Spring Harbor, NY: Cold Spring Harbor Laboratory Press.

Rampton, Sheldon, and Stauber, John C. 1997. *Mad Cow U.S.A.: Could the Nightmare Happen Here?* Monroe, ME: Common Courage Press.

Ratzan, Scott C. (Editor). 1998. *Mad Cow Crisis: Health and the Public Good*. New York University Press.

"Researchers Stress Link Between Deer Disease, Humans Remote." Associated Press, December 27, 1999.

Rhodes, Richard. 1998. *Deadly Feasts: The "Prion" Controversy and the Public's Health*. New York: Touchstone Books.

Ridley, Rosalind, and Baker, Harry F. 1998. *Fatal Protein: The Story of CJD, BSE, and Other Prion Diseases*. New York: Oxford University Press.

Scott, Elizabeth, and Sockett, Paul. 1998. *How to Prevent Food Poisoning: A Practical Guide to Safe Cooking, Eating, and Food Handling*. New York: John Wiley.

Shapiro, Roger L., et al. "Botulism surveillance and emergency response: a public health strategy for a global challenge." *Journal of the American Medical Assocation*, August 6, 1997.

Shell, Ellen R. "Could Mad-Cow Disease Happen Here?" *Atlantic Monthly*, September 1998.

Taormina, P.J., et al. "Infections Associated with Eating Seed Sprouts." *Emerging Infectious Diseases*, September–October 1999.

"Trichinosis—Maine, Alaska." *Morbidity and Mortality Weekly Report*, January 24, 1986, pp. 33–35.

"Waterborne *Campylobacter* Gastroenteritis." *Morbidity and Mortality Weekly Report*, Vol. 27, 1978, pp. 207 ff.

Watkins, W.E., Pollitt, E. "'Stupidity or Worms': Do Intestinal Worms Impair Mental Performance?" *Psychological Bulletin*, March 1997, pp. 171–187.

Wong, C.S., et al. "The Risk of Hemolytic-Uremic Syndrome after Antibiotic Treatment of *Escherichia coli* 0157:H7 Infections." *New England Journal of Medicine*, June 29, 2000, pp. 1930–36.

Zarranz, J.J., et al. "Kuru Plaques in the Brain of Two Cases with Creutzfeldt-Jakob Disease: A Common Origin for the Two Diseases?" *Journal of Neurological Science*, October 1979, pp. 291–300.

CHAPTER 4

Human Pathogens in Air

'Tis now the very witching time of night
When churchyards yawn and hell itself breathes out
Contagion to this world.
— William Shakespeare, *Hamlet, III, ii, 413*

People have always paid close attention to one another's respiratory behavior. The ancient Persians, for example, believed that any demons in residence were likely to exit the body during a sneeze. When someone sneezed, other people in the room feared that the liberated demons might colonize them by the same route; thus, they prayed for a blessing, and so do we still ("Bless you!"). In Medieval Europe, sneezing might mean the literal or figurative departure of the soul, as immortalized by the plague lyric:

Achoo, achoo,

All fall down.

The Ainu people of Sakhalin Island threw balls of nasal mucus at people they disliked; in Western cultures this practice is now largely restricted to third graders. The Ifugao of the northern Philippines believed that a committee of eight spirits of the dead, called Spitters, caused diseases such as leprosy and jungle rot by spitting on the living,

and that two other spirits protected the living from the Spitters by granting shade or invisibility. Even without microscopes, all these people had a fairly good idea how things worked.

The world's most prevalent and deadly infectious disease, tuberculosis, is mainly airborne. So is influenza, which has caused the largest and most deadly disease epidemics in recent history. While the purveyors of biological weapons study the properties of aerosol clouds, health agencies and pharmaceutical companies race to develop better vaccines and antiviral drugs.

CROSS-REFERENCE

The titles of Chapters 2–5 reflect the principal modes of disease transmission. Most pathogens, however, can be transmitted in more than one way. Microorganisms that travel through the air as droplet nuclei or spores may also spread by direct contact. A

Table 4.1
Cross-Reference: Other Airborne Diseases

Disease	Chapter	Notes
Buruli Ulcer	2	Probably waterborne (also as aerosol?)
Melioidosis	2	Waterborne, airborne, or contact
Chickenpox	5	Contact or airborne
Enterobiasis	5	Contact or airborne
Hand, Foot, and Mouth Disease	5	Contact or possibly airborne
Hib	5	Contact or airborne
Lassa Fever	5	Contact or rarely airborne
Machupo Fever	5	Contact or rarely airborne
Leprosy	5	Contact or possibly airborne
Listeriosis	5	Contact, food, or airborne
Meningitis	5	Contact or airborne
Rabies	5	Contact or (rarely) airborne
Rat-bite Fever	5	Contact, milk, or possibly airborne
Rotavirus	5	Contact, food, or possibly airborne
Rubella	5	Contact or airborne
Staphylococcal Disease	5	Contact or airborne
Tularemia	5	Contact, food, water, or rarely airborne
Typhus	5	Contact or rarely airborne
Brucellosis	6	Contact, food, airborne; mainly livestock
Wheat Rust Fungus	6	Spores cause lung damage; a plant disease

more ambiguous situation arises when a sneeze, for example, transfers larger droplets at close range; this, too, is defined as direct contact (see Chapter 5). For the reader's convenience, Table 4.1 provides a cross-reference for potentially airborne pathogens that are covered in other chapters.

EXAMPLES OF AIRBORNE BACTERIA

Anthrax or Woolsorter's Disease. Although anthrax spreads mainly by contact under natural conditions, recent media reports have focused attention on biological weapons—and postal envelopes—that re-

lease anthrax spores in aerosolized form and cause inhalation anthrax. The threat of such an epidemic is real enough, but it is primarily an artifact of the modern age, as discussed further in Chapter 9.

In its natural state, anthrax is mainly a skin disease of cattle, sheep, horses, and other mammals, caused by a bacterium called *Bacillus anthracis*. When people domesticated these animals thousands of years ago, they came in contact with the disease, which usually causes skin lesions (see Chapter 5) or foodborne illness (see Chapter 3). Inhalation anthrax can occur under natural conditions; in 1976, a California woman died of this disease after inhaling spores on wool imported from Pakistan, and a 1957 outbreak at a textile factory in Manchester, New Hampshire killed four workers. Most recent cases of inhalation anthrax in the literature, however, have been associated with accidental laboratory releases or terrorism.

Like most upper respiratory infections, inhalation anthrax starts with fatigue, fever, and a cough. After the first day or two, victims tend to improve, so they dismiss their illness as a slight cold. Next comes a sudden attack of respiratory distress, profuse sweating, shock, and death. Antibiotics such as ciprofloxacin or doxycycline would help, if taken at the first symptoms; but again, the early stages of this disease resemble the common cold or influenza, and all well-informed consumers and their doctors know that antibiotics are useless against colds and flu.

The October 2001 anthrax mailings, however despicable their intent, may have served a useful purpose by alerting the public and health-care providers to this ever-present biohazard. Diagnostic testing is available, and most doctors are now aware that the patient's chest X-ray is likely to show a widened mediastinum (the space between the lungs). Inhalation anthrax does not spread directly from one person to another, apparently because of the large infective dose required. The case fatality rate for inhalation anthrax, once estimated at 95 to 100 percent even with treatment, was 50 percent in the 2001 postal attack (assuming that all cases were recognized and reported).

Although recent events have made it more difficult for would-be terrorists to buy bacteria by mail order, they can still find the burial sites of cows that died of anthrax decades ago, dig up the carcasses, and harvest the spores. Some expertise is needed to convert the spores to aerosolized form; alternatively, weapons-grade anthrax may be available on the black market. These topics have received saturation coverage in the media.

An effective anthrax vaccine is available; as discussed in Chapter 9, it has been the focus of some controversy regarding the rights of military personnel and the safety of immunization in general. The vaccine requires six shots over an 18-month period, followed by annual boosters. The low risk of contracting inhalation anthrax, combined with the scarcity of the vaccine and some associated risk, makes mass immunization impractical at present. The long incubation period for this disease (45 to 90 days) suggests that an exposed population might be vaccinated after a mass attack—always assuming that the released bug was standard-issue and not genetically modified. A protective face mask with an appropriate filter might also protect against inhalation anthrax, given some advance warning of its presence. Other treatments include anthrax antitoxin (not widely available in the United States) and antibodies from the blood of persons previously vaccinated against anthrax.

Diphtheria. This disease, like smallpox and polio, has been "gone" just long enough for people in developed nations to imagine that it never existed. Although doctors developed a diphtheria vaccine as early as 1890, widespread immunization did not start until about 1950. Before that, thousands of children and adults died of diphtheria every year. At the time of the 1880

U.S. Census, for example, eight of every 10,000 deaths resulted from diphtheria; of all infectious diseases reported, only tuberculosis claimed more lives. In 1933, there were more than 50,000 cases of diphtheria in the United States, with a case fatality rate of about 10 percent.

The agent of diphtheria is the bacterium *Corynebacterium diphtheriae*, which lives only in humans. Like cholera and some other diseases, diphtheria results mainly from the effects of a toxin that the bacterium can produce only if it contains a virus. The disease starts like so many others with a fever and sore throat, but it has one unusual symptom that few of today's physicians have ever seen: a thick, tough gray membrane that grows in the throat, blocking the windpipe in at least 25 percent of cases. Death can result either from asphyxiation or from the effects of the diphtheria toxin, which can damage the heart and central nervous system. A second, less serious form of diphtheria causes lesions on the skin. Diphtheria usually responds to treatment with diphtheria antitoxin and some antibiotics, including penicillin and erythromycin.

Although diphtheria is now rare in developed nations, the disease is far from gone, and epidemics still occur wherever vaccination programs are neglected. There was a major epidemic in the former Soviet Union in the 1990s (Table 4.2). Worldwide, there were about 4,000 deaths from diph-

Table 4.2
Examples of Outbreaks of Airborne Disease

Disease	Date	Location	Est. Cases	Est. Deaths
Anthrax	1979	Soviet Union	100	70
Diphtheria	1880	Chicago, IL	NR	1,463
Diphtheria	1990–96	Former Soviet Union	140,000	4,000
Encephalitis	1916–27	Worldwide	5 million	1.6 million
Hantavirus	1993	SW United States	30	20
Influenza	1918–19	Worldwide	1 billion	25 million
Influenza	1957–58	Worldwide	NR	70,000
Influenza	1968–69	Worldwide	NR	34,000
Legionellosis	1976	Philadelphia, PA	221	34
Measles	1846	Faeroes	7,782	NR
Measles	1989–91	United States	55,000	135
Nipah Virus	1998	Malaysia	265	106
Pertussis	1977	Great Britain	99,000	23
Pertussis	1979	Japan	13,000	41
Smallpox	1721–22	Boston, MA	6,000	844
Smallpox	1781–84	Great Lakes area	NR	90% of Chippewa
Smallpox	1835–38	Great Plains area	NR	33% of Plains Indians
Smallpox	1882	Chicago, IL	NR	1,292
Valley Fever	1991–94	Kern County, CA	8,200	55

Sources: Yampolaska (1994); Chua et al. (2000); Menominee Nation, Web site <http://www.menominee.nsn.us/>; Crosby (1990); U.S. Centers for Disease Control and Prevention.

theria in 1999, most of them in Southeast Asia.

Legionellosis or Pontiac Fever. Until 1976, no one had ever heard of this highly lethal form of pneumonia. Its agent—a bacterium later described as *Legionella pneumophila*—had lived peacefully in freshwater ponds and similar habitats throughout human history without attracting enough attention even to receive a scientific name.

The reason for its emergence appears to be threefold. First, it can cause large outbreaks only when air bubbles break at the surface of the water where it lives, ejecting bacteria in aerosol droplets that many people are likely to inhale. The ancient Egyptians, for example, did not encounter legionellosis very often because they did not have air-conditioning systems. Second, until recently the human population did not include a high proportion of elderly and immunosuppressed persons, the main risk groups for this disease. Finally, pneumonia is such a common cause of death that many sporadic cases before 1976 probably went unrecognized.

The 1976 outbreak occurred in Philadelphia during an American Legion convention (hence the name) and was traced to contaminated water in the hotel's air-conditioning system. Men over 50 with underlying medical problems, persons with HIV/AIDS, or those taking immunosuppressant drugs are particularly vulnerable to legionellosis. Worldwide statistics are not available, but in the United States alone, some 25,000 people contract legionellosis every year and about 1000 die.

In 1999, several Europeans died of legionellosis contracted from showers in institutional settings, including 11 patients at an Italian hospital and four inmates of a German prison. Other outbreaks have been traced to contaminated fountains, humidifiers, and respiratory therapy equipment. The bacterium also is common in soil; in 2000, three people contracted legionellosis from potting soil in California, Oregon, and Washington, respectively. After the discovery of legionellosis and its mode of action, researchers found several earlier reports in the literature regarding outbreaks of respiratory disease associated with air conditioners. In 1997, researchers in France reported that a related species, *Legionella parisiensis*, also causes pneumonia.

The tragedy of legionellosis is that the people most likely to get it are those who need it least, such as retired people trying to enjoy their lives, premature infants on respirators, and children undergoing chemotherapy for cancer. In England in 1986, upon learning that he was HIV positive, a young man threw himself from a bridge into the River Thames—only to contract legionellosis from the contaminated water. (That, at least, was curable with antibiotics.)

Plague. This disease, like anthrax, is not primarily airborne under natural conditions. We include it here because of the publicity it has received as a potential biological weapon. To deploy such a weapon, one cannot simply infect a few rats and hope for the best; for maximum efficiency, it is necessary to disperse the agent in a cloud. Plague, like anthrax, unfortunately is a terrorist's dream in this respect.

The agent of plague is a bacterium called *Yersinia pestis*. The usual form of the disease, bubonic plague, causes large swellings (called buboes) to appear on the groin. In this form, plague does not spread directly from one person to another. But if the patient then develops a pneumonia called secondary pneumonic plague—secondary because the disease did not start in the lungs—his coughing may transmit the disease to others in a form called primary pneumonic plague. Without treatment, pneumonic plague is fatal in 90 percent of cases. This outcome is not inevitable; of the 10–15 cases of plague that now occur each year in the United States, only one or two progress to secondary pneumonic plague. An artificially produced aerosol, however, could jump-start an epidemic with a high incidence of pneumonic plague. As in most disease epidemics, some individuals would resist infection or become only mildly ill; this condition is called pestis minor.

Antibiotic treatment is effective if started early enough. At present, the available plague vaccine protects only against bubonic plague; it could help prevent secondary pneumonic plague, in the unlikely event of a bubonic plague epidemic, but it would not be useful in a battlefield situation. In 1999, the manufacturer reportedly stopped producing the vaccine. That same year, however, British scientists developed a genetically modified vaccine that is intended to protect military personnel who might be exposed to plague in aerosol form. At latest word, the new vaccine was still being tested.

Pneumonia. This is not a specific disease, but a general term that refers to an inflammation of the lungs. The symptoms include fever, chills, headache, coughing, and shortness of breath. Many different viral, bacterial, fungal, and nonliving agents can cause pneumonia. Some diseases described under other names in this chapter—hantavirus

pulmonary syndrome, legionellosis, pneumonic plague, psittacosis, Q fever, and the various airborne mycoses—are actually forms of pneumonia.

Aside from those pathogens, some of the most frequent agents of pneumonia are the bacteria *Streptococcus pneumoniae* (the pneumococcus), *Mycoplasma pneumoniae*, *Chlamydia pneumoniae*, *Haemophilus influenzae*, *Pseudomonas aeruginosa*, *Serratia marcescens*, and (especially in AIDS patients) *Pneumocystis carinii*; several viruses, including the respiratory syncytial virus (RSV), rhinoviruses, enteroviruses, and the agents of influenza and measles; and various nonliving materials, ranging from aspirated food to chemical weapons.

Penicillin was the drug of choice for treating pneumococcal pneumonia until drug-resistant strains appeared. At present, at least 20 percent of all patients with pneumococcal pneumonia have resistant serotypes. More powerful antibiotics are available, but vaccination is advisable for vulnerable persons, such as the elderly and those with medical conditions such as diabetes. The vaccine is reported to be about 90 percent effective in preventing pneumococcal disease. Other bacterial pneumonias usually respond to antibiotic treatment, but some of those agents also have become resistant. Viral pneumonias usually are less severe, and chemical pneumonias are beyond the scope of this book.

Psittacosis. This is one of several airborne respiratory infections associated with bird droppings. It is also called parrot fever, and most people who catch it work for poultry farms or pet shops. The agent is a bacterium called *Chlamydia psittaci*, and there are only about 100 reported cases in the United States each year. As the disease usually is mild, many cases probably go unreported. Some cases are severe, with fever, headache, loss of appetite, and attacks of coughing; endocarditis and hepatitis are rare complications. Relapses may occur, but most people recover. Tetracycline and related antibiotics usually are effective as treatment.

Q Fever. Farmers, veterinarians, dairy workers, and other people who work with large domestic animals are susceptible to this disease. The bacterial agent is a rickettsia (*Coxiella burneti*) that commonly infects cattle, sheep, goats, and certain wild mammals, such as the Australian bandicoot. Until 1935, when Australian scientists identified this organism, laboratories called it Q, which stood for "query"; the name evidently stuck. The disease now occurs worldwide, and it is not clear where it originated. It is primarily airborne, in dust or in contaminated areas, but people have also caught it from raw milk, contact with infected animals or humans, or contaminated objects, such as wool or soiled laundry.

Symptoms of Q fever are those of pneumonia, with a fever, headache, fatigue, and cough. Like psittacosis, it may lead to chronic endocarditis, hepatitis, or other complications; otherwise, the case fatality rate for untreated patients is less than 1 percent. The disease responds well to antibiotics such as tetracycline, and a person who recovers has permanent immunity.

Pertussis or *Whooping Cough*. Before the introduction of a pertussis vaccine in the 1950s, this disease claimed the lives of thousands of young children each year. In 1934, for example, there were about 265,000 reported cases in the United States, with nearly 8000 deaths. Even without the vaccine, however, the case fatality rate for pertussis today is very low in developed countries, owing to better methods of resuscitation and rehydration. In 1977, a British study reported 99,000 cases with 23 deaths. Worldwide, nearly 300,000 people died of pertussis in 1999, most of them children in Africa and Asia. The agent, *Bordetella pertussis*, is a bacterium that spreads either by contact or by droplet inhalation.

As discussed in Chapter 9, some parents are reluctant to have their children vaccinated against pertussis because of side effects in one out of every 1750 children. Also, the pertussis vaccine itself (usually given as a component of the DPT vaccine) is less than 80 percent effective in preventing the disease. As a result of both factors, pertussis still affects several thousand children each year in the United States (8000 in 1998). Other developed nations, such as New Zealand, have had pertussis epidemics in recent years.

People who survive pertussis, like those who receive their DPT shots in infancy, are temporarily immune to the disease. Second attacks often occur later in life; studies have shown, in fact, that about 25 percent of adults with a persistent cough (three weeks or longer) actually have pertussis. Thus, many doctors now believe that adults should receive a pertussis booster shot to ensure that they will not contract the disease and transmit it to infants. Contrary to popular belief, there is no evidence that immune mothers give their children even short-term immunity to pertussis.

In 1999, doctors in Tennessee reported that infants who received the antibiotic erythromycin as treatment for pertussis had a higher-than-expected incidence of a severe stomach disorder called pyloric stenosis. All recovered with surgery.

Tuberculosis (TB). This highly infectious disease, caused by the tubercle bacillus (*Mycobacterium tuberculosis*), has been a major cause of death and disability throughout human history. The English author John Bunyan (1628–1688) aptly called it "the captain of all these men of death."

Scientists have found traces of the TB bacterium in the remains of a South American woman who died some 500 years before Columbus' voyage, a fact suggesting that the disease already had a worldwide distribution before humans reached the New World. The most common form of TB today is pulmonary tuberculosis, which is airborne; a related bacterium found in cows (*Mycobacterium bovis*) once caused a different form of tuberculosis called scrofula in humans who drank raw milk, but the cattle industry has largely eliminated this problem. Other forms of TB affect the brain, joints, kidneys, or other organs.

Tuberculosis, unlike most diseases, was actually fashionable at one time. Victorians believed that pale, thin, "consumptive" people were artistically or intellectually gifted (Figure 4.1). The clientele of a tuberculosis spa was nothing like that of a leper colony; well-to-do people flocked to these resorts, where they associated freely with the community at large and with one another, despite the fact that TB is far more contagious than leprosy. "Going to California for one's health" was a perverse status symbol well into the twentieth century. The list of famous Victorians with tuberculosis is not really so astonishing in view of the high prevalence of that disease in the gen-

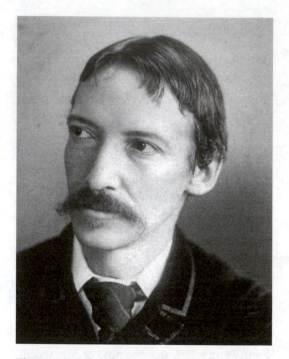

Figure 4.1. Robert Louis Stevenson (1850–1894). The author of *Treasure Island* and *Dr. Jekyll and Mr. Hyde* was among the many nineteenth-century writers and artists once believed to have succumbed to tuberculosis. Recent evidence suggests that Stevenson's illness was misdiagnosed (Chapter 3). (*Source*: The Stevenson House Collection, California State Parks, Monterey, California.)

eral population and the limited diagnostic skills of most physicians of the era. The cause was unknown until 1882, when Robert Koch discovered the TB bacterium.

At the start of the twentieth century, tuberculosis was listed as the cause of death for about one in every 200 people in Europe and the United States. At present, tuberculosis kills nearly two million people each year, more than any other single infectious disease (see Table 1.2, page 3, and Table 4.3).

**Table 4.3
Tuberculosis Deaths by WHO Region,
1999**

WHO Region	Deaths
All Member States	1,669,000
Africa	357,000
The Americas	59,000
Eastern Mediterranean	112,000
Europe	60,000
Southeast Asia	723,000
Western Pacific	359,000

Source: World Health Organization (numbers truncated to nearest thousand).

TB is now the leading killer of young women worldwide. The WHO estimates that about two billion people, or one-third of the human population, is infected with this disease. Of these, about 50 million harbor a strain of TB that is resistant to the usual drugs such as streptomycin, isoniazid, and rifampicin. More powerful drugs exist, but they are so expensive that most residents of developing nations cannot afford them.

Although most TB cases are in the developing world, the disease has made a recent comeback in the United States, where the pathogen now infects an estimated 10–15 million people. The number of new cases of active TB has declined since the peak in 1992, however, and there were only about 18,000 reported cases in this country in 1998, 40 percent of them in recent immigrants from countries where TB is common. In 1994, health officials reported that one-quarter of all students in a high school in Westminster, California had contracted a drug-resistant strain of tuberculosis. A similar problem occurred in West Virginia,

where a school bus driver infected at least 16 students. Worldwide, between 2 and 10 percent of all TB patients have multidrug-resistant strains. In Russia, the incidence of TB more than doubled between 1991 and 1997. In 1997 alone, nearly 25,000 people died from the disease in Russia, and somewhere between 108,000 and 150,000 new cases were reported, 20 percent of them multidrug-resistant.

A 2000 study at Johns Hopkins University showed that most private physicians in the United States do not know how to treat tuberculosis properly, and may even be making the drug resistance problem worse. There is some genetic variation within any population of bacterial cells; even if the TB patient is initially infected with a strain that is not drug-resistant, a few of his individual bacteria may tend in that direction. If a doctor prescribes the wrong drug regimen, it will kill only the susceptible cells, allowing the more resistant ones to survive and multiply. This process is called selection, and it happens not only in nature but in hospitals and doctors' offices all over the world. The end result is that the patient is infected entirely with drug-resistant bacteria, which pose a threat to others and require more complicated and expensive treatment. The Johns Hopkins team advised all TB patients to avoid doctors who are not experienced in treating this disease.

Testing laboratories also may fall short of the mark. In 1996, a boy from the Marshall Islands came to live with a family in North Dakota. He was tested for tuberculosis, as required by law; the result was negative. Unfortunately, the test was wrong. The boy, through no fault of his own, proceeded to infect 56 people in his new community.

The most widely administered vaccine in the world is the BCG tuberculosis vaccine, a live attenuated strain of the agent of bovine tuberculosis. BCG stands for bacille Calmette-Guérin, after Drs. Leon Calmette and Camille Guérin, who developed the vaccine in 1921. Doctors consider BCG safe for infants; it prevents TB of the brain and other serious forms of the disease in young children, and also helps protect health-care workers and residents of high-endemic areas. BCG occasionally causes skin abscesses or other complications, remains effective for only about five years, and does not reliably prevent all forms of tuberculosis. Despite these shortcomings, BCG vaccination has reduced the incidence of TB in some developing nations.

EXAMPLES OF AIRBORNE VIRUSES

This next group of pathogens causes some of the most familiar human diseases, including influenza and the common cold. Influenza was responsible for the largest disease epidemic in history, at least in terms of the absolute numbers of deaths; the Black Death of the Middle Ages killed fewer people, but the world's population was smaller then. More serious or fatal illnesses, including bacterial pneumonia, Reye's syndrome, and encephalomyelitis, sometimes follow even relatively minor viral infections.

Common Cold. This term represents a group of illnesses that are usually lumped together under the heading of "acute viral respiratory disease." Everyone knows the symptoms of a cold: rhinitis (runny nose), sore throat, coughing, and sneezing, in combination with a low-grade fever and general sick feeling. If the cold lasts more than a few days, usually there is a secondary bacterial infection, such as otitis media or sinusitis. A bad cold might be mistaken for influenza (q.v.) or vice versa. Seasonal allergies (see Chapter 7) may give the appearance of a cold that lasts for several weeks or months.

Typical agents of the common cold include several rhinoviruses (up to 35 percent of all adult colds), echoviruses, coronaviruses, coxsackieviruses, adenoviruses, myxoviruses, and enteroviruses, plus the parainfluenza virus and respiratory syncytial virus. A complete list of the viruses and serotypes associated with the common cold would far exceed the scope of this book, although it might help explain the absence of a vaccine. There is some disagreement in the literature regarding the mode of transmission of the common cold, but apparently it involves both airborne droplet inhalation and direct or indirect contact with respiratory discharges. Fecal-oral contamination also may be involved, depending on the virus.

Most readers probably are aware that wet, chilly weather does not cause colds, nor will megadoses of vitamin C prevent or cure colds. Warm or cold drinks may be soothing to the throat, but it makes little or no difference what is in the drink. Over-the-counter "cold pills" help control symptoms temporarily, but will not shorten the illness and may cause some side effects. Antibiotics are not helpful, unless there is a secondary bacterial infection. In general, a doctor's prescription is required for any cough suppressant strong enough to work, and it may be harmful to suppress a productive cough anyway. Preventive measures include handwashing, which appears to reduce transmission by contact, and avoiding crowded places.

Fifth Disease. In the early twentieth century, many doctors used a standard reference list of diseases, including several that caused a rash. The fifth disease on the list was erythema infectiosum (literally, "infectious redness"), which soon acquired the more pronounceable name "fifth disease." Its agent is a human parvovirus called B19—yet another impersonal name that implies a low level of public concern.

Normally, fifth disease is nothing more than a mild, flu-like illness of children between the ages of five and nine. It starts with red patches on the cheeks and ends with a rash on the arms, legs, and body, followed by a full recovery and lifelong immunity. Pregnant women who contract fifth disease, however, are believed to be at risk for miscarriage or stillbirth. This is not a frequent outcome, but no reliable statistics are available; so many pregnancies end in miscarriage for unknown reasons, and so many people are exposed to fifth disease, that it is hard to establish a connection.

Pregnant women are not the only population at risk. If a person with sickle-cell anemia or a weakened immune system contracts fifth disease, a life-threatening anemia and heart failure may result. Also, any adult with fifth disease may develop persistent joint pain, possibly leading to inappropriate treatment for arthritis, Lyme disease, or some other condition.

At present, there is no treatment for fifth disease, but a diagnostic blood test is available.

Hantavirus Pulmonary Syndrome (HPS). The sudden emergence of HPS in 1993 caught public health officials off guard. It was not only deadly, but appeared to be "new," despite centuries of close contact between its principal host—the deer mouse (*Peromyscus maniculatus*)—and human populations in North America. The tabloids went wild at first, claiming that a genetically engineered virus had escaped from an Army research laboratory or that terrorists were testing a secret weapon. The rumors were reminiscent of 1942, when California residents blamed the Japanese for an outbreak of bubonic plague in ground squirrels. (In fact, plague is endemic in California ground squirrel populations, and outbreaks occur every year.)

Scientists had known for many years that North American rodents, like their European and Asian counterparts, harbor a group of pathogens known as hantaviruses. The mystery lies not in the origin of the virus, but in its apparently new ability to cause respiratory illness in humans. There is still a great deal that we do not know about this disease, and the real story may ultimately prove to be stranger than any tabloid journalist could imagine.

The early conspiracy theories probably resulted from the striking symptoms of HPS and its high case fatality rate. Even with the best medical care, about half of all victims die within a few days after contracting the disease, literally drowning with a severe form of pneumonia. But if the virus really is a weapon, it is a remarkably inefficient one. Although tens of millions of Americans live near infected mice, there were only about 200 reported human cases between 1993 and 1999.

The 1993 outbreak began on May 14 when a young Navajo man in New Mexico died of severe pneumonia soon after reaching a hospital. During the next few weeks, about 20 more cases appeared, all in the Four Corners region of northern Arizona and New Mexico. CDC researchers soon identified the agent as a hantavirus found in deer mice. Elsewhere in the world, related hantaviruses cause hundreds of thousands of deaths each year—but from kidney failure, not from respiratory collapse. At some point, the new hantavirus was dubbed Sin Nombre ("without a name"), and the outbreak was attributed to unusually high rodent population densities following spring rains in the Southwest in 1993.

Later outbreaks of respiratory disease caused by Sin Nombre and related hantaviruses were not confined to the American Southwest, but also occurred in Canada, in the eastern United States, in Panama, and in several South American countries. A retrospective study turned up one HPS case as far back as 1975. At least four other North America hantaviruses, each with a rodent host, also appear to cause HPS: the New York virus in that state, the Black Creek Canal virus in Florida, the Bayou virus in Louisiana and Texas, and the Convict Creek virus in northern California.

All forms of HPS start with flu-like symptoms, followed by acute respiratory distress within 24 to 48 hours. The disease occurs mainly in rural areas, and the usual mode of transmission appears to be airborne. Doctors suspect that most victims inhale the pathogen in dust contaminated with rodent feces and urine; some cases also have been associated with rodent bites. It is unlikely that the virus can remain infectious outside the host for more than a few days. A typical high-risk situation might involve a person sweeping a closed space occupied by

deer mice, such as a barn or storage shed, thus raising a cloud of contaminated dust. In South America, but apparently not in the United States, HPS caused by a Sin Nombre-like virus has spread directly from person to person.

At first, some researchers guessed that the virus must cause inapparent infection in most exposed subjects, with only a small percentage becoming severely ill. This is the explanation for some other diseases with a high case fatality rate; most cases are so mild that the patient does not bother to see a doctor. The available data support this pattern in South America but not, for some reason, in North America. Limited sampling in endemic areas in the United States has shown that less than 1 percent of the general population has antibodies to hantavirus. In Paraguay and Argentina, by contrast, seroprevalence up to 66 percent has been reported.

An important clue to this puzzle comes from a 1999 study, which revealed hantavirus antibodies in 26 percent of North American patients with acute and chronic renal diseases, but in none of 100 healthy controls. A 1993 study had found a similar but less striking correlation. In other words, hantavirus antibodies are rare in the general population, but fairly common among people with severe kidney disease. This makes sense, as related hantaviruses in Europe and Asia cause a kidney disease called hemorrhagic fever with renal syndrome (HFRS), which affected over 3000 United Nations troops during the Korean War. Both viruses act by damaging epithelial cells of the capillaries and arterioles; apparently, the North American hantaviruses can attack either the lungs or the kidneys, whereas the

European virus focuses on the latter. But these findings fail to explain why so few Americans contract the disease in the first place.

One might expect to find a higher seroprevalence in occupational groups exposed to hantavirus, such as field biologists who handle mice. A study of mammalogists attending a meeting in Europe in 1995 revealed that 11 percent had hantavirus antibodies—but a 1994 study of 528 North American mammalogists and rodent workers found that only about 1 percent had Sin Nombre Virus antibodies.

One hypothesis is that the seroprevalence was high in the South American population because they were more recently or frequently exposed to the virus than the North American subjects. If the virus does not provoke a full immune response or cause disease in most people, the antibodies might disappear fairly quickly. In that case, the few North American subjects with antibodies and kidney disease, as well as those with HPS, might be victims of their own overzealous immune systems.

Treatment of HPS requires supplemental oxygen in an intensive care setting, but this is effective only if started within a few hours after the first signs of respiratory distress. An antiviral drug called ribavarin may be helpful. Early reports indicated that antibiotics also helped if given within the first few hours, an unexpected finding for a viral disease. It is not clear whether there was a secondary bacterial infection, or the treatment was unrelated to the patients' recovery.

Hendra Virus and Nipah Virus. In 2000, scientists announced the discovery of a new virus that had caused outbreaks of respiratory infections and encephalitis in Malaysia and Singapore (see Table 4.2). The agent, a paramyxovirus, had a 40 percent lethality rate and was called Nipah for the district where it was found. The same virus also infects dogs, cats, pigs, bats, and horses, and can spread to humans either as an aerosol (from the coughing of infected pigs) or by contact. Soldiers in Malaysia reportedly killed over one million pigs in an effort to stop the virus from spreading.

Nipah is closely related to another paramyxovirus called Hendra, formerly known as equine morbillivirus (see Chapter 6). There have been only three known human infections with Hendra, all in Australia in 1994; two were fatal. Fruit bats may be the natural reservoir host.

Influenza. This viral disease, more commonly known as the flu, is familiar to almost everyone. Hippocrates described the disease as early as 412 B.C. Formerly called "la grippe," it results from infection with any of three families of the influenza virus, designated as influenza A, B, and C. Influenza A also infects pigs and birds, and the human disease probably originated in one of these groups; influenza B occurs in humans and in harbor seals, but not in pigs or birds. Influenza C only infects humans and causes milder illness.

The influenza A virus apparently remains genetically stable in birds, because it does not make them sick, and their immune systems do not respond to its presence. When swine contract the virus from birds, however, the new host's immune system attacks the virus, causing an antigenic shift—a change in the frequencies of certain proteins found on the surface of the virus particle (Figure 4.2). For this reason, there is some concern that a deadly new strain might arise

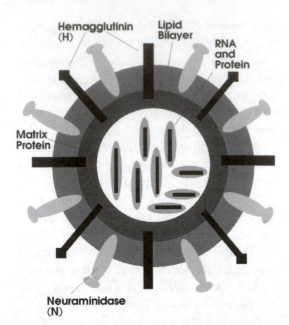

Hemagglutinin (H)

Lipid Bilayer

RNA and Protein

Matrix Protein

Neuraminidase (N)

Figure 4.2. Diagram of Influenza A Virion. A new influenza vaccine is needed every year because the surface proteins shown in this diagram mutate frequently, creating new flu strains. (Adapted from a drawing by Dr. John W. Kimball.)

in a country such as the Netherlands, which has the world's highest-density pig population (up to 9000 animals per square kilometer). Similarly, the practice of fish farming in Southeast Asia may promote the evolution of new strains of influenza by bringing humans into close contact with ducks and pigs, allowing the transfer of genetic material between human and animal influenza viruses.

People can catch a new, potentially deadly flu strain directly from live pigs, or they can catch an older strain from live chickens or other birds. Most often, however, humans catch the flu from one another. Two-thirds of all human influenza cases,

and the most severe ones that occur in large epidemics, are influenza A. Although most influenza strains have a low fatality rate, flu is the sixth most frequent cause of death in the United States. It rarely kills anyone directly, but it provides an opportunity for a secondary bacterial infection that can be dangerous for older persons or those with compromised immune systems. In a typical year, as many as 50 million Americans catch the flu, 100,000 require hospitalization for flu, and 20,000 die of related complications.

The strain known as Spanish flu, which caused the 1918–1919 pandemic, was unusual in that its victims sometimes died within a few hours. The overall case fatality rate, even among healthy young adults, was between 3 and 10 percent. That pandemic took the lives of 20 to 30 million people worldwide, including about 700,000 in the United States. In San Francisco alone, there were over 3500 deaths from influenza between September and December 1918. The strain apparently originated in the United States as a disease of swine, and American soldiers mobilized for World War I inadvertently spread the virus around the globe. Public health officials are well aware that the "Spanish Lady" might one day return, and researchers have spent decades identifying the strain and studying its properties. According to one recent study, however, a high percentage of deaths in the 1918 epidemic may have resulted from undetected tuberculosis in combination with the flu.

A U.S. Army private who died of influenza in 1918, at age 21, has done the world an inestimable service—ironically, by dying before bacteria had time to destroy both his lungs. One lung remained intact and sat in a block of paraffin for nearly 60 years, awaiting the invention of molecular biology. In 1997, researchers announced that they had successfully recovered and analyzed RNA from the virus that killed the soldier. Their work confirmed that the 1918 influenza was unlike the strains identified in more recent pandemics (1957 and 1968), and that it was more closely related to swine flu than to avian (bird) flu. This information will help researchers understand the origins of this strain and the reasons for its virulence, and might enable them to develop a vaccine to protect against future outbreaks.

Other influenza pandemics were minor by comparison, although the loss of life was still considerable. Some 70,000 Americans died in the 1957 Asian flu pandemic, and the 1968 Hong Kong flu claimed 34,000 more. Influenza usually starts abruptly, with a fever, chills, coughing and sneezing, headache, and severe muscle aches. Doctors sometimes prescribe antiviral drugs such as amantadine or rimantadine, but more often allow the bug to run its course.

Influenza immunization ("flu shots") are helpful, but people at risk need a new shot every winter, as the virus mutates frequently. The annual flu outbreak normally starts in Asia and heads east toward the United States, reaching Alaska first, then the West Coast, and finally the eastern states. International travelers can change this pattern; in 1997, an Australian visitor brought a new influenza strain to Montreal, where it caused a minor outbreak. Public health officials track the progress of each new flu virus and normally have an appropriate vaccine available by September or October of each year. Worrisome vaccine shortages

and delayed shipments occurred in October 2000 and 2001.

Many scientists believe the next influenza pandemic is long overdue, and the widespread fear of such an outbreak has led to some public health fiascos. The discovery of swine flu in a soldier in New Jersey, for example, prompted a nationwide swine flu vaccination campaign in 1976. There was no swine flu epidemic, but some people became ill from the shots. More recently, a bad batch of vaccine caused a small influenza outbreak in California. Epidemiology is a complicated business, and public health officials are doing the best they can.

According to the latest CDC estimates, the next influenza pandemic might cause between 89,000 and 207,000 deaths in the United States alone, plus 314,000 to 734,000 hospitalizations and major disruptions to commerce and society, at a total cost to the economy of $71.3–$166.5 billion. At present, the U.S. National Institute of Allergy and Infectious Diseases (NIAID) and a pharmaceutical company are working to develop an influenza vaccine that is administered in the form of a nasal spray. A 1998 study of children showed that the spray was 93 percent effective in preventing the flu; unexpectedly, it was also 98 percent effective in preventing a middle-ear infection called otitis media.

Measles or *Rubeola*. Many people confuse this disease with an entirely different one called German measles or rubella (see Chapter 5). Rubeola, also called red measles or hard measles, was once a major scourge of childhood; in 1941, there were 894,134 reported cases and 2279 deaths in the United States alone. The true incidence probably was in the millions, as virtually all children formerly contracted measles. Although now infrequent in the United States—there were 95 cases in 2001, none fatal—measles remains a far more serious disease than many Americans realize. In 1999, 875,000 people worldwide died of measles.

About one-third of all measles cases involve at least one complication, such as diarrhea, ear infections, pneumonia, or seizures. Serious complications, such as meningitis, occur in about one out of every 1000 cases. A rare complication called subacute sclerosing panencephalitis (SSP) can cause death or permanent neurological damage. In a pregnant woman, measles (like German measles) can cause miscarriage and possibly birth defects. Another problem with measles is that it can activate an existing tuberculosis infection. In 1552, 15-year-old Edward VI of England (son of Henry VIII) had an incredible run of bad luck: he caught measles and smallpox in rapid succession, followed by tuberculosis, which ended his life in 1553.

A measles vaccine has been available since 1963, but like most vaccines, it is not 100 percent effective. Also, during the first few years after its introduction, doctors did not realize that children who were vaccinated before their first birthday might not have full protection. In 1989, the United States had an unexpected measles epidemic, with about 55,000 cases nationwide (Table 4.2). Many were college students who had never been vaccinated, or whose childhood vaccinations had been given too early; younger children who caught measles in 1989 were mostly unvaccinated. Although this outbreak represented a tiny fraction of the annual incidence of measles before 1963,

opponents of immunization still point to the 1989 epidemic as proof of the vaccine's failure. On the contrary, the numbers from that outbreak and others show that the vaccine is about 95 percent successful.

Measles is one of the most readily transmitted communicable diseases, spreading both by airborne droplet inhalation and by direct or indirect contact. Two doses of the combined MMR (measles-mumps-rubella) vaccine are recommended, one at age 15 months and the second when the child starts school.

Mumps. This disease is rare in developed nations today, thanks to the combined MMR vaccine, but in earlier generations nearly every child caught it. Hippocrates described a mumps epidemic on the Greek island of Thasos in 410 B.C.

A person with a severe case of mumps finds it difficult to think about sour foods, such as lemons and pickles, because the virus causes inflammation and swelling of the salivary glands in the neck—the same glands that tend to contract in response to such thoughts. Other symptoms include fever, body aches, and headaches, sometimes with pain and swelling of the testicles. Mumps can cause infertility in males; one such victim was former U.S. President James Madison (1751–1836). Other long-term complications of mumps may include deafness, arthritis, and nervous disorders. There is some evidence that mumps may predispose to later diabetes.

Smallpox (Variola). This disease can spread either by contact or by airborne transmission. Sources do not agree on the primary mode of transmission; possibly, no one remembers, as the disease was eradicated in 1979. As recently as the first half of the twentieth century, however, smallpox killed an estimated 300 million people per year worldwide. In earlier centuries, the toll was even worse. Over 400,000 died of smallpox each year in Europe alone in the late eighteenth century, and one-third of the survivors became blind.

Europeans carried this disease to the New World in 1520, and in the centuries that followed, it decimated entire communities and tribes (see Table 4.2). Native Americans were highly susceptible to smallpox for several reasons. Their immune systems had never been exposed to it; they lacked blood type B, which confers some resistance; some of their traditional methods of treating sickness, such as jumping into a cold river, were inappropriate; and there is strong documentary evidence of a British campaign to infect Indians with gifts of blankets previously used by smallpox victims. Some tribes, however, developed effective countermeasures. One Cherokee custom was to hang a bag of skunk scent over the doorway of a family's home; during a severe epidemic, people even rubbed the scent on their skin. Although this might sound pointless, it was a polite way to discourage mass gatherings and to repel visitors who might carry the disease.

In China and the Middle East, people had already discovered a crude form of smallpox vaccination by the seventeenth century, but European doctors dismissed it as superstition. In one of history's least accurate predictions, an eighteenth-century British doctor named Wagstaffe described the Turkish practice of variation as "an Experiment practiced only by a few Ignorant Women, amongst an illiterate and unthinking People."

But Lady Mary Wortley Montagu, an Englishwoman and smallpox survivor who visited Istanbul in 1718, was so impressed by the method that she had her own son inoculated. The procedure involved scratching the arm and applying material taken from pustules of a smallpox patient with a mild case of the disease. Upon her return to England in 1721, Lady Montagu introduced variation, even persuading members of the Royal Family to try it. Soon afterward, the practice spread to North America.

Although this event revolutionized smallpox treatment and reduced the number of smallpox deaths by 90 percent, variation was risky. About 3 percent of variolated persons died of smallpox, transmitted smallpox to others, or caught unrelated diseases from the donor. The next advance came in 1796, when Dr. Edward Jenner followed the advice of local milkmaids, who knew their exposure to cows had somehow made them immune to smallpox. Although similar experiments had been tried before, Dr. Jenner was the first to vaccinate patients successfully with cowpox, a mild disease of cows caused by a poxvirus called vaccinia.

The rest of the story is well known. Despite some opposition, the new practice of vaccination spread rapidly to every continent. Less than 200 years later, the World Health Organization (WHO) declared the worldwide eradication of smallpox, and manufacturers stopped making the vaccine. The last known "wild" case, a Somali man named Ali Maow Maalin, contracted smallpox and recovered in 1977—but there were two more casualties in England in 1978: a photographer who died when smallpox virus escaped from a laboratory, and the director of that laboratory, who later committed suicide. Two known samples of the smallpox virus now reside in high-security laboratories in the United States and Russia, but other nations may have samples of their own.

Although smallpox itself is more or less gone, many animal species have closely related poxviruses, such as buffalopox, raccoonpox, and camelpox. An African disease called monkeypox has recently become the focus of media attention. Scientists have known about monkeypox since 1958, and there were several hundred known cases in Zaire in the 1980s, but most Westerners paid little attention. There were no major outbreaks, only sporadic cases in children who caught the disease while skinning infected animals caught in the forest.

In 1996, however, civil unrest in the Congo forced more people to hunt monkeys for food. New outbreaks of monkeypox occurred, and health officials noted that most cases were transmitted directly from one person to another. This new characteristic of the disease raised some concern about future outbreaks, and in fact monkeypox has continued to spread. Smallpox vaccination protects against both diseases, but as noted above, production of that vaccine ended with the eradication of smallpox.

There are two general forms of smallpox, variola minor and variola major, and both spread by airborne transmission as well as direct contact. The first disease is somewhat worse than a bad case of chickenpox, with many bumps, some scarring, and a fatality rate below 1 percent. The second, variola major, is what we usually mean by smallpox; and here the confusion starts. Depending on which sources one believes, variola major is either a severe pustular disease that kills about 20 percent of untreated patients and disfigures many more; or else it is a science-fiction nightmare that flays its victims into screaming puddles of glop.

Here is a description written before 1975, when smallpox still existed:

The 2 to 4 day pre-eruptive illness frequently resembles influenza. The temperature falls and a deep-seated rash appears. This rash passes through successive stage of macules, papules, vesicles, pustules and finally scabs, which fall off at the end of the third to fourth week; fever frequently intensifies after the rash has evolved to the pustular stage.[1]

Not our first choice, in other words, but not that much worse than some other diseases. Most patients recovered, but were badly scarred; others went blind or died. An unknown percentage of smallpox deaths, however, actually resulted from secondary bacterial infections that are now treatable, and many other patients simply became dehydrated because the lesions made it hard for them to swallow. But here is a 1999 description of the same disease:

The spots turn into blisters, called pustules, and the pustules enlarge, filling with pressurized opalescent pus. The eruption of pustules is sometimes called the splitting of the dermis. The skin doesn't break, but splits horizontally, tearing away from its underlayers. . . . In the bloody cases, the virus destroys the linings of the throat, the stomach, the intestines, the rectum, and the vagina, and these membranes disintegrate.[2]

---

[1]Abram S. Benenson, (Editor), *Control of Communicable Diseases in Man,* 12th ed. (Washington, DC: American Public Health Association, 1975), p. 288.
[2]Richard Preston, "The Demon in the Freezer" (*The New Yorker*, July 12, 1999, pp. 44–61).

And so on, for pages. Just since 1979, smallpox has receded so far into history that we can safely demonize it. Of course, it was a dreadful disease, but these words do not describe anything like a typical case. There were no hemorrhages in variola minor or in 98 percent of variola major cases.

For the final word on smallpox, we turn not to doctors or journalists, but to a Texas man named Charles Barber. In 1949, his mother Lillian became the last person to die of smallpox in the United States. His father and younger brother survived the disease, but the rest of the family did not contract it, although all were quarantined together:

I had to put socks on his hands so that he wouldn't scratch himself. And I would change his sheets, and each time I would burn a double handful of scabs that came off his body. . . . My brother was very sick, but he didn't break out, not in one solid scab like my daddy.[3]

EXAMPLES OF AIRBORNE FUNGAL DISEASES

The frequency of airborne fungal diseases in North America appears to have increased in the past 20 years. One likely reason is that the HIV/AIDS epidemic has created a large population of immune-compromised individuals who are particularly vulnerable to opportunistic infection. Some scientists also believe that global warming is contributing to a higher incidence of fungal diseases and allergies.

Acremonium or *Cephalosporium*. This fungus is a minor player in human illness, but it deserves mention because of its ability to produce trichothecene toxins (see Chapter 7) and to cause nausea, vomiting, and diarrhea in the occupants of houses where it grows. In recent years, several fungi have come under suspicion as sources of "sick building syndrome" and various illnesses. *Acremonium* also can infect the human fingernails and (like *Alternaria*, Chapter 5) the cornea of the eye.

Aspergillosis. The agent of this disease, an innocent-looking fungus called *Aspergillus flavus*, causes grief by an amazing variety of routes. When it grows on certain foods, notably peanuts, it produces aflatoxin, a potent cancer-causing chemical; when airborne, the fungus causes severe asthmatic attacks in susceptible persons. Both these topics are discussed in Chapter 7. But the same fungus also colonizes the human body, causing disease in several forms. It can invade an existing cavity in the lung, forming a large ball of gunk called an aspergilloma; it can infect the ear or sinus, or the site of a prosthetic heart valve; or it can cause a lethal form of pneumonia that may spread to the kidneys or brain.

Aspergillus grows in compost piles, stored hay, cereal grains, and many other places worldwide. Fortunately, despite its abundance in the environment, human aspergillosis is relatively rare. It occurs mainly as an opportunistic infection in people whose immune systems are weakened, either by HIV/AIDS or by immunosuppressive therapy after organ transplants. Even before the HIV/AIDS epidemic started, aspergillosis was a serious problem for this population; for example, it was responsible for one in every 200 hospital deaths in Germany between 1978 and 1982. To make matters worse, drug-resistant strains of *Aspergillus*

---

[3]"Family Recalls Last Smallpox Outbreak," Associated Press, December 17, 2001.

appeared in 1990, and their frequency is increasing.

Blastomycosis **or** *Gilchrist's Disease*. This name describes several different acute or chronic respiratory diseases caused by airborne fungi. The agent of North American blastomycosis is the fungus *Blastomyces dermatiditis*, which grows as a mold at room temperature and as a yeast in human or animal hosts. There is also South American blastomycosis, caused by the fungus *Paracoccidioides brasiliensis*; keloidal blastomycosis, another South American disease, caused by *Loboa loboi*; and European blastomycosis, another name for cryptococcosis (see below).

North American blastomycosis is not a nationally reportable disease, and its exact incidence apparently is not known. In 1992, it was listed as the cause of 44 deaths in the United States. As the case fatality rate is about 4 percent in Wisconsin (where the disease is reportable), we may estimate that there are about 1000 cases each year nationwide. Most reported cases are in the Ohio and Mississippi River valleys and in the southeastern states.

This disease also occurs in dogs, horses, cats, and other domestic animals, but people do not catch it from animals or from one another. The incidence is higher in adults than children, and higher in males than females. The risk appears greatest for men over 35 who have worked outdoors in endemic areas.

Systemic blastomycosis, in its most common form, causes a subacute or chronic lung disease with coughing and weight loss. The disease may also spread, forming abscesses in the skin, bone, prostate, or central nervous system. Cutaneous blastomycosis causes ulcers on the face, hands, or other exposed body parts. Treatment with antifungal drugs such as amphotericin B is usually effective for all forms of blastomycosis. Without treatment, the disease is often fatal.

Coccidioidomycosis **or** *Valley Fever*. This disease is common in dry, dusty regions, including the southwestern United States from California to west Texas and several countries in Central and South America. The agent, like those of several other diseases in this section, is a fungus (*Coccidioides immitis*) that can grow both in soil and in the human body. It releases airborne spores that can infect humans, domestic animals, and a number of wild mammal species.

About 60 percent of people who contract this disease have no symptoms, and most of the others have a flu-like respiratory infection that lasts several weeks but eventually resolves on its own. In about 4 percent of cases, however, the disease spreads beyond the lungs, causing serious complications such as meningitis, arthritis, or skin and bone infections. About 1 percent of such cases are fatal. At present, there is no vaccine for valley fever and no effective treatment. A vaccine is in development as of 2000; meanwhile, the available antifungal drugs (mostly the azoles) have unpleasant side effects and often do not work.

Cryptococcosis. Although sporadic cases of this disease occur worldwide, it rarely affects healthy people. It occurs most often in patients with immune disorders and in organ transplant recipients who are taking immunosuppressive drugs. The agent, *Cryptococcus neoformans*, commonly grows on the droppings of pigeons, canaries, and other birds. In 2000, a 72-year-old woman with a transplanted kidney died of cryptococcal meningitis after apparently inhaling dust from her pet cockatoo's cage. The same fungus causes about 6 percent of all infections in HIV/AIDS patients.

The symptoms and treatment are similar to most of the other airborne fungal diseases in this section. The fungus infects the lungs, often spreading to other organs, and also causing skin ulcers and other lesions. In many cases, lifelong treatment is necessary.

Histoplasmosis. This fungus (*Histoplasma capsulatum*) grows as a mold in deposits of bird feces or bat guano, or in soils with high organic content; it also grows as a yeast in human and animal hosts. Most outbreaks have been associated with contaminated areas near pigeon or starling roosts, chicken houses, or bat caves. Unlike cryptoccosis, however, this disease readily infects people with normal immune systems.

In a typical case in 1993, a maintenance worker at a paper factory swept bird guano from a roof, creating a dust cloud that infected 18 of 96 employees with histoplasmosis. All the subjects were otherwise in good health, and all recovered. Severe cases are treated with antifungal drugs such as amphotericin B.

A fairly frequent complication of histoplasmosis is pericarditis, an inflammation of the membrane surrounding the heart. This complication apparently results from the body's inflammatory response to the presence of the fungus, and it can be serious if untreated. Another unusual aspect of histoplasmosis is its apparent ability to lie dormant for long periods of time. In one case reported in 1998, an 81-year-old man had a recurrence of a histoplasmosis infection that he had contracted 50 years earlier while a prisoner of war in Sumatra.

EXAMPLES OF AIRBORNE MULTICELLULAR PARASITES

If a flying insect bites a person and injects a pathogen, the resulting disease is said to be vectorborne (see Chapter 5), not airborne. If the insect injects a venom, instead, the resulting illness is an intoxication or allergy (Chapter 7), depending on the circumstances. But if flying insects or their offspring actually take up residence in the human body, then the insect logically qualifies as an airborne multicellular parasite—although this usage, admittedly, is not quite standard.

In 1998, for example, an Alabama man returned from a vacation in the Brazilian rain forest and discovered that his scalp was infested with screwworm maggots. This unpleasant insect lays its eggs in open wounds, where the larvae emerge to find a limitless food supply. The event caused near panic in the public health community—not because of humanitarian concern about holes in the man's head, but because screwworm is also a costly livestock parasite that was eradicated in the United States in 1966 (see Chapter 6).

The maggots of some fly species have important uses in medicine, whatever one might think of them privately. In every major war, soldiers have figured out that it is better to allow maggots to eat dead tissue from their wounds rather than to die of gangrene. Today, "maggot therapy" is not some New-Age weirdness but a legitimate field of study. The University of California at Irvine currently has a Web site devoted to its maggot therapy project at http://www.ucihs.uci.edu/path/sherman/home_pg.htm.

OUTLOOK FOR THE TWENTY-FIRST CENTURY

The emergence and proliferation of drug-resistant bacterial strains will most likely continue to challenge physicians and pharmaceutical companies for many years to come. New antibiotics, although helpful, can only postpone the problem while new strains continue to evolve. Another promising approach is to treat bacterial infections with bacteriophages, viruses that attack specific bacteria but not humans. In 1999, doctors in Canada used this method successfully to treat a heart patient who had contracted an otherwise incurable staphylococcus infection during surgery. Within 20 hours, the bacterial infection was gone, although the woman succumbed to her heart problem a few months later.

Early diagnosis is another valuable tool in treating such infections, particularly in the case of drug-resistant tuberculosis (TB). In 1999, researchers at the U.S. Department of Energy's Argonne National Laboratory announced the development of a device to help diagnose TB patients with drug-resistant strains. Called a biochip, the device consists of a glass slide with thousands of tiny gel pads used to test samples of DNA from various TB strains. By 2000, the re-emergence of TB in the United States had attained the proportions of a crisis, and NIAID had established TB centers to coordinate research programs, study the mechanisms of antibiotic resistance, and test promising natural and synthetic compounds.

Nature is another potential source of new pharmaceuticals that may help in treating such infections, if the investigators use the same rigorous screening and testing protocols required for any drug. In 1999, an ethnobotanist from Louisiana State University found that extracts from several Peruvian plants appeared to inhibit the growth of the TB bacterium, at least under laboratory conditions.

Although the common cold and influenza might seem to be low-priority targets, their annual cost to the U.S. economy is immense. Promising new treatments include improved antiviral drugs, such as pleconaril for colds and zanamivir (Relenza®) and oseltamivir (Tamiflu®) for influenza. Since pharmaceutical companies must recover their investments, the already aggressive advertising campaigns for such drugs will most likely intensify, and the consumer must carefully investigate the benefits and risks of any new treatment.

The coming century may bring an effective HIV/AIDS vaccine (see Chapter 5), which will also help to limit the spread of airborne diseases such as tuberculosis and opportunistic respiratory infections among people with compromised immune systems.

Finally, the real and perceived risks associated with biological warfare and terrorism will continue to be major issues, as discussed further in Chapter 9. Public health agencies are responding to public concern by reviewing emergency response plans and sponsoring the development of improved vaccines and antibiotics. At the time this book went to press, the October 2001 anthrax mailings and their long-term implications were not yet fully understood. Suffice it to say that this unprecedented attack confirms the feasibility of large-scale bioterrorism by a foreign power—and yet the evidence to date suggests that the unknown mailer was most likely an American.

THE GOOD OLD DAYS

Until recent times, a strict quarantine was the only effective way to stop the spread of an airborne disease. People knew how to boil water and preserve food long before they understood the nature of the disease-bearing particles that can travel through the air from one person to another. The growth of cities, overcrowded slums, and unsanitary work environments favored the spread of diseases such as tuberculosis. Airborne epidemics could spread with astonishing speed, and some occupational diseases were unavoidable, as the following quotations illustrate.

The first is an excerpt from a letter by a physician who describes one of the most devastating epidemics in human history, the Spanish influenza pandemic of 1918.

Camp Devens is near Boston, and has about 50,000 men, or did have before this epidemic broke loose. It also has the Base Hospital for the Div. of the N. East. This epidemic started about four weeks ago, and has developed so rapidly that the camp is demoralized and all ordinary work is held up till it has passed. All assemblages of soldiers taboo.

These men start with what appears to be an ordinary attack of LaGrippe or Influenza, and when brought to the Hosp. they very rapidly develop the most viscous type of Pneumonia that has ever been seen. Two hours after admission they have the Mahogany spots over the cheek bones, and a few hours later you can begin to see the Cyanosis extending from their ears and spreading all over the face. . . . It is only a matter of a few hours then until death comes, and it is simply a struggle for air until they suffocate. It is horrible. One can stand it to see one, two or twenty men die, but to see these poor devils dropping like flies sort of gets on your nerves. We have been averaging about 100 deaths per day, and still keeping it up. There is no doubt in my mind that there is a new mixed infection here, but what I dont know. My total time is taken up hunting Rales, rales dry or moist, sibilant or crepitant or any other of the hundred things that one may find in the chest, they all mean but one thing here—Pneumonia—and that means in about all cases death.[4]

As the 1918 influenza epidemic progressed, it spread beyond the military to affect every segment of American society. The death rate in the United States was lower than in many other countries, thanks to better living conditions, but fear was prevalent. Schools and theaters were closed; people who refused to wear flu masks (gauze face masks, Figure 4.3) sometimes were jailed. Children on the streets chanted several versions of the popular "I opened the door and in flew Enza!" Nor was the trauma quickly forgotten. In the 1950s, parents who remembered the 1918 epidemic still encased their children in "flu jackets" at the first hint of a sniffle. (A flu jacket was a thick, quilted jacket of unbleached cotton, worn by patients in military hospitals during World War I.)

Next is a description of conditions in the guano mining industry of the mid-nineteenth century, when exposed workers suffered the full ravages of some of the airborne fungal diseases described in this chapter:

For many years the three Chinca Islands, 120 miles south of the major port of Callao, were the main focus of guano mining . . . as guano dust billowed out from the holds, crews often took to the rigging to avoid breathing it. The "trimmers" working to balance the load in the holds were

[4]Letter written by a physician at Camp Devens, Massachusetts dated September 29, 1918 (published by N.R. Quist in the *British Medical Journal*, December 1979).

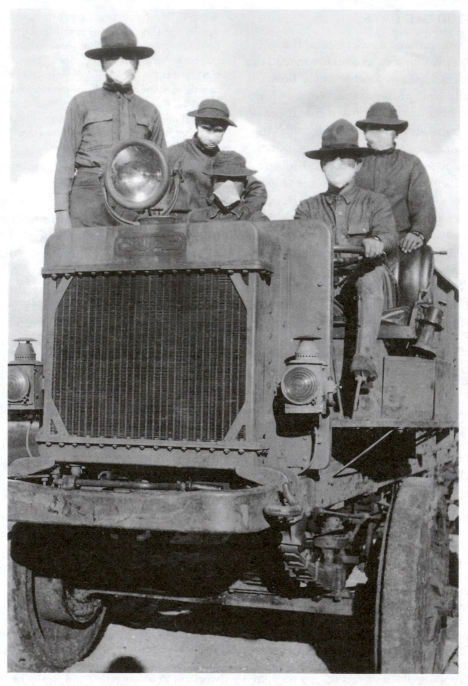

Figure 4.3. World War I soldiers wearing "Flu Masks." (*Source*: The San Diego Historical Society—Photograph Collection, www.sandiegohistory.org.)

not so lucky, and could only work 20 minutes at a time. A ghastly array of occupational diseases continually thinned the work force. The Peruvian government used convicts, indentured Chinese, and kidnapped Polynesians as laborers in these terrible conditions. The Peruvians and Chileans practically depopulated Easter Island and Tongareva in this way, before international outcry stopped the virtual slavery.[5]

Last, there are flies. Infestation with fly larvae is a problem that most Westerners expect to find in cows, not people, but here is a nineteenth-century account:

There are forms of nasal disorder caused by [fly] larvae, which some native surgeons in India regard as a chronic and malignant ulceration of the mucous membranes of the nose and adjacent sinuses in the debilitated and the scrofulous. Worms lodging in the cribriform plate of the ethmoid feed on the soft tissues of that region. Eventually their ravages destroy the olfactory nerves, with subsequent loss of the sense of smell, and they finally eat away the bridge of the nose. The head of the victim droops, and he complains of crawling of worms in the interior of the nose. The eyelids swell so that the patient cannot see, and a deformity arises which exceeds that produced by syphilis. . . . Flies deposit their ova in the nasal discharges, and from their infection maggots eventually arise.[6]

FROM THE AUTHOR'S FILE CABINET

About ten years ago, the author worked for a small environmental consulting office in a semidesert region of southern California. One day, the staff decided it was necessary to check something in the attic; so the author stood on a chair and opened the trapdoor, releasing a large accumulation of dried pigeon droppings onto her head. As the birds scattered and dust filled the small room, everyone began to cough. Two weeks later, we were still coughing.

Most of us recovered quickly without treatment, and assumed we had caught the flu. But after a few weeks, the oldest staff member, a woman in her sixties, developed a more serious respiratory illness, accompanied by a heart problem that landed her in the hospital. The author told the woman's husband about the incident with the trapdoor, and explained that outbreaks of histoplasmosis have occurred under similar circumstances, since the fungus grows on bird droppings. He wrote "histoplasmosis" on a piece of paper and took it to his wife's physician.

The next day, he reported the outcome: The doctor had assured him that the illness could not be histoplasmosis because, he said, that was another name for valley fever, which did not occur in California! In other words, the doctor had confused histoplasmosis with coccidioidomycosis, and was not aware that both diseases are endemic in southern California. The woman eventually recovered, although her illness was never identified.

Regardless of whether this woman had histoplasmosis or not, the point is clear: Some infectious diseases may seem rare only because few doctors are familiar with them, and because most patients recover without treatment. After such a disease receives some publicity, there may appear to be a sudden outbreak of cases.

[5]R. Cowen, Geology 115 Lecture Notes, Chapter 16 (University of California at Davis Web site, 1999).
[6]G. M. Gould and W.L. Pyle, *Anomalies and Curiosities of Medicine* (New York: Bell Publishing Co., 1896).

REFERENCES AND RECOMMENDED READING

Allegra, L., and Blasi, F. (Editors). 1999. Chlamydia pneumoniae: *The Lung and the Heart*. New York: Springer Verlag.

Amos, D. "Disease by Cruise Ship: Infectious Illnesses Are Being Transported to the United States by Travelers." ABCNEWS.com, November 9, 1997.

Andrews, R. "Developer of Recombinant BCG Vaccine Wins Infectious Disease Research Award." *The Scientist*, January 6, 1992.

Armstrong, L.R., et al. "Occupational Exposure to Hantavirus in Mammalogists and Rodent Workers." *American Journal of Tropical Medicine and Hygiene*, 51 (1994 Supplement): 94.

Barquet, Nicolau, and Domingo, Pere. "Smallpox: The Triumph Over the Most Terrible of the Ministers of Death." *Annals of Internal Medicine*, October 15, 1997, pp. 635–642.

Beveridge, William I.B. 1977. *Influenza, the Last Great Plague: An Unfinished Story of Discovery*. New York: Prodist.

"Blastomycosis—Wisconsin, 1986–1995." *Morbidity and Mortality Weekly Report*, July 19, 1996, pp. 601–603.

"California School Becomes Notorious for Epidemic of TB." *New York Times*, July 18, 1994.

Chua, K.B., et al. "Nipah Virus: A Recently Emergent Deadly Paramyxovirus." *Science*, May 26, 2000, pp. 1432–1435.

Cliff, A.D., Haggett, A.D., and Ord, J.K. 1986. *Spatial Aspects of Influenza Epidemics*. London: Pion Ltd.

Coker, Richard J. 2000. *From Chaos to Coercion: Detention and the Control of Tuberculosis*. New York: St. Martin's Press.

Collier, Richard. 1974. *The Plague of the Spanish Lady: The Influenza Pandemic of 1918–1919*. New York: Scribner.

Crosby, Alfred W. 1990. *America's Forgotten Pandemic: The Influenza of 1918*. New York: Cambridge University Press.

Daniel, Thomas M. 1999. *Captain of Death: The Story of Tuberculosis*. Rochester, NY: Boydell & Brewer.

Dubos, Rene J. 1987. *The White Plague: Tuberculosis, Man, and Society*. New Brunswick, NJ: Rutgers University Press.

Ferrer, J.F., et al. "High Prevalence of Hantavirus Infection in Indian Communities of the Paraguayan and Argentinean Gran Chaco." *American Journal of Tropical Medicine and Hygiene*, September 1998, pp. 438–444.

Fritz, Curtis L., et al. 1996. "Surveillance for Pneumonic Plague in the United States During an International Emergency: a Model for Control of Imported Emerging Diseases." *Emerging Infectious Diseases* 2(1), Jan.–Mar. 1996, pp. 30–36.

Gladwell, Malcolm. "The Dead Zone." *New Yorker*, September 29, 1997.

Godfrey, Simon, and Wilson, Robert. 1996. *Pneumonia*. Boston, MA: Blackwell Science Inc.

Guillemin, Jeanne. 1999. *Anthrax: The Investigation of a Deadly Outbreak*. Berkeley: University of California Press.

Henig, Robin M. "Flu Pandemic." *New York Times Magazine*, November 1992, pp. 28–31.

Holmes, Grace, et al. "The Death of Young King Edward VI." *New England Journal of Medicine*, July 5, 2001, pp. 60–62.

Howson, Christopher P., et al. 1991. *Adverse Effects of Pertussis and Rubella Vaccines*. Washington, DC: National Academy Press.

Kazemi, A. H. "Spontaneous Rupture of the Spleen due to Q Fever." *Southern Medical Journal*, June 2000, pp. 609–610.

"Kern County Leads Effort to Avert Valley Fever Peril." Associated Press, November 6, 1997.

Lambert, Bengt. 1951. *The Frequency of Mumps and of Mumps Orchitis and the Consequences for Sexuality and Fertility*. Basel: Karger.

Larone, D.H. 1995. *Medically Important Fungi: A Guide to Identification*. Washington, DC: American Society for Microbiology.

"Legionnaires' Disease Associated with Potting Soil." *Morbidity and Mortality Weekly Report*, September 1, 2000.

"Legionnaires' Scare Closes California School." Reuters News Service, October 11, 1999.

Luckingham, Bradford. 1984. *Epidemic in the Southwest, 1918–1919*. Southwestern Studies, Monograph no. 72. El Paso, TX: Texas Western Press.

MacKenzie, Debora. "This Little Piggy Fell Ill." *New Scientist*, September 12, 1998, p. 18.

Mead, G.E., et al. "Oral Histoplasmosis: A Case Report." *Journal of Infection*, July 1998, pp. 73–75.

Meyer, Andrea. 1999. *Of Mice, Men, and Microbes: Hantavirus*. San Diego, CA: Academic Press.

Morell, Virginia. "Mummy Settles TB Antiquity Debate." *Science*, March 25, 1994, pp. 1686–1687.

Morgan-Capner, P., and Caul, E.O. "The Risk of Acquiring Q Fever on Farms: A Seroepidemiological Study." *Occupational and Environmental Medicine*, October 1995, pp. 644–647.

Noymer, Andrew, and Garenne, M. "The 1918 Influenza Epidemic's Effects on Sex Differentials in Mortality in the United States." *Population and Development Review*, September 2000, pp. 565–581.

Ott, Katherine. 1999. *Fevered Lives: Tuberculosis in American Culture Since 1870*. Cambridge, MA: Harvard University Press.

Pan American Health Organization. 1999. *Hantavirus in the Americas: Guidelines for Diagnosis, Treatment, Prevention, and Control* (available in English and Spanish). Washington, DC: Pan American Health Organization.

Patnaik, M., et al. "Hantavirus-Specific IgG, IgM, and IgA in Acute and Chronic Renal Disease Versus Congenital Renal Disease in the United States." *American Journal of Kidney Diseases*, April 1999, pp. 734–737.

Patriarca, Peter A., et al. 1999. *Pandemic Influenza: A Planning Guide for State and Local Officials (Draft 2.1)*. Atlanta, GA: U.S. Department of Health and Human Services, Public Health Service, Centers for Disease Control and Prevention.

Patterson, K. David. 1986. *Pandemic Influenza, 1700–1900: A Study in Historical Epidemiology*. Lanham, MA: Rowman & Littlefield.

Pettigrew, Eileen. 1983. *Silent Enemy: Canada and the Deadly Flu of 1918*. Saskatoon, Saskatchewan: Western Producer Prairie Books.

Phillips, John L. "Urologic Histories of 11 U.S. Presidents, 1789–1972." Abstract, 1999 Annual Meeting, American Urological Association.

"Resurgence of Pertussis—United States, 1993." *Morbidity and Mortality Weekly Report*, December 17, 1993.

Rosa, Frank. 1993. *Legionnaires' Disease: Prevention and Control*. Mansfield, OH: Bookmasters.

Rothman, Sheila M. 1995. *Living in the Shadow of Death: Tuberculosis and the Social Experience of Illness in American History*. Baltimore, MD: Johns Hopkins.

Sacks, Oliver. 1973. *Awakenings*. New York: HarperCollins.

Scholtissek, C. "Cultivating a Killer Virus." *Natural History*, January 1992, p. 2 ff.

Sekura, Ronald D., et al. 1985. *Pertussis Toxin*. Orlando, FL: Academic Press.

Selzer, Richard. 1995. *Raising the Dead*. Toronto: Penguin.

Smith, Everett, et al. 1996. *Medical Mycology and Human Mycoses*. Belmont, CA: Star Publishing Co.

Stobierski, M.G., et al. "Outbreak of Histoplasmosis Among Employees in a Paper Factory—Michigan, 1993." *Journal of Clinical Microbiology*, May 1996, pp. 1220–1223.

Taubenberger, J.K., et al. "Initial Genetic Characterization of the 1918 "Spanish" Influenza Virus." *Science*, March 21, 1997, pp. 1793–1796.

"Traveler's Exposure to Screwworm Raises Concerns of Possible Infestation." Associated Press, August 8, 1998.

"U.S. Study Criticizes Private Doctors' TB Treatment." Reuters News Service, March 15, 2000.

Van Hartesveldt, Fred R. 1993. *The 1918–1919 Pandemic of Influenza: The Urban Experience in the Western World*. Lewiston, NY: Edwin Mellen Press.

Vanden Bossche, Hugo (Editor). 1990. *Mycoses in AIDS Patients*. New York: Plenum Publishing.

Walzer, Peter D. 1994. Pneumocystis carinii *Pneumonia*. 2nd edition. New York: Marcel Dekker.

Wardlaw, Alastair C. 1988. *Pathogenesis and Immunity in Pertussis*. New York: John Wiley.

Wheat, L.J., et al. "Pericarditis as a Manifestation of Histoplasmosis During Two Large Urban Outbreaks." *Medicine* (Baltimore), March 1983, pp. 110–119.

Yampolaska, Olga. "The Sverdlovsk Anthrax Outbreak of 1979." *Science*, November 18, 1994, pp. 1202–1208.

CHAPTER 5

Human Pathogens Transmitted by Contact

> For before what is sudden, unexpected, and least within calcula-
> tion, the spirit quails; and putting all else aside, the plague has cer-
> tainly been an emergency of this kind.
> —Thucydides, *The History of the Peloponnesian War, Second Book,*
> *Chapter VII: The Plague of Athens* (430 B.C.)

The 1956 motion picture *Ben Hur* contains a poignant scene that is only a few seconds long. Juda Ben Hur arrives at the gates of Jerusalem with his dying sister and mother, hoping for a glimpse of the Messiah, only to learn of His imminent crucifixion. They converse with a blind beggar, to whom they give a coin; the man, of course, cannot see that the two women are both in the advanced stages of leprosy. Then a crowd approaches, shouting "Lepers!", and begins hurling stones at the family. The blind man, realizing his mistake, inverts his cup and drops the coin on the ground.

In the context of this book, the coin was a **fomite**—a contaminated object that can spread disease. More accurately, it was a perceived fomite. Today, we know that leprosy (an old name for Hansen's disease) is very hard to catch; the beggar need not have worried about the coin. But the scene vividly depicts the ancient fear of contagion.

Long before doctors learned how water, air, and food can transmit disease pathogens, the general public knew enough to avoid touching anyone who appeared to be sick. A plague destroys much more than individual lives. It can destroy entire communities, by making people fear and abandon one another.

CROSS-REFERENCE

The titles of Chapters 2–5 reflect the principal modes of disease transmission. Most pathogens, however, can be transmitted in more than one way. Microorganisms in blood may pass from one person to another by direct contact or during a medical procedure, but a patient who is coughing blood may also produce a cloud of airborne droplets for others to inhale. If the droplets land immediately on a nearby person's face, the exchange is still a form of contact. But if the pathogen is one that can survive longer, as a smaller suspended aerosol, the disease is airborne (see Chapter 4). For the reader's convenience, Table 5.1 provides a cross-reference for pathogens in other chapters that are potentially transmissible by contact.

MAJOR SEXUALLY TRANSMITTED DISEASES (STDs)

In 2000, the U.S. Centers for Disease Control and Prevention (CDC) announced that more than 15 million new cases of sexually transmitted diseases (STDs) are reported in the United States each year. This country has a higher incidence of STDs than any other industrialized nation in the world. In 1998, the city of Baltimore, Maryland had the nation's highest incidence of syphilis, gonorrhea, and other STDs.

Lovers can share almost any infectious disease, from measles to athlete's foot. STDs are unique only in the sense that their transmission requires prolonged physical contact with a direct transfer of body fluids. While this excludes casual conversation, such a

Table 5.1
Cross-Reference: Other Diseases Transmitted by Contact

Disease	Chapter	Notes
Buruli Ulcer	2	Waterborne or vectorborne
Leptospirosis	2	Water, food, or contact
Melioidosis	2	Waterborne, airborne, or contact
Shigellosis	2	Water, food, or STD in male homosexuals
CJD/BSE	3	May be transferable by blood transfusions
Clostridium perfringens	3	Causes both gas gangrene and food poisoning
E. coli	3	Foodborne, waterborne, or contact
Hepatitis A	3	Foodborne or contact
Pork Tapeworm	3	Foodborne, waterborne, or contact
Toxoplasmosis	3	Foodborne or contact
Yersiniosis	3	Foodborne or contact
Diphtheria	4	Airborne or contact
Fifth Disease	4	Airborne or contact
Hantavirus	4	Airborne or possibly contact
Hendra and Nipah Viruses	4	Airborne or contact
Influenza	4	Airborne or contact
Measles	4	Airborne or contact
Mumps	4	Airborne or contact
Pertussis	4	Airborne or contact
Pneumonia	4	Airborne or contact
Psittacosis	4	Airborne or contact
Alternaria Fungus	6	Can infect the human eye
Brucellosis	6	Foodborne or contact; mainly in livestock
Rift Valley Fever	6	Vectorborne; mainly in livestock

transfer might occur not only during sex, but also through gestation, birth, or breast-feeding, or the sharing of contaminated hypodermic needles, tattooing equipment, or ear-piercing devices. Some people have contracted STDs (and other diseases) during medical procedures such as vaccinations, transfusions, and organ transplants. Since the start of the HIV epidemic, hundreds of health care workers reportedly have died of AIDS as a result of needlestick injuries. The annual cost of treating STDs in the United States, not including HIV/AIDS, is $10 billion.

STDs have an extensive mythology, for obvious reasons. Until recently, most people were reluctant to admit engaging in the types of behavior that spread such infections. Suffice it to say that a few STDs are transmissible via contaminated towels or toilet seats, but most are not. Mosquitoes do not transmit HIV, nor can you catch gonorrhea by swimming in the same pool with an infected person. The local zoo is no help either; as explained below, camels do not carry or transmit syphilis, despite an urban legend that has survived for over 500 years.

Bacterial STDs

In the 1960s and 1970s, the "Love Generation" did not worry much about STDs, for the most prevalent ones were caused by bacteria and responded well to antibiotic treatment. In 1969, a celebrity physician proposed that syphilis could be eradicated worldwide in a single day, just by giving simultaneous penicillin shots to everyone. In 1975, an article in *Scientific American* stated that U.S. residents no longer needed to worry about infectious disease in general.

We may scoff at these statements, but Monday-morning quarterbacking is easy. A generation hence, our own predictions will sound equally naive.

Chancroid. This disease occurs mainly in the tropics. The agent (*Haemophilus ducreyi*) causes painful, oozing ulcers at the site where it enters through a scrape or crack in the skin or mucous membrane. Regional lymph nodes on one side of the body may swell. Although chancroid is primarily an STD, nurses caring for patients with the disease have developed lesions on their hands. Antibiotic treatment usually is effective against chancroid.

Chlamydia. This sexually transmitted infection is now the most frequently reported of all infectious diseases in the United States, with over 700,000 new cases in 2000 alone (see Table 10.1, page 286). This is only the number of reported cases; by some estimates, the true incidence may be three to four million per year.

The agent, a small bacterium called *Chlamydia trachomatis*, now infects up to one-fourth of all young women in the United States. It can cause pelvic inflammatory disease and infertility; a 2001 study showed that some chlamydia strains increase the risk of cervical cancer. Men also get chlamydia infections in the form of nongonococcal urethritis (NGU), which means inflammation of the urethra resulting from some infection other than gonorrhea.

If one sex partner is infected with chlamydia, both must be treated, or they will simply play ping-pong with the bacterium. Patients may also need eye drops, since the same bacterium causes a common eye infection called conjunctivitis or "sticky eye." The eye infection itself is not dangerous, but can easily reinfect the urethra via contaminated towels or other contact. Well-documented outbreaks have even occurred in public swimming pools.

As if these facts were not bad enough, chlamydia can infect a baby during birth, sometimes causing a dangerous form of neonatal pneumonia, and it can invade the joints of adults, causing arthritis and possibly temporomandibular joint dysfunction (TJD). The disease can even be fatal. In 1999, some 16,000 women in Africa and Southeast Asia reportedly died of chlamydia infections.

There is still a great deal that we do not know about this disease. Chlamydia is one of several pathogens that have been tentatively linked to later development of multiple sclerosis (MS). Also, the same bacterium has other strains that cause far more devastating diseases: trachoma, the world's leading cause of preventable blindness, and lymphogranuloma venereum (LV), a sexually transmitted disease that can cause ulceration and massive swelling and scarring of the genitalia. At present, trachoma and LV occur mostly in the tropics, but both are among the diseases that might expand their ranges into the Earth's temperate zones if the present global warming trend continues.

Every woman, regardless of personal habits, should be tested for chlamydia. At present, it responds well to treatment with antibiotics.

Gardnerella. Many cases of so-called nonspecific vaginitis (inflammation of the vagina, often with an unpleasant odor and discharge) result from infection with a bacterium called *Gardnerella vaginalis*. Like yeast (see below), this is not exactly a sexually transmitted disease, but most sources describe it in that context. The *Gardnerella* bacterium is a normal occupant of the human vagina, causing symptoms only if its numbers increase abnormally. Douching, cigarette smoking, and certain medications all appear to kill lactobacilli ("good" vaginal bacteria), thus allowing certain pathogens to multiply out of control.

Regardless of its origin, such an infection requires treatment, or it may lead to pelvic inflammatory disease and possible infertility. *Gardnerella*, like some other pathogens, also can cause NGU in men. The infection usually responds to broad-spectrum antibiotics. Increasing the population of lactobacilli in the vagina also may be effective.

Syphilis. Until AIDS appeared in 1982, syphilis was the most feared of all STDs. Although it was treatable by the twentieth century, and considerably less severe than in the past, people remembered the highly virulent strains that swept Europe in the sixteenth and seventeenth centuries. It is not clear how the "Great Pox" epidemic started, but it often caused massive disfigurement and killed its victims in a few months. One theory is that Europeans lacked resistance to a strain of syphilis found in the West Indies. Its ravages continued for centuries, later inspiring a verse by William Blake (note the reference to placental transfer):

> But most thro' midnight streets I hear
> How the youthful Harlot's curse
> Blasts the newborn Infant's tear,
> And blights with plagues the Marriage
>   hearse.[1]

---

[1]William Blake, *Songs of Experience* (New York: Dover, 1984, reprint of 1794 edition).

Every nation claimed that this dreadful disease originated somewhere else. The English called it the French Disease, and the French called it the Italian Disease. Europeans returning from the New World claimed to have caught it from the Indians or, strangest of all, from their llamas.

According to a popular urban legend that survives to the present day, camels (and their New World relatives, the llamas and alpacas) are carriers of syphilis and can transmit this disease by spitting on unwary humans. The story usually ends with the hapless victim trying to explain to a public health officer (or a clergyman or spouse) how he or she managed to catch syphilis from a camel. The origins of most urban legends are obscure, but this one is an exception: the Spanish Conquistadores started the rumor in the sixteenth century, as part of a campaign to promote sheep as a better source of wool than alpacas. Tending flocks has always been a lonely job, and historical documents show that bestiality was a social concern in Peru long before Cortez arrived. Thus, according to one interpretation, the Europeans exploited this issue to their own economic benefit, by convincing the Native people to slaughter their alpacas and raise sheep instead.

Until recently, most scientists and historians believed that syphilis originated in the New World, and those who bought the Spanish rumor probably assumed llama drivers were the source. Later, when evidence of syphilis turned up in northern European skeletons that predated Columbus' voyage, the rumor had to adapt or die; so it attached itself to Old World camels and their drivers, instead. It is true that we owe many of our diseases to nonhuman species—influenza was once a disease of birds and pigs, and we may thank the chimpanzee for AIDS—but there is no evidence of syphilis in llamas, alpacas, or other camels today. In fact, scientists have never found syphilis in any species other than our own.

Syphilis is actually one of several closely related diseases caused by similar bacteria. The sexually transmitted form of syphilis, and a second, nonvenereal disease called bejel, both result from infection with the spirochete *Treponema pallidum*. Syphilis per se is worldwide, but bejel occurs only in parts of Africa, Asia, and the eastern Mediterranean. The closely related bacterium *Treponema pertenue* causes a tropical disease called yaws, which is common in South America and the Caribbean as well as in Africa and Southeast Asia. A fourth disease, pinta, occurs in Central and South America and is associated with *Treponema carateum*. All these forms may have evolved from an ancestral disease similar to yaws. Researchers have reported evidence of yaws lesions on a 1.5-million-year-old *Homo erectus* skeleton from Africa.

All four diseases are transmitted mainly by direct contact with exudates from open skin lesions. Syphilis is transmitted either by sexual contact or by placental transfer (rarely by fomites) and is sometimes lethal. The case fatality rate is hard to estimate, as most patients now receive medical treatment and the late complications rarely appear. The other three diseases usually result from casual contact, often under conditions of poor hygiene, and are less severe. Otherwise, all follow a similar course, in that they start with skin lesions near the site of the original infection, followed by a secondary eruption that eventually disappears. Years later, destructive lesions may invade the skin, mucous membranes, nasopharynx, or bones. In venereal syphilis, these lesions sometimes progress to the central nervous system or heart, causing dementia and death. Severe cases of syphilis were once confused with leprosy. In both syphilis and leprosy, much of the damage appears to result from the host's immune response rather than from the pathogen itself.

Before antibiotics were available, doctors resorted to extreme measures to cure syphilis. In 1927, J. Wagner von Jauregg received the Nobel Prize in Medicine for his innovative work in this field. His method was to infect syphilis patients with malaria, thus inducing a high fever that destroyed the syphilis spirochetes; then he used quinine to cure the malaria. This method remained in use until the 1950s.

In 1999, the CDC announced a new initiative to eliminate syphilis. The plan has focused on areas with a high incidence of the disease, by providing closer monitoring, more community involvement, faster response to outbreaks, and greater access to health care. As of 2001, this effort appeared to be succeeding; the rate of new syphilis cases in the United States had reached an all-time low, with fewer than 6000 new cases in 2000. As recently as 1990, there were over 50,000 new cases per year. The 1999 incidence was highest in the southern states, and it was three times as high among African Americans as in Caucasians. These differences largely reflect unequal access to health care, but they are still a great improvement over 1990, when the rate of syphilis was 64 times as high in African Americans. (For information on the infamous Tuskegee study, see Chapter 10.)

Some other countries, by contrast, have seen a resurgence of syphilis in recent years. In 1998, the Russian Health Ministry announced that the former Soviet Union had over 450,000 new cases of syphilis in 1997 alone, as compared with 7900 new cases in 1990. To be effective, STD prevention programs must take into account new lifestyles and social patterns; the Russian government attributed its problem to increased prostitution. Other epidemics have been traced to less obvious sources in specific communities. In 2000, for example, the source of a syphilis outbreak in San Francisco was an America Online chat room for gay men. Of course, HIV cannot spread electronically, but people often meet in this way. On the bright side, the same medium that promotes disease transmission can be equally effective in promoting caution.

Gonorrhea. With so much publicity focused on HIV/AIDS and other emerging STDs, this old standby—once common enough to need a half-dozen nicknames—has tended to fade from public awareness. Gonorrhea is still a serious public health concern, however, with an estimated 650,000 new cases in the United States each year; the actual number of reported cases in 2000 was 358,995. The reported incidence varies considerably from state to state, from a low of 5.4 cases per 100,000 in Maine to a high of 391.5 cases per 100,000 in Mississippi (1997 data). Overall, the frequency of gonorrhea in the United States is about ten times as high as in Canada and 50 times as high as in Sweden.

The incidence of this disease fell by 64 percent between 1985 and 1997, apparently owing to condom use resulting from the fear of HIV/AIDS. Now that the latter disease is so common as to seem almost normal, and pharmaceutical companies have prolonged its victims' lives, many people have become careless and complacent again. As a result, gonorrhea and other STDs have rebounded.

The agent of gonorrhea, a bacterium called *Neisseria gonorrhoeae*, occurs only in humans. The mode of transmission is sexual contact or, in rare cases, contact with a contaminated object. The most frequent symptoms are a urethral discharge and pain during urination, although the throat or anus may also become infected. About 50 percent of infected women have no symptoms. The disease is often self-limiting, but sometimes persists in a chronic carrier state. Although gonorrhea rarely causes death, occasionally there are serious complications such as arthritis, endocarditis, or meningitis. In women, the infection often causes pelvic inflammatory disease and infertility. Doctors believe that persons infected with gonorrhea are more likely than others to contract HIV/AIDS if exposed.

The same bacterium also causes two types of infection in children, called gonococcal vulvovaginitis and gonococcal ophthalmia neonatorum. The first, an inflammation of the urogenital tract of young girls, was once common in children's institutions and may result from sexual abuse or other causes (such as contaminated fomites, sex play with other children, simple misdiagnosis, or even birth itself). The second disease is a severe eye infection that often occurs in newborns whose mothers are infected with gonorrhea. All babies born in the United States routinely receive protective eye drops from the birth attendant.

Until recently, gonorrhea responded well to penicillin treatment, but a drug-resistant strain called PPNG (penicillinase-producing *Neisseria* gonorrhea) has evolved. Other antibiotics, such as ceftriaxone or ciprofloxacin, are effective against this strain.

Viral STDs

Until the 1980s, most well-known sexually transmitted diseases were caused by bacteria and could be treated with antibiotics. The exceptions were herpes and genital warts, which no one took seriously until researchers discovered their link to cervical cancer in the early 1990s. By that time, HIV had arrived on the scene and effectively changed the world.

AIDS and *HIV Disease*. At the time this book went to press, the last great plague of the twentieth century had infected over 60 million people worldwide and had killed over 19 million. Nearly six million new cases were reported during 1998; in Africa alone, HIV kills over 5000 people every day. In sub-Saharan Africa and parts of Asia, the epidemic is essentially out of control, with 20–30 percent of some populations infected. Skeptics note correctly that these estimates vary and may be inflated, but such quibbling will not make the disease vanish. (Underreporting has also occurred in some countries; in 2001, the Thailand Health Ministry discovered that most AIDS deaths in that country were recorded incorrectly as heart disease.)

The chief modes of HIV transmission are well known, but bear repeating: sexual contact (either homosexual or heterosexual) with exchange of body fluids; needle sharing; blood transfusions or other medical procedures; laboratory transfer, such as needlestick injuries or splashing of contaminated body fluids on a skin lesion; or transfer during pregnancy or birth. The virus cannot replicate itself in mosquitoes, bedbugs, or ticks, so it is unlikely that these insects can serve as vectors. The virus can, however, survive for eight days in a bedbug or ten days in a tick.

Many readers will remember the early 1980s, when the media and the public tended to dismiss AIDS as a problem unique to patrons of gay bars. Even serious researchers speculated that the disease resulted from lifestyle factors such as promiscuity and drug abuse.[2] This view has largely yielded to the newest statistics, which show the disease spreading rapidly among heterosexuals and their children (Figure 5.1). A few journalists still insist that HIV does not cause AIDS, and that the entire issue is bogus.

During the first ten years or so after the discovery of AIDS, the condom industry boomed. Every middle-school student was suddenly an expert on safe sex, and the tabloids "outed" one dead celebrity after another. But the scare campaign was effective; the number of new HIV cases reported each year fell steadily, as did the incidence of other STDs. There were an estimated 6000 new HIV infections in San Francisco in 1982, but only about 500 per year during the 1990s. In 1994, only 23 percent of gay men in San Francisco said they had unprotected sex with more than one partner. By 1999, however, that rate had jumped again to 43 percent; and by 2000, the incidence of HIV infection (and gonorrhea) had also doubled.

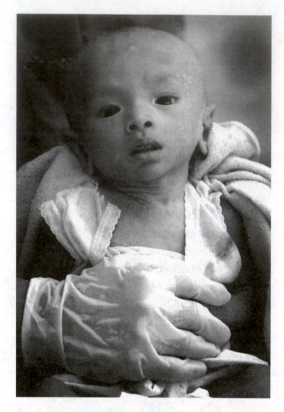

Figure 5.1. AIDS orphan in Cambodia. A gloved nurse carefully handles a six-month-old child with AIDS whose parents abandoned him at birth. (*Source*: AP/Wide World Photos/David Longstreath.)

Thus, the HIV/AIDS epidemic had entered a new phase. Not only was the rate rising again, but about one-third of the new HIV infections (at least in San Francisco) were among heterosexuals.

Doctors attribute these trends to the public's perception that new drugs have virtually brought HIV disease under control. Protease inhibitors, when used in com-

---

[2]Similarly, during the Black Death of 1348, early measures to fight bubonic plague included massacring Jews, selling herbal poultices, and barring the import of figs to the city of Florence.

bination with other AIDS drugs, can reduce the amount of HIV in an infected person's blood to undetectable levels and can prolong life. But HIV already is becoming resistant to available treatments, and the viral load quickly climbs again in 10–50 percent of patients. Many of these patients continue to spread the disease, as it is human nature to enjoy life while it lasts. Another factor contributing to the spread of HIV is the unsafe blood supply in many countries. Worldwide, an estimated 80,000–160,000 new HIV infections result from this source each year.

During the early years of the HIV/AIDS epidemic, most doctors believed that the disease was 100 percent fatal and that susceptibility was universal. More recently, studies have identified people who seem resistant or even immune to HIV. Several prostitutes in Kenya, for example, have remained HIV-negative for many years, despite frequent unprotected sex with a largely HIV-positive clientele. The reason for their immunity is unknown, but many of these women are related to one another, a fact that suggests a possible genetic factor. In 1997, scientists reported a genetic mutation that prevents AIDS in about 10 percent of people of European descent, by blocking the virus from entering macrophages (a type of white blood cell produced by the immune system). As of 2001, no comparable mutation had been found in Africans, although genes were found that delay or accelerate the onset of AIDS.

Genetic analysis has shown that the European mutation arose about 700 years ago, and researchers believe that its bearers might have survived a major epidemic, most likely either plague or smallpox. Both diseases were ravaging Europe at about that time, and both pathogens act by invading certain cells of the immune system, just as HIV does. Of course, a mutation does not arise magically to solve a problem; but if a few families already had that particular mutant gene when the epidemic happened, they would have survived and left more descendants than their neighbors. Thus, the gene would also have survived.[3]

There are actually two known AIDS viruses that infect humans. HIV-1, which has caused most cases of HIV disease and AIDS, may have originated in chimpanzees in about 1931 (see also Chapter 9). No one knows exactly when or how it made the leap to humans, but it now exists in several forms. The HIV-1 viruses responsible for the worldwide epidemic are known as Group M; within that group, the A strain is most prevalent in Africa and the B strain in the United States. Other strains called C, D, and E also occur in Africa and Asia. A second AIDS virus, called HIV-2, may have come from the sooty mangabey monkey.

On August 31, 2000, British Parliamentarian Dr. Evan Harris became the first human injected with a new experimental AIDS vaccine. He is one of 18 healthy volunteers who will determine the vaccine's safety. The next phases of the study will involve Africans and high-risk populations. Even if the vaccine is safe, however, scientists do not expect it to be available for global use until at least 2010. In 2001, Microsoft Corporation chairman Bill Gates pledged $50 million to support this effort. At about the same time,

---

[3]It is not the author's intention to patronize readers who already understand how natural selection works or to offend those whose beliefs dictate another interpretation of these events.

the Bush administration announced the closure or downsizing of the U.S. Office of National AIDS Policy.

A review of alternative and experimental treatments for HIV would exceed the scope of this book; herbal remedies, marijuana, acupuncture, antioxidant supplements, massage, and spiritual healing all have improved quality of life for some patients. In 2001, researchers in Iowa reported that AIDS patients survived longer if they were concurrently infected with the little-known, apparently harmless hepatitis G virus (HGV or GBV-C).

Genital Herpes. The human herpesvirus (HHV) exists in several different forms, with more appearing in the literature every year. HHV-2 (also called HSV-2) is the primary agent of genital herpes, but some cases result from HHV-1, which normally causes fever blisters on the face. Closely related herpesviruses cause chickenpox, mononucleosis, roseola, Kaposi's sarcoma, and other diseases.

According to recent studies,[4] about 22 percent of U.S. adults—more than one in five— have genital herpes and can transmit the disease to sex partners or other contacts, even when no lesions are present. The virus lies dormant in nerves at the base of the spinal cord, producing occasional flareups of painful, oozing blisters. Besides being unpleasant, these open sores make it easier for an infected person to contract HIV or other diseases. Herpes infection appears to be a risk factor for cervical cancer, possibly because infected women are more likely than others to contract HPV (next section) or because the herpesvirus modifies the HPV

genome. If transmitted to a newborn infant, herpes can cause a fatal generalized infection. Placental transfer of the virus may also cause birth defects.

At present, genital herpes is incurable. Some over-the-counter drugs offer temporary relief from symptoms. Tests of a new herpes vaccine in 2000 showed that it was less than 50 percent effective, and worked only for women.

Human Papillomavirus (HPV). In the United States alone, some 20 million people are already infected with HPV, and as many as five million new cases occur every year. The infection often leads to cervical cancer, a disease that kills about 250,000 women per year worldwide. People who have an STD with open lesions, such as herpes, seem more likely than others to contract HPV. One of the most promising strategies for controlling this disease is the development of an HPV vaccine based on proteins from the human papillomavirus. In 2001, clinical trials by the U.S. National Cancer Institute demonstrated the safety of a new HPV vaccine and its ability to elicit an immune response in human volunteers.

A papilloma is a wart, and HPV, as its name implies, can also cause genital warts, usually on the penis or vulva or near the anus. These unsightly cone-shaped growths may sprout singly or in groups, and the overall effect is reminiscent of bracket fungi on a log. The usual treatment is to remove individual warts by electrodesiccation and then treat the mucous membrane with chemicals that denature the viruses. Thick masses of warts may require treatment with

---

[4]D.T. Fleming, et al., "Herpes Simplex Virus Type 2 in the United States, 1976 to 1994" (*New England Journal of Medicine*, October 16, 1997, pp. 1105–1111).

harsh chemicals that cause the diseased epidermis to slough.

Molluscum Contagiosum. This disease is most often, but not always, transmitted by sexual contact. Usually it takes the form of numerous small pink or whitish bumps in the genital area, each with a prominent central pore. Children also catch the disease, possibly from contaminated towels or other fomites, and the lesions may appear anywhere on their bodies. These lesions often heal on their own after several months; a doctor can also freeze them or remove them with a needle. More than 90 percent of adults have antibodies to the poxvirus that causes this disease, and its distribution is worldwide.

STDs Caused by Protozoans

At least two protozoal diseases, amebiasis and giardiasis, can be transmitted by male homosexual activity. Since these are primarily waterborne diseases rather than STDs, their accounts appear in Chapter 2. One protozoal disease remains in this category.

Trichomoniasis. There are two to five million new cases of trichomoniasis (trich) each year in the United States and at least 170 million worldwide. The agent is a protozoan called *Trichomonas vaginalis*; despite the name, it lives not only in the vagina but also in the male urethra and prostate gland. Like most protozoa, this one cannot live long outside the body, and no one on record has caught trich from a toilet seat. Infants can, however, contract the disease from their mothers at birth.

In women, the symptoms (if any) usually include a discharge and itching, sometimes with abdominal pain. Men with trich usually have no symptoms, but may need to urinate frequently. The drugs of choice are metronidazole (Flagyl®) or tinidazole, but resistant strains have recently appeared.

Fungal STDs

Any interpersonal contact, sexual or otherwise, can transmit fungal diseases such as ringworm and athlete's foot. The only common fungal infection that is often associated with sexual contact is candidiasis or yeast. Most people are familiar with this infection, if only from watching endless television commercials for yeast infection remedies.

Candidiasis or Moniliasis. This common fungal infection has many names, depending on where the yeast (*Candida albicans* or related species) happens to grow. These fungi are part of the normal flora of the mouth, GI tract, vagina, and skin. They cause disease only when some change in the body (HIV/AIDS, diabetes, antibiotic therapy, pregnancy, birth, or even new dentures) provides an opportunity for increased growth. Thus, yeast is not exactly a sexually transmitted disease, except in the sense that any irritation in a damp region of the body is likely to set it off.

Oral thrush is a common infection of the mouth of newborn infants, who contract it during birth and recover within a few weeks. Adults with HIV/AIDS also get oral thrush due to their weakened immune response. Intertrigo occurs when yeast infects a body crevice that remains damp much of the time, such as a baby's diaper area, a skin fold on an obese person, or the skin between the fingers of a dishwasher. Paronychia is a similar infection that occurs at the base of the fingernail. The most common and occasionally disabling form of candidiasis, however, infects the vagina of women or the anus of male homosexuals. The symptoms may include a profuse whitish discharge, itching, and pain during intercourse. In rare cases, particularly in drug addicts or diabetics, the fungi may enter the bloodstream and invade the kidney, lung, brain, or heart.

Antifungal drugs are available, but are not always effective unless the underlying cause of the infection can be resolved. Topical anesthetics are used to relieve the pain of oral thrush in adults, but it is best to use them at least an hour before meals to avoid aspiration of food.

Multicellular Parasites Transmitted by Sexual Contact

Crab Louse **(Phthirus pubis).** This parasite is similar to the head louse (described later in this chapter), except that it lives in the pubic area and often colonizes a new host during sexual contact. Symptoms include itching and louse eggs (nits) attached to pubic hairs. Over-the-counter and prescription drugs are more or less effective, but the lice and eggs also can live for a while on clothing, so it is also important to wash and change clothes.

Pork Tapeworm **(Taenia solium).** This is usually a foodborne parasite (see Chapter 3), but it has been transmitted on occasion by male homosexual activity or other direct contact.

REFERENCES AND RECOMMENDED READING

"AIDS Leading Cause of Death in Thailand." Associated Press, August 31, 2001.

Anttila, T., et al. "Serotypes of *Chlamydia trachomatis* and Risk for Development of Cervical Squamous Cell Carcinoma. *Journal of the American Medical Association*, January 3, 2001, pp. 47–51.

Barr, Robert. "Tracing Syphilis: Medieval English Skeletons Had Syphilis Before Columbus." Associated Press, August 29, 2000.

Brandt, Allan M. 1987. *No Magic Bullet: A Social History of Venereal Disease in the United States Since 1880*. New York: Oxford University Press.

Carmichael, Cynthia G. 1999. *AIDS and HIV Essentials*. Pompano Beach, FL: Health Studies Institute.

Christie-Dever, Barbara, et al. 1996. *AIDS: What Teens Need to Know*. Huntington Beach, CA: Learning Works.

de Balogh, Katinka. "Is There a Future for Llama and Alpaca Meat?" *European Consortium for Continuing Education in Advanced Meat Science and Technology Newsletter*, Vol. 32, September 1999.

Fabricius, Johannes. 1994. *Syphilis in Shakespeare's England*. London: Taylor and Francis.

Fox, Maggie. "Herpes Vaccine Works for Women, Not Men." Reuters News Service, September 17, 2000.

Gallo, Robert. 1993. *Virus Hunting: AIDS, Cancer, and the Human Retrovirus: A Story of Scientific Discovery*. New York: Basic Books.

Gray, Fred D. 1998. *The Tuskegee Syphilis Study: The Real Story and Beyond*. Montgomery, AL: Black Belt Press.

Hara, Y. "Effect of Herpes Simplex Virus on the DNA of Human Papillomavirus 18." *Journal of Medical Virology*, September 1997, pp. 4–12.

Harro, C.D., et al. "Safety and Immunogenicity Trial in Adult Volunteers of a Human Papillomavirus 16 L1 Virus-Like Particle Vaccine." *Journal of the National Cancer Institute*, February 21, 2001, pp. 284–292.

Kelland, Kate. "AIDS Vaccine Trial: British Parliamentarian to be First Human Injected." Reuters News Service, August 31, 2000.

King, K., et al. 1998. *Sexually Transmitted Diseases*. 3rd ed. New York: McGraw-Hill.

Kolata, Gina. "Scientists Discover Similarity in HIV and Black Death." *New York Times* News Service, June 3, 1998.

Lalani, Alshad, et al. "Use of Chemokine Receptors by Poxviruses." *Science*, December 3, 1999, pp. 1968–1971.

Murakami, M., et al. "Human Papillomavirus Vaccines for Cervical Cancer." *Journal of Immunotherapy*, May 1999, pp. 212–218.

"Nairobi Prostitutes May Hold Key to AIDS Vaccine." CNN/Associated Press, October 25, 1997.

Powell, J., and Bourdeau, A. 1996. *AIDS and HIV-Related Diseases: An Educational Guide for Professionals and the Public*. Reading, MA: Perseus Press.

Reitman, Judith. 1998. *Bad Blood: Crisis in the American Red Cross*. Los Angeles, CA: Pinnacle Books.

Reverby, Susan, and Jones, James H. 2000. *Tuskegee's Truths: Rethinking the Tuskegee Syphilis Study*. Chapel Hill, NC: University of North Carolina Press.

Schoub, Barry D. 1999. *AIDS and HIV in Perspective: A Guide to Understanding the Virus and its Consequences*. 2nd ed. New York: Cambridge University Press.

Smith, Everett, et al. 1996. *Medical Mycology and Human Mycoses*. Belmont, CA: Star Publishing Co.

Stine, Gerald J. 1999. *AIDS Update 2000*. Englewood Cliffs, NJ: Prentice-Hall.

U.S. Public Health Service, Centers for Disease Control and Prevention. "Sexually Transmitted Disease Sweeps the Former Soviet Union." *HIV/STD/TB Prevention News Update*, May 28, 1998.

U.S. Public Health Service, Centers for Disease Control and Prevention. 1998. *1998 Guidelines for Treatment of Sexually Transmitted Diseases*. Washington, DC: Reiter's Scientific and Professional Books.

Watstein, Sarah B., and Chandler, Karen. 1998. *The AIDS Dictionary*. New York: Checkmark Books.

Xiang, J., et al. "Effect of Coinfection with GB Virus C on Survival Among Patients with HIV Infection." *New England Journal of Medicine*, September 6, 2001, pp. 707–714.

"Yaws Origin." *Archaeology Newsbriefs*, May–June 1996.

EXAMPLES OF DISEASES TRANSMITTED BY INSECTS OR OTHER VECTORS

A vector is a small animal, usually an arthropod, that can transmit an infectious agent directly to a vertebrate host. Some sources define a vector as any organism that transmits disease; but if a dog bites you, for example, and the wound becomes infected with bacteria from the dog's teeth, we will not call the dog a vector.

Mosquitoes transmit some of the most serious human diseases, such as malaria and yellow fever. Other important vectors are flies, fleas, lice, ticks, and kissing bugs. The relative roles of these vectors in various parts of the world depend largely on climate, terrain, and personal hygiene. It is possible to control some diseases by targeting the vectors and their habitats, but in practice it is often difficult to kill vectors without causing severe environmental damage. Earlier generations drained wetlands, hoping to reduce mosquito populations and stop the malaria and yellow fever epidemics that once killed thousands every year in North America—and it worked so well that few wetlands remain.

Some of the most reviled environmental impacts, from the Tennessee Valley Authority's dams to the cattle industry's mass production of substitute hosts, have largely eliminated malaria and yellow fever in the United States. In the process, however, these changes harmed many native species and disrupted important ecological cycles. Today's environmental planners, having largely forgotten why their grandparents destroyed wetlands in the first place, now labor to restore these ecosystems. Meanwhile, in less developed nations, one to two million people die of malaria each year.

Mosquitoes cause occasional small outbreaks of encephalitis in North America, but major epidemics of mosquito-borne diseases now occur mainly in the tropics. Most people in the Western world no longer have fleas or body lice, which once served as vectors for major epidemics of plague and typhus. Thus, in the United States and most developed nations today, ticks are the most important arthropod vectors.

Vectorborne Bacterial Diseases

Bubonic Plague. This is the most common form of an ancient disease, plague, whose name is now synonymous with any great epidemic or tragedy. "Bubonic" refers to the large swellings or buboes that appear on the groin; these are inflamed lymph nodes that drain the site of the original infection. Chapter 4 describes the airborne form of plague, but most cases result either from the bites of infective fleas—fleas that have previously bitten infected rodents—or from contact with infected animal tissues. Several recent cases of bubonic plague in the United States have resulted when hunters skinned or dressed infected animals. The fatality rate without treatment is about 50 percent.

In A.D. 541, the first recorded plague pandemic (now called Justinian's Plague) struck the Mediterranean region, where it raged for two centuries and killed an estimated 40 million people. Scientists who study tree rings have found evidence of a worldwide catastrophe or climate change in about A.D. 540, but the connection (if any) is unknown. The more famous Black Death of the fourteenth century killed about 25 million Europeans, then one-third of the continent's population, in less than four years (Table 5.2). An estimated two-thirds of China's population died in the same plague. In the late nineteenth century, a third plague pandemic spread the disease worldwide, finally bringing it to North America.

Some historians now interpret the Black Death as a windfall that relieved population pressure in Europe, overturned the feudal system, reduced the authority of the church, inspired the invention of various labor-saving devices, and put the population through a genetic bottleneck that may have imparted HIV resistance to modern Europeans. Although this sounds inspiring, it is undoubtedly better to live after a major plague than during one:

In the year of the Lord 1348 there was a very great pestilence in the city and district of Florence. . . . The symptoms were the following: a bubo in the groin, where the thigh meets the trunk; or a small swelling under the armpit; sudden fever; spitting blood and saliva (and no one who spit blood survived it). . . . So they remained in their beds until they stank. And the neighbors, if there were any, having smelled the stench, placed them in a shroud and sent for burial. The house remained open and yet there was no one daring enough to touch anything because it seemed that things remained poisoned and that whoever used them picked up the illness. . . . And then more bodies were put on top of them, with a little more dirt over those; they put layer on layer just like one puts layers of cheese in a lasagna.[5]

It is not entirely clear when plague reached the New World, but most historians believe it arrived in San Francisco on a

[5]Marchione di Coppo Stefani, *The Florentine Chronicle*, Rubric 643 (ca. 1380).

Table 5.2
Examples of Epidemics of Diseases Transmitted Primarily by Direct Contact or Vectors

Disease	Date	Location	Est. Cases	Est. Deaths
Chlamydia	1990s	United States	600,000/year	None
HIV/AIDS	1982–99	Worldwide	50 million	17 million
Dengue	1972	Cuba	300,000	150+
Dengue	1972	New Caledonia	40% of pop.	NR
Plague	A.D. 542–543	Constantinople	NR	70,000
Plague	1346–52	Europe and China	NR	25 to 50 million
Plague	1665–66	London	NR	17,440
Plague	1898–1905	India	NR	10 million
Plague	1924–25	Los Angeles, CA	32	31
Typhus	1918–22	Soviet Union	12 million	Over 2 million
W. Nile Encephalitis	1999	New York State	68	6
Yellow Fever	1853	New Orleans	NR	9000
Yellow Fever	1878	Mississippi Valley	NR	20,000
Anthrax	1978–79	Zimbabwe	10,738	182
Ebola Fever	1976	Zaire	318	280
Ebola Fever	1995	Zaire	315	245
Ebola Fever	1997	Gabon	NR	10
Ebola Fever	2000	Uganda	288	96
Enterovirus 71	1975	Bulgaria	705	44
Meningitis	1996	Ivory Coast	100,000+	10,000+
Poliomyelitis	1916	Northeast U.S.	NR	6,000
Poliomyelitis	1952	North America	57,000	NR
Poliomyelitis	1996	Albania	138	14
Poliomyelitis	1992–93	Netherlands	71	NR
Poliomyelitis	2000	Cape Verde	44	17
Scarlet Fever	1877	Chicago, IL	NR	819
Unidentified	430 B.C.	Athens, Greece	NR	1/3 of population

Sources: J. Diamond, "The Arrow of Disease" (*Discover*, October 1992, pp. 64–73); World Health Organization; U.S. Public Health Service.

steamship from China in about 1900. It is now endemic in the western one-third of the United States and in parts of South America. Urban plague has been largely eliminated, but sylvatic plague in wild rodent populations is here to stay. Despite opportunities for contact, however, only 10 to 15 people contract plague each year in the United States. The disease is so rare that a single case makes headline news, and most vic-

tims survive with treatment. Plague, like leprosy, is a crisis that has outstayed its welcome.

Every year, public health officials in the western states announce that they have found plague in ground squirrels in some campground. Then they close the campground, kill some squirrels, and open it again. Although monitoring is important, these announcements serve mainly to reassure the public. A 2000 study showed that large-scale extermination of infected rodents can actually trigger plague outbreaks in humans.

A vaccine is available that confers short-term protection against the bubonic form of plague; it has some side effects and requires an annual booster. Few people obtain it because of the rarity of the disease in the United States and the high cost and unavailability of the vaccine elsewhere, and the manufacturer reportedly stopped production in 1999. In that same year, British scientists developed an improved plague vaccine that is intended to protect military personnel who might be exposed to pneumonic plague on the battlefield.

At least until recently, treatment of plague with tetracycline, streptomycin, or other antibiotics was highly effective if started early enough. In 1997, however, scientists reported that an antibiotic-resistant strain of plague had appeared in Madagascar.

Ehrlichiosis. This so-called emerging disease has only recently gained the attention of the medical community, as it was not known to affect humans until the 1980s. At present, there are four known forms of human ehrlichiosis, all vectored by ticks.

Sennetsu fever, which occurs only in Japan and Southeast Asia, causes fever and swollen lymph nodes; in 1953, scientists identified its agent as a rickettsia called *Ehrlichia sennetsu*. More recently, three forms of human ehrlichiosis have turned up in the United States. The first, monocytic ehrlichiosis, was identified in 1987. It occurs mainly in the southeastern and south central states, and its agent is *Ehrlichia chaffeensis*. In 1994, the agent of human granulocytic ehrlichiosis was tentatively identified as *Ehrlichia equi*, which also infects horses. Another rickettsia, *Ehrlichia ewingii*, later turned up in a few immunosuppressed patients, but its status is uncertain.

These bacteria attack the white blood cells, causing sudden onset of fever, headache, vomiting, diarrhea, joint pains, and other symptoms. Blood tests may show a low white blood cell count or a low platelet count. Tetracycline and related antibiotics usually are effective.

Lyme Disease. Like most "emerging" diseases, this one has been with us for a long time but has only recently attracted attention. European doctors described a similar disease before 1900 and associated it with tick bites in 1909, but the disease did not receive a name until 1975, after an outbreak of juvenile rheumatoid arthritis in the town of Lyme, Connecticut.

The vectors of Lyme disease are deer ticks (*Ixodes*, Figure 5.2), which have become more numerous as North American deer herds have grown larger (a trend that appears related to predator control). At least in the laboratory, mosquitoes and biting flies also may transmit the disease. The agent is a spirochete called *Borrelia burgdorferi*. Recent studies have shown that up to 24 percent of people in some endemic areas test positive for exposure to Lyme disease. A pregnant woman infected with Lyme disease can transmit it to her fetus.

Today, nearly everyone has heard of Lyme disease, thanks to an aggressive publicity campaign. In fairness, however, the Lyme movement also has contributed its share to the confusion that surrounds any emerging disease. Although Lyme is real and potentially devastating, its myriad

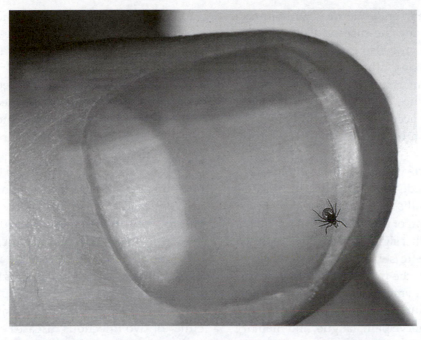

Figure 5.2. Deer Tick (*Ixodes* sp.). (*Source*: U.S. National Institute of Allergy and Infectious Diseases.)

symptoms and the difficulty of diagnosis have attracted a population of chronic patients who feel sick and believe they must have Lyme. As discussed below, when tested more carefully, many of these patients turn out to have some other disease, or none.

Uncritically reviewed records show that Lyme is now the most common tickborne disease in the United States, with about 16,000 new cases reported each year and an estimated annual price tag of over $1 billion. As of 1998, the average cost of treating each patient was over $61,000. Lyme is also, however, the only tickborne disease known to most family practice physicians. A 1998 study showed that Lyme disease is vastly overdiagnosed in Oklahoma due to reliance on false-positive test results. Many cases turned out to be either ehrlichiosis or Rocky Mountain spotted fever; the investigators were unable to confirm even one case of true Lyme disease in Oklahoma. A 1998 study at Yale University reevaluated 209 patients who were diagnosed with Lyme disease elsewhere, and found that 60 percent showed no evidence of current or past infection. Thus, the true distribution and prevalence of Lyme disease is hard to estimate.

Diagnosis requires a blood test, but at the time this book was published, none of the widely available diagnostic tests actually detected the presence of *Borrelia burgdorferi*. Most tests simply detect antibodies to the bacterium, and many people are likely to be seropositive in endemic areas without necessarily having the disease. False-positive results for Lyme also can result from antibodies to many other diseases, and false negatives may result if the body has not had time to produce Lyme antibodies. The latest protocol for accurate Lyme testing requires confirmation by two different test procedures.

Lyme starts with flu-like symptoms, usually low-grade fever, fatigue, and muscle aches. A "bull's-eye" rash may also appear at the location of the tick bite, but not all patients have this sign. In at least one reported case, epileptic seizures in an adolescent turned out to be the first sign of Lyme disease. Some Lyme patients develop chronic symptoms including musculoskeletal and peripheral nerve pain, fatigue, and memory impairment. The Lyme Foundation Web site presents an astonishing list of other symptoms attributed to Lyme disease, affecting the jaw, bladder, lungs, ears, eyes, throat, central nervous system, stomach, heart, joints, liver, spleen, testicles, endocrine system, and skin. Lyme is appropriately called "The Great Imitator," but at least one scientist has dubbed it "The Easy Answer."

Studies have shown that long-term antibiotic treatment of Lyme disease is often ineffective. If administered within three days after a tick bite, however, doxycycline is 87 percent effective. Again, it is important to determine if the person really has Lyme disease or some other tickborne disease such as ehrlichiosis or babesiosis, since a different antibiotic might be needed. If it turns out to be a viral disease, such as Colorado tick fever, no antibiotic will help.

In 2000, the U.S. Food and Drug Administration approved the first Lyme disease vaccine for human use. The vaccine requires a series of three shots and provides about 80 percent protection. At the time this book went to press, however, safety trials were not yet complete. Not unexpectedly, early tests of the vaccine in 1995 caused serious side effects in some volunteers, and the first lawsuits against the manufacturer are already in progress.

Deer ticks infest animals other than deer and humans; one host, the western fence lizard (*Sceloporus occidentalis*), may hold the clue to a new treatment for Lyme disease. In 1998, researchers reported that these lizards are immune to Lyme disease because their blood contains a protein that kills the Lyme bacterium.

Relapsing Fever. This name may refer to either of two infectious diseases caused by *Borrelia recurrentis* and related spirochetes. Although they are in the same genus as the agent of Lyme disease, these spirochetes behave differently, and the diseases are not particularly similar to Lyme (except to the extent that almost everything starts "like flu"). Human body lice and several species of ticks all can spread relapsing fever.

Outbreaks of louseborne relapsing fever usually occur during wars, famines, and mass migrations; no outbreak has occurred in the United States in over a century. Tickborne relapsing fever, however, is reasonably common in North, Central, and South America, as well as in Africa, Asia, and the Middle East. It can occur either sporadically or in small outbreaks. In the western United States, such outbreaks often occur in rodent-infested mountain cabins. Unlike the ticks that transmit Lyme, the relapsing fever vectors typically do not embed themselves in the skin; thus, they can feed at night and depart before morning, leaving the victim none the wiser.

Both forms of relapsing fever start, as the name suggests, with a very high fever (often 105°F) that drops after several days and then returns once or twice. Other symptoms include headache, severe muscle and joint pains, diarrhea, vomiting, coughing, and sometimes a rash. Complications may include pneumonia, bronchitis, or damage to the heart, kidney, or central nervous system. The fatality rate for tickborne relapsing fever usually is between 2 and 10 percent, but in louseborne epidemics it may exceed 50 percent.

Either tetracycline or penicillin usually is effective, but should not be given at the peak of the patient's fever. The death of large numbers of spirochetes can release toxic by-products that cause severe symptoms resembling toxic shock. Chloramphenicol is effective for resistant strains, but may cause serious side effects such as anemia.

Rickettsialpox. Although this disease was once common in New York City and elsewhere in the United States, public health officials in the 1970s thought it was eradicated in this country. Several cases appeared in New York in the 1980s, however, and a 1999 study showed that 16 percent of intravenous drug users in Baltimore were seropositive for this disease. It also occurs in the Mediterranean region and in the former Soviet Union.

Rickettsialpox is a disease of the house mouse (*Mus musculus*), an Old World rodent that is well established in urban areas worldwide. The vector, a mite called *Allodermanyssus sanguineus*, bites infected mice and then bites humans, transmitting the disease. The high seroprevalence among drug users suggests that it also spreads from one person to another by needle sharing. The agent, *Rickettsia akari*, is a member of the spotted fever group.

The disease starts with a skin lesion or eschar, followed by a high fever, chills, and a rash similar to that of chickenpox—so similar, in fact, that the apparent decline of rickettsialpox may result partly from the fact that it is often mistaken for chickenpox (and thus left untreated). Tetracycline is effective against rickettsialpox, but the case fatality rate even without treatment is less than 1 percent.

Rocky Mountain Spotted Fever. This tickborne rickettsial fever occurs mainly in the United States, although there are similar diseases elsewhere in the world (Boutonneuse fever in Africa and the Mediterranean, Queensland fever in Australia). The agent of Rocky Mountain spotted fever, *Rickettsia rickettsi*, owes its repetitive name to the fact that it was the first rickettsia ever discovered.

Several species of ticks serve as vectors for this disease, which causes high fever, severe headache, fatigue, deep muscle pain, chills, and a skin rash that usually starts on the arms or legs and spreads to the rest of the body. The fatality rate without treatment is about 20 percent, but treatment with tetracycline or chloramphenicol usually is effective.

Tularemia. This disease is remarkably uncommon in the United States, considering how many animals carry it and how many different ways there are to catch it. Deerflies (Figure 5.3), ticks, and (in Scandinavia) mosquitoes all serve as vectors, but people more often contract the disease from animal

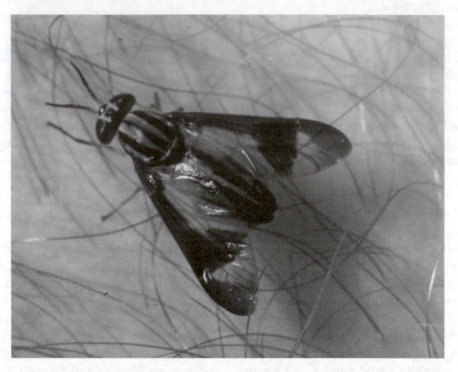

Figure 5.3. Deerfly (*Chrysops* sp.). This insect serves as a vector for several diseases and also has a painful bite. (*Source*: Dr. John A. Jackman, Texas A&M University.)

bites, from contact with body fluids, or by eating undercooked meat or drinking contaminated water. Under unusual circumstances, it can even spread as an aerosol.

This disease is also known as rabbit fever, because hunters sometimes catch it when skinning rabbits. The agent is a bacterium, *Francisella tularensis*, and the disease has a wide distribution in North America, Europe, and Asia. As the symptoms are highly variable and often mild, most cases probably go unreported. There were 2291 reported cases in the United States in 1939, but only 291 in 1984 and 142 in 2000.

Tularemia usually "starts like the flu" (to coin a phrase), and milder cases also end like the flu. Symptoms of vectorborne tula-

remia may also include an ulcer-like lesion and swollen lymph nodes. Other forms of tularemia are designated as typhoidal (similar to typhoid fever), pulmonary (similar to pneumonia), and ocular (similar to conjunctivitis). If recognized in time, the disease responds well to several antibiotics, including streptomycin and ciprofloxacin. Survivors have lifelong immunity.

Tularemia can be serious, and the fatality rate for recognized cases is about 5 percent without treatment. A 58-year-old Massachusetts woman, for example, died of the disease in 1996. As she was incoherent when found, no one knows how she caught it. In a more recent case, an unlucky Long Island yardman ran his lawnmower over a dead rabbit and contracted pulmonary tularemia. Doctors initially treated the case as an infection resulting from intravenous drug abuse, which the patient denied. When the blood culture finally revealed *Francisella tularensis*, appropriate antibiotics were given, and the man survived.

Typhus Fever. Typhus is really three different diseases: epidemic typhus, endemic typhus, and scrub typhus. All are vector-borne diseases with similar symptoms, and the agents are closely related rickettsiae.

The agent of epidemic typhus is *Rickettsia prowazeki*, and the usual vector is the human body louse; sporadic cases also result from flea bites. Outbreaks tend to occur under crowded, unsanitary conditions. Some historians believe that epidemic typhus caused at least some of five major disease epidemics that occurred in the New World before Columbus' voyage. Aztec documents show that each of these epidemics followed a natural disaster and famine. Other historians, however, maintain that Europeans brought typhus to the Americas.

The early symptoms are like those of many other acute infectious diseases: severe headache, chills, high fever, confusion, and muscle pains. After a few days, reddish spots appear on the shoulders and armpits, later spreading to other parts of the body. Other symptoms may include severe nightmares, loss of hearing, low blood pressure, and kidney failure. Without treatment, the case fatality rate is as high as 40 percent in some epidemics. Tetracycline and other antibiotics are effective. An insecticide is also necessary to destroy the lice that transmit the disease.

Epidemic typhus in its typical form no longer occurs in the United States, although there are occasional reports of Brill-Zinsser disease, a mild relapse of epidemic typhus in a previously infected person. Between 1976 and 1982, however, there were at least 30 sporadic cases of typhus in the United States, all traced to *Rickettsia prowazekii*. None of these patients had body lice; all apparently contracted the disease from flying squirrels (*Glaucomys volans* and *G. sabrinus*) or their ectoparasites. Flying squirrels are a reservoir host for epidemic typhus, and their fleas bite people on occasion, but cannot live on the human body; thus, as the disease cannot spread from person to person without the help of vectors, no outbreaks resulted. All the patients survived, whether treated or not.

Endemic typhus, a milder but otherwise similar disease, occurs sporadically worldwide. In the United States, the incidence has declined from 5400 cases in 1944 to about 50 cases per year at present. Fleas transmit the pathogen (*Rickettsia typhi*), and the reservoir hosts include rats, opossums, and possibly domestic cats.

Scrub typhus presently occurs only in Asia and Australia; the agent is *Rickettsia tsutsugamushi*, and the vectors are larval mites (chiggers). Depending on the strain and the affected population, the case fatality rate for scrub typhus may range from 1 to 40 percent.

Vectorborne Viral Diseases

Colorado Tick Fever (CTF). The agent is a reovirus (CTF, coltivirus, or Eyach virus) found in the tick *Dermacentor andersoni*, which is also the vector of Rocky Mountain spotted fever and other serious bacterial infections. In the past decade, Lyme disease has tended to knock Colorado tick fever off the front pages, so to speak, and there are few recent reports. In 1994, CTF turned up in a Manhattan resident who had recently visited Colorado. The disease is not communicable from one person to another, and no outbreak resulted.

CTF is not restricted to Colorado, but occurs from western Canada through the Pacific and Rocky Mountain states to New Mexico. Closely related diseases occur in Africa and Indonesia. The disease starts unremarkably with a fever and sometimes a rash. There is often a short remission, followed by the return of fever a few days later. The disease is usually short, and the death rate is very low. We mention Colorado tick fever mainly because it is one of several diseases that may be mistaken for Lyme disease.

Congo Hemorrhagic Fever. The agent of this disease, an African bunyavirus called the Congo virus, also causes Crimean hemorrhagic fever in Asia and eastern Europe. The vectors are ticks, and the reservoir hosts include various wild and domestic mammals. Most cases start abruptly with fever, weakness, headache, and nausea, followed by a rash, jaundice, and some bleeding from the mouth, nose, and/or gastrointestinal tract. Congo fever may cause extensive liver damage and death, with case fatality rates sometimes exceeding 60 percent.

Recent outbreaks of this disease have occurred in Saudi Arabia, Pakistan, the United Arab Emirates, South Africa, Senegal, Mauritania, and Egypt. In September 2000, a small outbreak in Iran was attributed to smuggling of livestock into the country; at least six of 13 known patients died. Preliminary data suggest that the antiviral drug ribavirin is effective against Congo fever. Florence Nightingale, the founder of modern nursing practice, contracted a similar illness during her service in the Crimean War (1854–1856),[6] but some medical historians have identified it instead as chronic brucellosis (see Chapter 6).

Dengue Fever and Dengue Hemorrhagic Fever (DHF). The agent is a flavivirus, closely related to the virus that causes yellow fever; the same mosquito vectors (*Aedes aegyptii* and relatives) transmit both the dengue and yellow fever viruses. The dengue virus has four serotypes, called DEN-1, DEN-2, DEN-3, and DEN-4. All four serotypes can cause either dengue fever or the more severe DHF. There is no cross-protective immunity, so one person can catch dengue at least four times.

The usual form of dengue fever has a wide distribution in the southeastern United States, Mexico, Central and South America, the islands of the South Pacific, Asia, and Africa. The only major dengue outbreak in the continental United States occurred in Philadelphia in 1780, when the disease arrived on a ship during an exceptionally hot summer. A doctor who treated patients during that outbreak called dengue "breakbone fever" because of the severe joint pain it causes. For unknown reasons, DHF, once found only in Asia, has expanded its range since the 1980s to include the Pacific region and the Americas.

Dengue and DHF together have emerged as the most important mosquitoborne viral disease of humans, with tens of millions of

---

[6]J.K. Farley, "My Bout with Crimean Fever—Florence Nightingale" (*Nursing News*, April 1990, pp. 10–11).

cases each year worldwide. The case fatality rate for dengue is low, with about 13,000 reported deaths in 1999, most of them in Asia; untreated DHF, however, may be fatal in 50 percent of cases. Between 1977 and 1994, there were a total of 2248 reported cases of dengue in the United States.

Recommended measures to fight the spread of dengue include better mosquito control in endemic areas; more funding to support surveillance programs and public health infrastructure in developing nations; and continued research to develop a dengue vaccine. Dengue is one of several diseases that might become established in the Earth's temperate zones if the present global warming trend continues. The Asian tiger mosquito (*Aedes albopictus*), a potential vector of dengue, became established in the United States in the 1980s.

Encephalitis, Arthropod-Borne. Encephalitis means an inflammation of the brain, irrespective of the agent. Many different viruses and bacteria can cause encephalitis; this section focuses on vectorborne viral diseases that actually have the word encephalitis in their names. Some books refer to the agents as arboviruses, a generic term that simply means an arthropod-borne virus.

The names of these diseases are somewhat confusing, and the diseases themselves vary greatly in severity. In North America, mosquitoes are the usual vectors; some less familiar Asian and European forms of encephalitis are mainly tickborne, but occasionally transmitted in milk. Most American forms of encephalitis are named for their original locations or hosts, but California encephalitis is not restricted to California, nor are the three "equine" species uniquely associated with horses.

In alphabetical order, the most common U.S. forms are California, eastern equine, LaCrosse, Saint Louis, Venezuelan equine, western equine, and—most famous of all in recent years—West Nile encephalitis, an Old World disease that reached our shores in 1998. Mosquitoes are the vectors for all these diseases, and birds and other animals serve as reservoir hosts, giving the virus a place to overwinter when no mosquitoes are active. The agents belong to a group of RNA viruses called togaviruses. In all forms, the illness begins 5 to 15 days after the mosquito bite with a sudden high fever and headache, often accompanied by a stiff neck and disorientation. Severe cases may involve convulsions, coma, paralysis, or dementia; in 2000, an Alaska Airlines passenger who stripped off his clothes and attacked the pilot later turned out to have encephalitis. Although the symptoms of this disease are alarming and require immediate hospital treatment, most healthy adults eventually make a full recovery.

In the first North American outbreak of West Nile encephalitis in summer 1999, six of the 68 reported cases (about 9 percent) were fatal; most of these patients were over 80 years old. Public health officials believe, however, that the actual number of cases was about 8200. Thus, the case fatality rate was very low, with most infected people showing no symptoms. In eastern equine encephalitis, by contrast, the case fatality rate may be as high as 60 percent. Unusual hazards also are associated with some forms of encephalitis. Reports indicate, for example, that Venezuelan equine encephalitis (VEE) can cause birth defects. Although VEE has not occurred in the United States since 1971, it remains a serious problem in South America.

Some of the mosquitoes that spread these forms of encephalitis breed in small pools of stagnant water, such as birdbaths and rain gutters. Others favor piles of discarded automobile tires, tree holes, and other habitats. The relationship between encephalitis outbreaks and climate change is not entirely clear; more rain should mean more places for mosquitoes to breed, but drought forces large numbers of birds to aggregate at a few watering holes, where encephalitis is likely to spread.

Despite the controversy over "new" diseases such as West Nile (see Chapter 9), there is no need for panic. Large-scale bombardment with pesticides may impress the public, but it has proven ineffective and may endanger public health and the environment. Reasonable preventive measures, depending on the location, might include recycling stockpiled tires, changing the water in the birdbath every few days, and stocking larger ponds with mosquito fish. In 2001, Yale researchers successfully immunized mice against the West Nile virus.

Sandfly Fever. This hemorrhagic fever occurs in tropical and subtropical areas of southern Europe, Asia, and Central and South America. The vectors are sandflies (*Phlebotomus papatasii* and related species), and the agents include at least five different bunyaviruses, related to the virus that causes Rift Valley fever (see Chapter 6). Symptoms include fever, headache, backache, nausea, vomiting, and jaundice. Meningitis, encephalitis, hemorrhaging from the nose or mouth, and mental depression may also occur. The reported case fatality rate is as low as 5 percent in indigenous populations of areas where the disease is endemic, but among foreigners or in epidemics it may

reach 50 percent. A 1999 study showed that about one-fourth of a sample of middle-aged adults in Israel were seropositive for the sandfly fever viruses, although no outbreak had occurred in more than 50 years.

The distribution of sandfly fever is highly dependent on the distribution of its vector, which needs a warm, humid climate. Some environmental scientists believe that this disease, like several others, may extend its geographic and seasonal range if the present worldwide warming trend continues. Sandflies also transmit an unrelated protozoal disease called leishmaniasis, discussed later in this chapter. Some sources refer to leishmaniasis as sandfly fever.

Yellow Fever. Ever since the discovery of the Ebola virus in Zaire, hemorrhagic fevers have been high on the American public's list of things to avoid. Yellow fever is one of the worst diseases in this category; although largely eradicated in developed nations today, it caused large epidemics in North America as recently as the nineteenth century. Ships docking at ports on the Gulf of Mexico afflicted entire towns with the dreaded "yellow jack," a colorful disease whose victims typically had red eyes, yellow skin, and black vomit. The infection damaged or destroyed the liver, and the case fatality rate ranged from 5 percent to over 50 percent.

For centuries, people believed that vapors from swamps caused yellow fever (and other diseases such as malaria). Draining wetlands was, indeed, an effective way to control yellow fever, but it was a costly measure; undefined vapors are harder to fight than mosquitoes. In 1849, Louisiana Senator Solomon Downs, testifying on the Swamp Act, stated:

If there is any fact which may be supposed to be known by everybody and therefore by the courts, it is that swamps and stagnant waters are the cause of malaria and malignant fevers and that public power is never more legitimately exercised than in removing such nuisances.[7]

In the late 1880s, the prevalence of yellow fever in Central America nearly stopped the construction of the Panama Canal. Thousands of workers on that project lost their lives before an Army physician named William Crawford Gorgas arrived on the scene. Like many scientists, he already knew that mosquitoes transmitted yellow fever and malaria, but it was rather like the earlier notion of the earth being round; it was not a fact until everyone knew it. Gorgas managed to eliminate yellow fever and malaria from the vicinity of the canal by covering standing water with an oil-based insecticide, by draining some marshes and ponds, and by isolating infected patients. Another Army doctor, Walter Reed, conducted a landmark study of yellow fever in Cuba in 1900. His work established control measures that enabled American cities to eliminate this disease once and for all. The last outbreak in the United States occurred in New Orleans in 1905.

There are two general forms of yellow fever: urban yellow fever, transmitted by the mosquito *Aedes aegypti*, and jungle yellow fever, which has several different mosquito vectors. Outbreaks of urban yellow fever still occur in Africa, but not in the New World. Jungle yellow fever is endemic and enzootic both in South America and in Africa, where mosquitoes transmit the disease to humans from monkeys, the main reservoir.

[7]From the Farm Bill Network Web site, 1998.

Yellow fever vaccination is required for all travelers to endemic areas of Africa and South America. The vaccine is considered highly effective and safe.

Vectorborne Protozoan Diseases

Only a few common diseases belong in the section, but they are among the worst diseases that afflict human beings. All result when a specific insect vector bites a person, injecting single-celled parasites into the bloodstream. At present, all these diseases occur mainly in the tropics.

African Sleeping Sickness. The agents of African sleeping sickness are two flagellated protozoans called *Trypanosoma gambiense* and *T. rhodesiense*, and their vector is the tsetse fly (*Glossina* sp.). For thousands of years, African farmers controlled this disease simply by staying out of areas where tsetse flies were numerous. They did not need to fund a study, such as the Walter Reed Commission, to prove cause and effect; they simply figured out that people who were bitten by tsetse flies tended to become horribly sick. Most slipped into comas and died, while others emerged from their comas but were permanently demented. Avoidance was the prudent course.

Then Europeans arrived in the nineteenth century and sliced Africa into colonies, forcing people to abandon their traditional patterns and to work in places they would normally avoid. The result was catastrophic. By 1906, African sleeping sickness had reduced the population of Uganda from 6.5 million to 2.5 million. These man-made epidemics raged until the 1940s and 1950s, when new anti-trypanosome drugs and tsetse fly traps appeared to be solving the problem. The World Health Organization (WHO) even hoped to eliminate the disease from Africa by the 1960s.

In the 1990s, however, there was a tremendous resurgence of sleeping sickness in the southern Sudan, the Central African Republic, the Democratic Republic of Congo, and other countries. This disease, once nearly conquered, now kills an estimated 300,000 people each year. Reports indicate that half the people in some villages are infected, and that other villages have disappeared altogether.

Drug treatment of African sleeping sickness is fairly effective if started early enough, but the side effects can be severe or even lethal. The drugs are also expensive, and doctors can afford to treat only a small fraction of the infected population.

Babesiosis. This disease occurs mainly in cattle and other livestock (see Chapter 6). The agents of human babesiosis, *Babesia microti* and related tickborne protozoa, reproduce in red blood cells and rupture them, causing a disease that resembles malaria (and has sometimes been mistaken for it). Symptoms include chills and fever, with jaundice, dark urine, nausea, vomiting, and mild enlargement of the spleen and liver. Recovery may take several weeks. In North America, the disease occurs mainly in the northeastern coastal states. People contract it from tick bites or, occasionally, from blood transfusions or transplacental or perinatal transmission.

Although rare, human babesiosis can be a serious disease, particularly in adult patients who have had their spleens removed. The disease tends to be milder in children than in adults. Of 139 human cases of babesiosis in New York State between 1982 and 1993, nine died, 35 required admission to the intensive care unit, and 35 were in the hospital longer than 14 days. Clindamycin and quinine sulfate in combination for five to ten days usually are effective, but a newer treatment with atovaquone and azithromycin appears to cause fewer side effects. Blood transfusions also may be necessary in severe cases.

Chagas' Disease. The agent of this disease, the protozoan *Trypanosoma cruzi*, is similar to the one that causes African sleeping sickness. Its vector, however, is not a fly but a wingless insect called a cone-nosed bug or kissing bug (Figure 5.4). Several related species of bugs can transmit the disease. Although they bite humans, they do not exactly inject the parasite; instead, they defecate after each meal, and the contaminated fecal material enters the body through any existing break in the skin. Transmission by contaminated blood transfusions, laboratory accidents, and placental transfer also occur. In laboratory experiments, the disease also has been transmitted in contaminated food and milk.

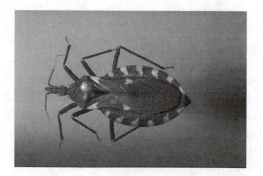

Figure 5.4. Kissing Bug (*Triatoma infestans*). (*Source*: Texas A&M University.)

Soon after infestation occurs, there is an acute disease that lasts up to eight weeks, with fever and swollen lymph nodes. Serious complications may occur, such as myocarditis or meningitis. The infestation often is lifelong, with chronic effects including serious damage to the heart and gastrointestinal tract. At present, Chagas' disease affects an estimated 18 million people in rural Mexico and in Central and South America. No effective treatment is available, and in 1999 alone, at least 21,000 people died from this disease. Some historians believe that biologist Charles Darwin contracted Chagas' disease in South America in the 1830s and suffered chronic ill health as a result.

Leishmaniasis. Several forms of this disease occur in most tropical regions throughout the world. For all, the pathogenic agents are flagellated protozoans in the genus *Leishmania*, and the vectors are sandflies (*Phlebotomus papatasii* and related species). The disease does not presently occur in the United States.

The main forms are American cutaneous leishmaniasis, which causes a chronic, destructive skin lesion, typically on the ear, but sometimes leading to a fatal infection of the oral or nasal mucosa; and visceral leishmaniasis or kala-azar, a chronic systemic disease with fever, sweating, diarrhea, and darkening of the skin. Although both diseases respond to treatment with a combination of several drugs, the side effects can be serious. Control of sandfly populations in endemic areas is essential to controlling this and other sandfly-borne diseases.

Malaria. The name of this disease, which means literally "bad air," reflects the ancient belief that marshes breathed evil influences at night—as of course they do, in the form of mosquitoes that carry disease. Malaria originated in Africa and spread to Europe and Asia early in human history; Alexander the Great died of this disease—or typhoid or poison, by some accounts—in 323 B.C. Much later, the slave trade brought malaria to the New World. By some estimates, malaria has killed half of all the human beings who have ever lived. This pattern held true at least until the 1940s, when public health programs, possibly aided by a short-term cooling trend, eliminated the disease from most temperate-zone countries. The disease has persisted in tropical areas, where there are at least 400 million new cases and one to two million deaths each year (Table 5.3). Poor people are especially hard hit, because their homes often lack window screens and they cannot afford insecticides.

The importance of this disease in human prehistory apparently accounts for the prevalence of two genetic disorders, sickle-cell anemia and thalassemia, in regions where malaria is endemic. One copy of the sickle-cell or thalassemia gene, in combination with a normal gene, protects a person against malaria; individuals who inherit two copies of the sickle-cell or thalassemia gene, however, develop a serious illness. Apparently, people who possessed one of these mutant genes were more likely than others to survive malaria and leave descendants, and thus the genes increased in frequency.

The United States had 1800 reported cases of malaria in 1997, most of them in travelers returning from endemic areas. Local transmission of malaria has, however, occurred in several states in recent years. In the late 1980s, four outbreaks occurred in San Diego County, California; in August 1999, there

Table 5.3
Malaria Deaths and Incidence, 1998

	Both Sexes	Males	Females
Deaths:			
All Member States	1,110,000	571,000	537,000
Africa	961,000	498,000	465,000
The Americas	4,000	1,000	1,000
Eastern Mediterranean	53,000	26,000	25,000
Europe	0	0	0
Southeast Asia	73,000	37,000	36,000
Western Pacific	20,000	11,000	9,000
Incidence:			
All Member States	272,925,000	136,572,000	136,354,000
Africa	237,647,000	118,858,000	118,789,000
The Americas	2,043,000	1,038,000	1,005,000
Eastern Mediterranean	13,693,000	6,870,000	6,822,000
Europe	0	0	0
Southeast Asia	15,791,000	7,862,000	7,928,000
Western Pacific	3,751,000	1,943,000	1,809,000

Source: World Health Organization (numbers truncated to nearest thousand).

were two cases at a children's summer camp on Long Island, New York. Malaria is one of several human diseases that may expand their range, or reclaim part of a former range, in response to global climate change.

Malaria is actually four different diseases. The one usually called malaria is the most serious, also known as falciparum or malignant tertian malaria. Its agent is a parasitic protozoan, *Plasmodium falciparum*. A mosquito acquires the parasite by biting an infected person and later injects it into a new host's blood or lymphatic circulation, which carries it to the liver. There it goes through a series of transformations that result in the release of thousands of parasites back into the bloodstream. Each of these invades a red blood cell (RBC), feeds on hemoglobin, and continues multiplying. The blood cells rup-

ture, releasing the parasites to invade more RBCs, return to the liver, or be picked up by the next mosquito bite. Typical symptoms include a severe headache, a fever as high as 107°F, chills, vomiting, and convulsions, in some cases followed by coma and multiple organ failure. The disease may instead become chronic, causing repeated attacks of symptoms for years.

The other forms of malaria, which usually are not life-threatening, are benign tertian malaria, quartan malaria, and ovale malaria, caused by *Plasmodium vivax*, *P. malariae*, and *P. ovale*, respectively. The first three forms are endemic in tropical regions of Africa, Asia, and the Americas, whereas ovale is limited to West Africa.

Although malaria today is almost exclusively a mosquitoborne disease, at one time in U.S. history a different pattern emerged. After World War II, intravenous drug use became prevalent in large cities. In some of these cities, particularly in the Northeast, malaria began to spread rapidly from one user to another because of needle sharing, just as HIV and hepatitis spread by the same route today.

When New York heroin dealers in the 1940s realized that their customer base was in danger, they came to the rescue by adding quinine to their product to kill the malaria parasite. As a result, New York junkies and dealers learned to recognize "real" heroin by its bitter taste, even though the taste had nothing to do with the heroin. According to an apocryphal-sounding story, some Los Angeles heroin dealers once tried to peddle their wares in New York. Their heroin contained no quinine, since malaria was not a problem in California; thus, when their eastern counterparts tasted a sample and found it was not bitter, they decided it must be counterfeit and executed the traveling salesmen.

One of the oldest treatments for malaria was a crude form of quinine obtained from the bark of South American evergreen trees in the genus *Cinchona*. This drug was called "the Jesuit powder" because missionary priests were among the first Europeans to recognize its value. Not everyone accepted this cure; Oliver Cromwell, Lord Protector of England, Scotland, and Ireland, contracted malaria in the marshes of Kent in his native England, but refused treatment on religious grounds and died of the disease in 1658.

Today, chloroquine and mefloquine (synthetic quinine) are the drugs of choice, but drug-resistant strains of the parasite have emerged and now account for 80 percent of all cases. Mosquitoes are not immune to the forces of natural selection either, and have become increasingly resistant to pesticides. Resistance, in a different sense, describes the reaction of many travelers, who report that mefloquine makes them feel nauseated and "spacey." Mosquito repellents and netting provide some protection in endemic areas. In 2000, British scientists began clinical trials of a promising new malaria vaccine in west Africa.

Vectorborne Multicellular Parasites

Filariasis. This term refers to any of several diseases that result when a flying insect, usually a mosquito, bites a person and injects nematode larvae. In most references to filariasis, the nematode is either *Wuchereria bancrofti* or *Brugia malayi*. The first species lives in warm regions on every continent, but in North America it does not occur farther north than Mexico. The second species is restricted to India, Southeast Asia, and Indonesia. Both worms take up residence in the lymphatics, where they eventually produce embryos (called microfilariae) that reach the bloodstream to be sucked up by another mosquito. Effective drugs are available for treatment of this disease, and the case fatality rate is low, but it affects an estimated 120 million people worldwide and is a major cause of poverty and long-term disability.

Readers may know this disease by another name, which refers to one of its symptoms: elephantiasis. When the nematode larvae block the lymphatic vessels, they can cause massive overgrowth of a limb or other body part, such as the scrotum. In the following nineteenth-century description of such a case, "mortification" means necrosis, not embarrassment:

Although elephantiasis is met with in all climates, it is more common in the tropics, and its occurrence has been repeatedly demonstrated in these localities to be dependent on the presence in the lymphatics of the filaria sanguinis hominis . . . [a man] had successive attacks of glandular swelling of the scrotum, until finally the scrotum was two feet long and six feet in circumference. It is mentioned that mortification of the part caused this patient's ultimate death.[8]

In 2001, a Gates Foundation grant created a $20 million World Bank trust fund to support the work of the Global Alliance for the Elimination of Lymphatic Filariasis.

Mansonella. A tiny nematode worm (*Mansonella ozzardi*) causes this obscure form of filariasis. It is not exactly a disease, as it rarely causes any symptoms, but few people like the idea of tiny worms living under their skin; thus, mansonella is a prime candidate for delusional parasitosis (see Chapter 9). In Mexico, Central America, and the Caribbean, the main vectors are tiny flying insects called biting midges (*Culicoides*), which also transmit related forms of filariasis in Africa. Blackflies (*Simulium*) are vectors for mansonella in South America.

River Blindness. This severe, chronic filarial disease occurs in Mexico, Central and South America, several African countries, and Yemen. The agent is a nematode called *Onchocerca volvulus*, and the vectors are blackflies (*Simulium*). As in other types of filariasis, the symptoms result from the migration of millions of parasites through the skin. Observers report that the itching is often so severe that victims mutilate themselves by frenzied scratching. The name, river blindness, refers to the fact that the adult worms often reach the retina and die there, causing infection and eventual blindness. Early treatments aimed at killing the parasites actually did more harm than good, by increasing the number of decomposing dead worms in the eye.

As of 1998, about 18 million Africans suffer from this infestation, which has already blinded about 270,000 of them. Within the next ten or 20 years, however, river blindness might actually be eradicated in Africa, thanks to a drug called ivermectin, which appears to kill the parasites without causing infections. The disease has already been nearly eliminated from several West African countries.

REFERENCES AND RECOMMENDED READING

Bastien, Joseph W. 1998. *The Kiss of Death: Chagas' Disease in the Americas*. Salt Lake City: University of Utah Press.

Bergen, M.S. "Malaria: Gone but Not Forgotten." *Brigham Young Magazine*, Winter 1997.

Blassingame, Wyatt. 1975. *The Little Killers: Fleas, Lice, Mosquitoes*. New York: Putnam.

Bloom, K.J. 1993. *The Mississippi Valley's Great Yellow Fever Epidemic of 1878*. Baton Rouge: Louisiana State University Press.

Calvo-Mendez, M.L., et al. "Infección Experimental con *Trypanosoma cruzi* a través de Agua y Alimentos Contaminados [Experimental Infection with *T. cruzi* by means of contaminated water and food]." *Revista*

[8] G.M. Gould and W.L. Pyle, *Anomalies and Curiosities of Medicine* (New York: Bell Publishing Co., 1896).

Latinoamericana de Microbiología, January–March 1994, pp. 67–69.

Cockrum, E. Lendell. 1997. *Rabies, Lyme Disease, Hanta Virus, and Other Animal-borne Human Diseases in the United States and Canada.* Cambridge, MA: Fisher Books.

Comer, J.A., et al. "Serologic Evidence of Rickettsialpox (*Rickettsia akari*) Infection among Intravenous Drug Users in Inner-City Baltimore, Maryland." *American Journal of Tropical Medicine and Hygiene*, June 1999, pp. 894–898.

"Common Source Outbreak of Relapsing Fever—California." *Morbidity and Mortality Weekly Report*, August 31, 1990, pp. 579–586.

Dalmat, Herbert T. 1955. *The Black Flies (Diptera, Simuliidae) of Guatemala and their Role as Vectors of Onchocerciasis.* Washington, DC: Smithsonian Institution.

Dansky, Martin. "Malaria in Yemen on the Rise." *Yemen Times*, December 22–28, 1997.

Desowitz, Robert S. 1993. *The Malaria Capers: Tales of Parasites and People.* New York: W.W. Norton.

Drummond, Roger. 1998. *Ticks and What You Can Do About Them.* 2nd ed. Berkeley, CA: Wilderness Press.

Duplaix, Nicole. "Fleas: The Lethal Leapers." *National Geographic*, May 1988, pp. 673–694.

Ellis, John H. 1992. *Yellow Fever and Public Health in the New South.* Lexington, KY: University Press of Kentucky.

Epstein, Paul R. "Is Global Warming Harmful to Health?" *Scientific American*, August 2000, pp. 50–57.

Fisher-Hock, S. P., et al. "Crimean Congo-Haemorrhagic Fever Treated with Oral Ribavirin." *Lancet*, August 19, 1995, pp. 472–475.

Gallagher, Nancy. "Public Health and Social Medicine: The Historical Legacy of the English Plague Experience." *University of Vermont History Review*, December 1994.

Goodpasture, H.C., et al. "Colorado Tick Fever: Clinical, Epidemiologic, and Laboratory Aspects of 228 Cases in Colorado in 1973–74." *Annals of Internal Medicine*, Vol. 88, 1978, pp. 303–310.

Gottfried, Robert S. 1985. *The Black Death: Natural and Human Disaster in Medieval Europe.* New York: Free Press.

Greenburg, Bernard. 1973. *Flies and Disease, Volume 2: Biology and Disease Transmission.* Princeton, NJ: Princeton University Press.

Gregg, C.T. 1985. *Plague: An Ancient Disease in the Twentieth Century.* Revised ed. Albuquerque: University of New Mexico Press.

Gubler, D.J., and Clark, G.G. "Dengue/Dengue Hemorrhagic Fever: The Emergence of a Global Health Problem." *Emerging Infectious Diseases*, April–June 1995, pp. 55–57.

Humphreys, Margaret. 1999. *Yellow Fever and the South.* Baltimore, MD: Johns Hopkins University Press.

Kaplan, Raymond. "Testing for Lyme Disease." *SmithKline Beecham Balanced Health Report*, October 1998, p. 2.

Kass, E.M., et al. "Rickettsialpox in a New York City Hospital, 1980 to 1989." *New England Journal of Medicine*, December 15, 1994, pp. 1612–1617.

Keeling, Matthew, and Gilligan, C.A. "Metapopulation Dynamics of Bubonic Plague." *Nature*, October 19, 2000, pp. 903–906.

Klempner, M.S., et al. "Two Controlled Trials of Antibiotic Treatment in Patients with Persistent Symptoms and a History of Lyme Disease." *New England Journal of Medicine*, July 12, 2001, pp. 85–92.

Lang, Denise, Lant, Denise V., and Territo, Joseph. 1997. *Coping With Lyme Disease: A Practical Guide to Dealing With Diagnosis and Treatment.* New York: Henry Holt.

Livni, Ephrat. "Vaccine Victims? The Controversy Surrounding SmithKline Beecham's LYMErix." ABCNews.com, May 17, 2000.

Mee, Charles L. "How a Mysterious Disease Laid Low Europe's Masses." *Smithsonian*, February 1990, pp. 66–74.

Midoneck, S.R., et al. "Colorado Tick Fever in a Resident of New York City." *Archives of Family Medicine*, August 1994, pp. 731–732.

Moody, E.K., et al. "Ticks and Tick-Borne Diseases in Oklahoma." *Journal of the Oklahoma State Medical Association*, November 1998, pp. 438–445.

Moore, C.G., and Mitchell, C.J. "*Aedes albopictus* in the United States: Ten-Year Presence and Public Health Implications." *Emerging Infectious Diseases*, July–September 1997, pp. 329–334.

Mostashari, F., et al. "Epidemic West Nile Encephalitis, New York, 1999: Results of a Household-based Seroepidemiological Survey." *Lancet*, July 28, 2001, pp. 261–264.

Mourin, S., et al. "Epilepsie Revelatrice d'une Neuroborreliose [Epilepsy Disclosing Neuroborreliosis]." *Review of Neurology* (Paris), Vol. 149, 1993, pp. 489–491.

Murray, Polly. 1996. *The Widening Circle: A Lyme Disease Pioneer Tells Her Story*. New York: St. Martin's Press.

Pan American Sanitary Bureau. 1994. *Dengue and Dengue Hemorrhagic Fever in the Americas: Guidelines for Prevention and Control*. Washington, DC: Pan American Health Organization.

Parshall, Gerald. "The End of a World." *U.S. News and World Report*, April 22, 1991, pp. 56–57.

Peterson, R.K.D. "Insects, disease, and military history." *American Entomologist* 41(3): 147–160, 1995.

Poser, Charles M., and Bruyn, G.W. 2000. *An Illustrated History of Malaria*. London: Parthenon Publishing Group.

Powell, J.H., et al. 1993. *Bring Out Your Dead: The Great Plague of Yellow Fever in Philadelphia in 1793*. Philadelphia: University of Pennsylvania Press.

Reid, M.C., et al. "The Consequences of Overdiagnosis and Overtreatment of Lyme Disease: An Observational Study." *Annals of Internal Medicine*, March 1998, pp. 354–362.

Rigau-Perez, J.G., et al. "Dengue and Dengue Hemorrhagic Fever." *Lancet*, Vol. 352, 1998, pp. 971–77.

Roberts, Richard B. "Pulmonary Case 14 [Tularemia]." Downloaded in July 2001 from the Web site of Cornell University Medical College, <http://edcenter.med.cornell.edu>.

"Trials of New Malaria Vaccine Start in Gambia." Reuters News Service, September 18, 2000.

Underwood, Ann. "The Winged Menace." *Newsweek*, September 20, 1999, p. 37.

Walker, D.H., and Dumler, J.S. "Emergence of the Ehrlichiosis as Human Health Problems." *Emerging Infectious Diseases*, Vol. 2, 1996, p. 18 ff.

Walker, D.H., and Fishbein, D.B. "Epidemiology of Rickettsial Diseases." *European Journal of Epidemiology*, May 1991, pp. 237–245.

WHO Expert Committee on Onchocerciasis Control. 1995. *Onchocerciasis and Its Control*. 1995. Geneva: World Health Organization, Technical Report Series.

White, D.J., et al. "Human Babesiosis in New York State." *Archives of Internal Medicine*, October 26, 1998, pp. 2149–2154.

Young, David G. 1991. *Phlebotomine Sandflies in the Americas*. Washington, DC: Pan American Health Organization.

Zimmer, Carl. "A Sleeping Storm." *Discover*, August 1998.

EXAMPLES OF DISEASES TRANSMITTED BY OTHER CONTACT

The diseases in this section commonly result from contact that does not involve either a vector or sexual activity, including the following:

- *Direct contact other than sex.* A babysitter with herpes blisters picks up a baby; or a child kisses her pet frog; or someone with a respiratory infection coughs in your face.

- *Indirect contact.* A person picks up an object (fomite) that has infectious material on its surface, such as discarded medical waste from a dumpster, or a toy at a preschool.

- *Injuries.* An infectious agent enters the body through a break in the skin resulting from an animal bite, an injection with a dirty hypodermic needle, or even a minor scratch.

- *Maternal transmission.* A woman catches a disease and then transmits it to her fetus via the placenta, to the newborn during birth, or to the baby during breastfeeding. (These diseases appear in various sections and chapters, depending on how the mother catches them.)

Bacterial Diseases Transmitted by Other Contact

Anthrax (Cutaneous). As explained in earlier chapters, this disease takes three forms: cutaneous, gastrointestinal, and inhalation. Cutaneous anthrax, the most common form, usually spreads by direct contact with contaminated animal tissues, hair, or soil. Contaminated surfaces also may transmit the disease, as seen in the October 2001 postal outbreak. Vectors such as deerflies (Figure 5.3) and vultures may play a role in some outbreaks. On average, there are about 7000 reported cases of human anthrax each year worldwide, most of them cutaneous.

If *Bacillus anthracis* spores infect a scratch on the skin, the result is an itchy bump that becomes an ugly, painless ulcer with a black center. Nearby lymph nodes may swell, and without antibiotic treatment about 20 percent of cases end in septicemia and death. The word anthrax in Greek means "malignant pustule."

The largest recorded outbreak of human cutaneous anthrax occurred in Zimbabwe between 1979 and 1980 during that country's civil war. Over 10,000 cases were reported, with at least 182 deaths (Table 5.2). As expected, there was also a major epizootic among cattle in Zimbabwe at the same time; however, a detailed analysis of the temporal and geographic distribution of cases, published in 1992, offered the startling conclusion that the outbreak might have been a biological warfare event. Other local outbreaks of anthrax may follow droughts or floods, as both can increase the contact between people, livestock, and contaminated soil.

For more information on anthrax, see Chapters 3, 4, 6, and 9.

Cat-Scratch Fever (Benign Lymphoreticulosis, Cat-Scratch Disease, or CSD). Although its symptoms may be alarming, this disease is self-limiting and nearly all patients survive. The agent for most cases of cat-scratch fever is the bacterium *Bartonella henselae* (a close relative of the agent of trench fever), but other bacteria have also been implicated. The disease is transmitted by a scratch from a cat, or occasionally by a flea or tick bite; in some cases, the mode of transmission is unknown. The Cat Fanciers' Association has proposed changing the name to bartonellosis.

The CDC estimates that about 6000 Americans contract this disease each year. Symptoms include fever, swollen lymph nodes, a generally sick feeling, a rash, and in some cases encephalitis. A 1991 study of 76 patients with neurological complications of this disease showed that nearly half had convulsions and 40 percent became aggressive. All patients made a full recovery within 12 months, and 78 percent within 1 to 12 weeks. Several antibiotics are effective as treatment, including rifamin and ciprofloxacin.

Hansen's Disease (Leprosy). At the time this book was published, science had not yet determined the exact mode of transmission for Hansen's disease, but apparently it requires physical contact or possibly droplet spread. Some researchers suspect that bedbugs and mosquitoes serve as vectors. Flies can contaminate food with the Hansen's bacterium—in the unlikely circumstance that the fly's feet have recently come in contact with the lesions of an untreated Hansen's patient—but there is no evidence that the disease is foodborne. The incubation period in some cases may be as long as 40 years.

For many reasons, Hansen's is a difficult disease to study. The bacterium is hard to grow in culture media, and it will not infect laboratory rats or mice. Researchers can grow it only in weird places, such as the footpads of dogs and the ears of armadillos. Epidemiological studies also are problematical; only about 5 percent of humans are susceptible to Hansen's, and even for those few, catching it seems to require many years of exposure. The disease then progresses slowly, deforming its victims by causing tissue destruction and scarring. In 1999, there were about 6000 Hansen's patients in the United States, most of them responding well to medication and leading normal lives. Thanks to the efforts of WHO, the worldwide incidence of the disease has decreased by 85 percent in the past ten years.

Why, then, is so much attention focused on Hansen's disease? The reasons are largely historical. Since Biblical times, no disease has inspired more fear than Hansen's, also known as leprosy. Until the twentieth century, Hansen's patients were outcasts who led lives of unimaginable horror. On the day science eradicates leprosy from the world, a great debt will be repaid. Leviticus 13:45–46:

And the leper in whom the plague is, his clothes shall be rent, and his head bare, and he shall put a covering upon his upper lip, and shall cry, Unclean, Unclean.
All the days wherein the plague shall be in him he shall be defiled; he is unclean: he shall

dwell alone; without the camp shall his habitation be.

The early Christian church continued this tradition, shoveling dirt onto the leper's feet in a mock funeral called a Leper Mass, and expelling him from society with the words: "Be thou dead to the world, but live again unto God." Scholars have argued that diagnosis was imprecise in that era, and that "leprosy" might have meant not only Hansen's disease, but also the advanced stages of syphilis. In 1994, however, science confirmed at least one diagnosis made in A.D. 600, by exhuming and testing bones from an alleged leper colony. The bones did, indeed, contain traces of *Mycobacterium leprae*. Even if some lepers were mislabeled in their day, the sentiment is clear: people who resembled lepers for any reason were not well liked.

Although other diseases were far more prevalent, more contagious, and more deadly, people have always feared leprosy because it made its victims unattractive. Tuberculosis made a Victorian lady pale and interesting (briefly), but leprosy was another matter. To understand what the word meant as recently as a century ago, we must turn not to science, but to literature:

Their hands, when they possessed them, were like harpy-claws. Their faces were the misfits and slips, crushed and bruised by some mad god at play in the machinery of life. Here and there were features which the mad god had smeared half away, and one woman wept scalding tears from twin pits of horror, where her eyes once had been. Some were in pain and groaned from their chests. Others coughed, making sounds like the tearing of tissue.[9]

[9]Jack London, "Koolau the Leper," in *The House of Pride and Other Tales of Hawaii* (New York: Macmillan, 1912).

By the early 1900s, Hansen's patients in the United States no longer had to beg for alms with a bucket on the end of a pole, as in the Middle Ages; yet society still confined them to group homes called leprosariums, where they passed their lives without hope of a cure. Finally, in 1941, Dr. Guy H. Faget developed sulfone therapy, and lepers began to emerge from their prisons. Some were understandably angry; in 2001, 127 Hansen's survivors won a class action lawsuit against the Japanese government for human rights violations, and groups in other countries are expected to follow suit. Hansen's patients are no longer quarantined, but simply take three drugs—rifampin, dapsone, and clofazamine—for at least two years. In milder forms of the disease, the first two drugs are used for six months.

In the 1970s, Hansen's research received a boost when scientists discovered a suitable laboratory animal in the armadillo. Efforts to develop a vaccine are now in progress. Wild armadillos apparently are not an important reservoir for this disease; on the contrary, it appears that armadillos may catch leprosy from humans. In a few cases, people who handled an infected armadillo have contracted the disease. In 1984, scientists traced a small outbreak of six cases of leprosy in southeastern Texas to an armadillo.

There are actually two forms of leprosy, plus intermediate or borderline cases. Lepromatous leprosy, the most severe form, affects the nerves in the hands and feet and also the skin. It causes ulcerating skin lesions and nodules that invade the mucous membranes of the upper respiratory tract, giving the patient a chronic stuffy nose in addition to everything else. Patients with tuberculoid leprosy, by contrast, usually have only a few well-defined lesions that are numb and may heal spontaneously.

A genetically engineered version of the BCG vaccine (see Chapter 4) is now used in treating leprosy. Its inventor, Dr. Barry R. Bloom, in 1992 won the first annual Bristol-Myers Squibb Award for Distinguished Achievement in Infectious Disease Research.

Hib (*Haemophilus influenzae type B*). This infection spreads by contact with mucus or by droplet inhalation. It usually occurs in children between the ages of three months and three years, and its effects may include meningitis, blood infections, pneumonia, arthritis, or even death. The case fatality rate for Hib bacterial meningitis is about 5 percent, and 25–35 percent of survivors have serious complications. A vaccine has been available since 1985, and most toddlers now receive it.

Some opponents of vaccination have raised the concern that children who receive the Hib vaccination may be more likely than others to develop diabetes, but a 1999 study of over 200,000 children found no such correlation. Diabetes itself has reached epidemic proportions during the same time interval since introduction of Hib, but it is more likely related to obesity or environmental factors.

Listeriosis. The main account of this foodborne disease appears in Chapter 3. As noted there, listeriosis in a pregnant woman may be transmitted to the fetus via the placenta, causing birth defects, miscarriage, or stillbirth.

Meningitis (Bacterial). Several different bacteria and viruses can cause meningitis, an inflammation of the membranes that surround the brain and spinal cord. When the press refers to an epidemic of meningitis, however, usually it means the disease associated with the meningococcus, *Neisseria meningitidis*. This bacterium cannot survive long outside the body, and appears to spread mainly by casual contact among people in crowded conditions.

There are about 3000 reported cases of bacterial meningitis in the United States each year, resulting in about 300 deaths. College students living in dormitories are at highest risk, with nearly five cases per 100,000. The disease starts with a headache and stiff neck, and a coma may follow within hours. Gangrene and other complications may occur. About 10 percent of reported cases are fatal, and another 10 percent of survivors have serious disabilities such as deafness, brain damage, or loss of limbs. These numbers may be misleading, however, as they refer only to reported cases. During large epidemics of meningitis, in Army barracks or other crowded situations, up to 25 percent of the entire population is infected with this bacterium but shows no symptoms. Even an inapparent infection results in type-specific immunity.

Every time a college student dies of meningitis—there are about ten such deaths every year—the press and the pharmaceutical industry recommend universal vaccination for this age group. At latest report, however, the vaccine available in the United States is partly effective against only four of the seven most common meningitis serotypes (A, C, Y, and W135). It offers no protection against serotype B, which has caused nearly half of all recent cases of bacterial meningitis in the United States. As the immunity is type-specific, the vaccine is better than nothing, but may confer a false sense of security. Add to that fact the low virulence of the virus, and the potential for side effects in any vaccine, and the result is a low rate of participation. New Zealand has the highest rate of meningitis in the developed world, but as of 2000, no vaccine was available for that nation's most common serotype either.

Treatment of meningococcal meningitis is controversial. Most doctors recommend early antibiotic treatment, but a Danish study showed that such treatment actually increased the fatality rate. Early admission to an intensive care unit seems to be the most important factor in treatment. People at risk are advised to have the vaccine if they wish, but not to rely on it, and to be aware of the symptoms of meningitis. Students should bear in mind that at least one 1999 college outbreak was linked to marijuana smoking, apparently because of the practice of sharing cigarettes. Secondhand exposure to tobacco smoke also is a risk factor, for unknown reasons.

Pasteurellosis. Several nasty bacterial infections can result from cat and dog bites. Two of the most frequent agents of such infections are the bacteria *Pasteurella multocida* and *P. haemolytica*. Although these organisms are part of the normal oral flora of cats and dogs, they can sometimes cause serious consequences in humans, including meningitis and arthritis.

Another bacterium recently associated with dog bites, called *Capnocytophaga canimorsus*, has caused at least one case of kidney failure following a dog bite. All these bacteria usually respond well to treatment with penicillin or other antibiotics.

Rat-bite Fever. Rat bites, like bites of any animal or human, can transmit a number of infectious diseases, including tetanus. A study of 622 rat bites in Philadelphia between 1974 and 1996 showed that children between ages five and nine were the most frequent victims, although most did not contract disease.

Rat-bite fever per se results from infection with either of two pathogens, *Streptobacillus moniliformis* or *Spirillum minor*. The first disease (also called Haverhill fever) is worldwide, and sporadic cases or small outbreaks have occurred in the United States. The second disease seems restricted to Japan and the Far East. Both forms of rat-bite fever are rare enough (or go unrecognized often enough) that individual cases often become the subject of medical journal articles.

These diseases spread by bites or other contact, by ingestion of rat-contaminated milk, or possibly by inhalation of contaminated dust in rat-infested buildings. Both diseases start, like so many others, with a sudden high fever, headache, and muscle pain, followed by a rash and (in Haverhill fever only) swollen joints. The infection may progress to abscesses or endocarditis; if untreated, the case fatality rate is about 10 percent, but antibiotic treatment usually is effective if started early enough.

Salmonellosis. Chapter 3 discusses *Salmonella* food poisoning, but as noted there, many infections result instead from contact with reptiles. In an unusual 1996 case, at least 50 people contracted salmonellosis after touching a fence surrounding an exhibit of Komodo dragons at a zoo in Denver, Colorado.

In the early 1970s, some 280,000 cases of human salmonellosis in the United States were traced to the ownership of baby turtles. These cases represented about 14 percent of all reported *Salmonella* infections. At the time, pet shops sold 15 million baby turtles each year, and about 5 percent of all American households owned one or more turtles. In 1975, the U.S. Congress reacted to these statistics by authorizing the Food and Drug Administration to regulate the turtle industry (21 CFR Sec. 1240.62). As a result, pet dealers no longer sell native species such as the red-eared slider turtle in the United States, but instead export them to foreign countries.

Staphylococcal Disease. Chapter 3 discusses the staphylococci in the context of food poisoning, but related bacteria also infect wounds and cause diseases ranging in severity from acne to brain abscess. In general, staphylococci produce some type of lesion that contains pus.

Most people have staph bacteria living on their skin or in their nostrils, and about one-third of infections result from the person's own bacteria gaining access to a place where they have no business. For example, nearly every parent has warned teenagers not to squeeze pimples on their noses, because the bacteria in the pus—often these are staphylococci—might enter the bloodstream and reach the brain, causing meningitis. Although this scenario sounds contrived (not to mention disgusting), it can actually happen.

Staphylococci also are among the many bacteria that can reach the heart after a dental procedure, causing endocarditis in susceptible persons. Both staphylococci and streptococci (see next section) can cause impetigo, a common, occasionally serious skin infection of children. Other staphylococcal diseases include pneumonia, septicemia, and osteomyelitis. In the 1980s, an epidemic of a severe toxicosis called toxic shock syndrome resulted from the growth of toxigenic staphylococci in superabsorbent tampons (which were later taken off the market).

Drug-resistant strains of staphylococci have been a major source of worry in hospitals for many years. About half of all staph bacteria in hospitals are now resistant to the antibiotic methicillin. Another antibiotic called vancomycin usually works against even the most stubborn staph infections, but vancomycin-resistant strains have recently appeared. The development of better antibiotics is now a major priority for several major pharmaceutical companies. In 2000, doctors announced successful clinical trials of the first effective staph vaccine for use in high-risk populations, such as dialysis patients.

Streptococcal Disease, Group A. Many serious diseases, and a few minor ones, can result from infection with *Streptococcus pyogenes* and related Group A streptococci. Some of these diseases are the familiar "strep throat" and its formerly lethal variant scarlet fever; acute rheumatic fever, which causes inflammation of the heart, central nervous system, or joints, sometimes with long-term consequences; erysipelas, a severe skin lesion that can spread and invade the bloodstream; otitis media, a common infection of the middle ear; impetigo, a skin infection of children, with vesicles and crusting; pneumonia, an inflammation of the lungs; nephritis, an inflammation of the kidneys; puerperal fever, an infection that killed many women after childbirth until attendants learned to wash their hands; and the famous "flesh-eating bacterial disease," or necrotizing fasciitis, a recent favorite of tabloids and shock TV, in which bacterial toxins destroy a person's flesh at the rate of about one inch per hour. (Other bacteria also can cause several of these diseases, but the culprit often is a Group A streptococcus.)

It is not entirely clear how one group of bacteria can cause so many different diseases. About 15–30 percent of all people in the United States carry Group A streptococci without symptoms, and in others the bacteria cause minor illness. Necrotizing fasciitis, however, can occur only when the bacterium itself is infected with a virus that makes it produce a toxin. Between 500 and 1500 infections identified as necrotizing fasciitis occur each year in the United States, with a case fatality rate of 20 percent.

Until recently, streptococcal infections responded quickly to antibiotic treatment, but drug-resistant strains have recently appeared. As with other bacteria, the main cause appears to be the overuse of antibiotics. In Finland, concerns about erythromycin-resistant streptococcus A led to a campaign to reduce erythromycin prescriptions. The result was a reduction in resistance levels from 19 to 9 percent in only three years.

Another problem with strep infection is diagnosis. If, for example, a person arrives at a hospital emergency room with a small scratch and claims to feel sick and confused, the overworked staff is unlikely to show much interest. These might be the symptoms of a drunken person who has fallen down; or a hypochondriac who wants attention; or a person who is mistaken about the severity of her illness; or a desperately ill person in the first stages of necrotizing fasciitis. But by the time the patient is in shock, and has lost half her leg, it may be too late to decide.

One of the strangest streptococcal infections is Sydenham's chorea, also known as St. Vitus' dance. It occurs most often in children, who may spend all their waking hours for six or eight months engaged in apparently senseless movements and facial grimacing that disappears when they fall asleep. The disease eventually passes, with antibiotic treatment and time, but if misdiagnosed it can be the source of serious misunderstandings with teachers and psychologists.

Streptococcus Group A infections also may occur as a secondary invasion following a viral disease. In California in 1994, for example, such an infection took the lives of five California children with chickenpox.

Tetanus or Lockjaw. The agent of this disease is the anaerobic bacterium *Clostridium tetani*, a relative of the bacteria that cause botulism and other foodborne illnesses (Chapter 3). Like those bacteria, it causes illness by releasing a toxin that acts on the nervous system. The traditional way to contract tetanus is by stepping on a rusty nail, but the nail's only role is to drive the attached soil and its resident bacteria deep into the person's foot.

Before effective treatment was available, farm workers and soldiers injured on the battlefield were highly susceptible to this infection, which has a fatality rate as high as 70 percent. Even today, tetanus kills about half of the 100 or so people who contract it in the United States each year. Dog bites and puncture wounds are frequent sources of tetanus infection. In some developing nations, tetanus is also a frequent cause of neonatal death, as the bacteria may enter through the unhealed umbilical cord. Early symptoms include a headache, fever, convulsions, difficulty in swallowing, and stiffness of the jaw.

Most residents of the United States receive tetanus immunization in the childhood DPT (diphtheria, pertussis, and tetanus) vaccine. For continued protection, booster shots are necessary every ten years. In 2001, however, Wyeth-Ayerst Laboratories decided to stop making the tetanus vaccine, and nationwide shortages resulted.

Trachoma. As discussed earlier in this chapter, the same bacterium that causes this disease also causes sexually transmitted chlamydial infections and other conditions. Any organism that causes so much unnecessary suffering, however, deserves a second look.

Although trachoma does not occur in the United States and receives little media attention here, it is the world's leading cause of preventable blindness. In the nineteenth century, European immigrants arriving in this country were carefully inspected for trachoma at Ellis Island; infected persons were turned away or required to undergo crude surgical treatment.

Trachoma causes the margins of the eyelids to become swollen and rolled inward (a condition called trichiasis), so that the embedded eyelashes scratch the cornea of the eye. When this happens, in the absence of medical care or antibiotics, the best response is to pull out the offending eyelash with a tweezer. Thus, victims of trachoma in Third World nations often wear a tweezer on a string around their necks. It can be hard to retrieve every eyelash, however, and the cumulative damage to the cornea eventually may cause blindness.

Trench Fever. More than one million soldiers contracted this disease during the first World War as a result of the crowded, unsanitary conditions in trenches (hence the name). The agent is a bacterium called *Bartonella quintana*, and the vector is the human body louse. The louse does not actually inject the bacterium; like the cone-nose bug, it excretes the pathogens in its feces, which enter the bite when the host scratches.

This disease now occurs sporadically in North America, Europe, Asia, and Africa. The symptoms include fever, rash, bone pain, and an enlarged spleen; relapses may occur. A related bacterium, *Bartonella bacilliformis*, occurs only in the mountains of South America and causes an often-fatal infection called bartonellosis.

Until the 1980s, trench fever was rare in North America, but it has reemerged in two high-risk groups: HIV-infected persons, and HIV-negative homeless persons. At least 20 percent of the homeless population of Seattle, Washington tests positive for trench fever. Treatment with erythromycin usually is effective.

Viral Diseases Transmitted by Other Contact

Astrovirus. Several different viruses can cause viral gastroenteritis, commonly called "stomach flu" (although it is not a form of influenza). Some of these pathogens, such as the Norwalk virus, are mainly foodborne (see Chapter 3). Astrovirus, however, is foodborne in only about 1 percent of cases; the rest are attributed to contact. The symptoms are watery diarrhea and vomiting, sometimes with a headache, fever, and abdominal cramps. The illness rarely lasts longer than ten days. Young children and disabled or elderly persons may become severely dehydrated and require hospitalization.

Chickenpox or *Varicella*. Before the introduction of the chickenpox vaccine in 1995, nearly everyone in the United States caught this disease in childhood, and those who had it good and hard would begin to itch years later at the mere mention of the name. The agent is a herpesvirus called varicella-zoster virus or HHV-3.

Chickenpox usually starts with an itchy rash that forms several hundred blisters and scabs after a few days. Family members then follow the patients around the house, telling them not to pick the scabs. In many cases, there is also a fever and general ill feeling. Although a severe case of chickenpox superficially resembles smallpox (and can leave scars), the two viruses are not closely related.

Chickenpox is rarely fatal unless viral pneumonia or a secondary bacterial infection results. It can be dangerous in infants younger than four weeks if their mothers are not immune. In the United States, about 100 children die of such complications each year, and another 5000 to 9000 require hospitalization. People who catch chickenpox as infants or as adults are more likely than healthy children to suffer complications; in a pregnant woman, the virus may even cause birth defects. Children with weakened immune systems are vulnerable to a dangerous form of chickenpox called disseminated varicella, which has a case fatality rate as high as 20 percent.

The double-whammy of chickenpox is shingles, a disease that occurs in adulthood when the chickenpox virus becomes reactivated after hiding for decades in a spinal nerve root. Reactivation may result from a decline of cell-mediated immunity due to aging or from a chronic disease, including HIV infection. The usual symptoms of shingles (also called zoster) are fever, headache, and skin blisters that cause an intense burning sensation. There are about 600,000 to one million cases of shingles each year in the United States. Antiviral drugs such as acyclovir may reduce the symptoms and duration of the disease. Postherpetic neuralgia, a major complication of shingles, may cause continued pain even after the blisters heal.

Cytomegalovirus (CMV). Infection with this virus usually causes no symptoms, or at most a mild illness with fatigue and swollen glands. CMV is important because it can cause serious illness in AIDS patients and because it can damage unborn infants. About 10 percent of babies born in the United States have CMV, and of these, 10 percent have brain damage or developmental disabilities. The infection can spread by direct contact, by blood transfusions and organ transplants, or by transmission from an infected woman to her fetus or newborn. There is no treatment and no vaccine; by adulthood, most people have been exposed to this virus.

Ebola Hemorrhagic Fever. Why is the Western press so fascinated with the Ebola virus, while millions die every year from more common diseases? Here is one possible explanation:

His personality was being wiped away by brain damage. . . . Then came a sound like a bed sheet being torn in half, the sound of his bowels opening and venting blood from his anus. The blood was mixed with intestinal lining. He had sloughed his gut. Monet had crashed and was bleeding out. Having destroyed its host, the virus was now coming out of every orifice, trying to find a new host.[10]

Ebola, in other words, has emerged as the "Jaws" of the unseen world of microbiology. In fairness, more people die from Ebola hemorrhagic fever than from shark attacks. Ebola killed several hundred people in 2000, while sharks killed a total of ten worldwide (and malaria claimed millions more).

At the time this book was written, no one knew exactly how an Ebola outbreak starts. One or more persons contract the disease from an unknown source—not a big help—and then spread it to others by direct contact with body fluids or by contaminated needles in a hospital setting. A few reports indicate that Ebola and other hemorrhagic fevers can spread by airborne transmission, although contact is more usual. To date, all known outbreaks have been small, but some doctors predict that larger epidemics will occur when more Africans have access to Western-style hospitals. Ironically, concentrating patients in a hospital setting may contribute to the interpersonal spread of a disease, although it may reduce the fatality rate.

The Ebola virus exists in at least four different forms: Ebola-Zaire, Ebola-Sudan, Ebola–Ivory Coast, and Ebola-Reston. The

[10]R. Preston, *The Hot Zone* (New York: Random House, 1994), excerpt published in the *Seattle Post-Intelligencer*.

first three affect humans and apparently occur only in Africa. Ebola-Reston is endemic to the Philippines, where it causes a similar hemorrhagic fever in monkeys; it is also transmissible to chimpanzees. This form was named for the famous 1989 incident at Reston, Virginia, when monkeys imported from the Philippines died of an Ebola-like disease in a quarantine facility. No one who came in contact with those monkeys became ill, but neither did the caretakers who handled Marburg-infected monkeys in Germany in 1967 (see below).

Scientists have not yet identified a vector or reservoir for the filoviruses that cause the Ebola and Marburg hemorrhagic fevers in humans. Ebola has a very high case fatality rate, on the order of 70 percent in many outbreaks. Studies have also demonstrated a high seroprevalence in endemic areas; apparently, many people are somehow exposed to the virus. In 2000, doctors in Gabon reported that some contacts of Ebola patients developed antibodies and a strong inflammatory response, but no symptoms of the disease. In the Central African Republic, the seroprevalence in male hunter-gatherers is over 37 percent, but in farmers it is only 13 percent. Surprisingly, about 7 percent of people in Germany also are seropositive for at least one filovirus, although no related diseases are known to occur there.

Extensive trapping and testing programs in Zaire and other endemic areas have revealed no infected bats, rodents, or other likely reservoir hosts. Perhaps the most intriguing theory is that the filoviruses may originate in plants, and that plant-feeding insects or other arthropods transmit the virus to humans by some accidental form of contact, as when the insect is swallowed in food. One study has detected the presence of filovirus-like particles in insects called leafhoppers.

Although the Ebola virus is considered "new," there is some circumstantial evidence of past outbreaks. Historians have long sought an explanation for the Plague of Athens, which appeared in Athens in 430 B.C. and killed an estimated one-third of the population in a few years. Thucydides, who survived the plague, has left a vivid account:

People in good health were all of a sudden attacked by violent heats in the head, and redness and inflammation in the eyes, the inward parts, such as the throat or tongue, becoming bloody and emitting an unnatural and fetid breath. These symptoms were followed by sneezing and hoarseness, after which the pain soon reached the chest, and produced a hard cough. . . . In most cases also an ineffectual retching [also translated as hiccup] followed, producing violent spasms, which in some cases ceased soon after, in others much later. Externally the body was not very hot to the touch, nor pale in its appearance, but reddish, livid, and breaking out into small pustules and ulcers. But internally it burned so that the patient could not bear to have on him clothing or linen even of the very lightest description . . . when they succumbed, as in most cases, on the seventh or eighth day to the internal inflammation, they had still some strength in them. But if they passed this stage, and the disease descended further into the bowels, inducing a violent ulceration there accompanied by severe diarrhoea, this brought on a weakness which was generally fatal.[11]

Although the prevailing view is that Thucydides was describing a smallpox epi-

---

[11]Thucydides, *The Peloponnesian War*, Second Book, Chapter VII, translated by Richard Crawley (New York: Modern Library, 1951).

demic, an alternative theory attributes the Plague of Athens to an Ebola-like disease. The hemorrhaging, diarrhea, and persistent hiccuping, plus the observer's unfamiliarity with the disease, seem more consistent with Ebola than with smallpox. Also, Thucydides wrote that the disease originated in Ethiopia and spread through Egypt and Libya before reaching Greece. Although the mystery may be unsolvable, it would be helpful to know if Ebola and related diseases can actually spread in this manner.

In 2000, researchers at the U.S. National Institutes of Health reported that an experimental vaccine protected a small sample of monkeys from contracting Ebola. To date, however, no Ebola vaccine is available for use on humans. Herbal remedies used by the Igbo and other African tribes have shown some promise in clinical trials; for example, compounds extracted from twigs of a tree called *Garcinia kola* have stopped the replication of the Ebola virus without killing the host cells. Certain other traditional practices, such as the Gabonese customs of washing the dead and eating ape meat, have favored the spread of Ebola. At present, the only known effective treatment is aggressive rehydration, which in some outbreaks has reduced mortality to less than 40 percent.

Hand, Foot, and Mouth Disease or *Herpangina*. This acute viral disease occurs only in humans and is not related to foot-and-mouth disease of livestock (see Chapter 6). The agent is a coxsackie virus called enterovirus 71. Most cases are mild, causing several days of fever and vomiting with a blister-like rash on the hands, feet, and mouth. It spreads mainly by contact, but also by droplet inhalation.

Complications are rare in most outbreaks, but may include pneumonia, meningitis, encephalomyelitis, or even paralysis similar to that caused by polio. In one outbreak in Australia in 1986, more than half of all patients admitted to hospitals with enterovirus 71 infection had central nervous system involvement. In 1975, an outbreak of 705 cases in Bulgaria caused 149 cases of paralysis and 44 deaths, mostly among infants and small children. In Taiwan in 1998, an estimated one million people contracted enterovirus 71; there were 405 severe cases and 78 deaths. At present, no effective antiviral drugs are available.

Hepatitis B. An estimated 140,000–320,000 new cases of hepatitis B occur each year in the United States, about half of them with no symptoms. Only about 25 percent of these cases are sexually transmitted. Over one million Americans now have this infection, which causes more than 6000 deaths per year in the United States, mostly from cirrhosis and liver cancer.

Worldwide, between eight million and 16 million people contract hepatitis B each year from unsafe blood transfusions alone. The blood supply in developed nations is relatively safe, but the virus is also transmissible by personal contact, sexual activity, wound infection, needle sharing by intravenous drug users, laboratory accidents, and (in Africa) possibly by mosquito bites. Symptoms include fatigue, loss of appetite, fever, nausea, vomiting, diarrhea, joint pain, and rash. The urine may become darker in color, and jaundice may appear.

There is no specific treatment for hepatitis B, and the virus remains in the blood for at least several months; about 10 percent of infected people become long-term carriers who must be careful not to infect others. An effective hepatitis B vaccine is available, and is recommended for all children and for high-risk adults, such as IV drug users and travelers to endemic areas. A hepatitis B immune globulin also is available for people who have been exposed to the virus.

Hepatitis C. This form of hepatitis, first discovered in 1989, causes about 20 percent of all cases of acute viral hepatitis in the United States. About 85 percent of people who contract the virus become chronic carriers, who not only transmit the disease to others, but are also at risk for cirrhosis and liver cancer. As of 2000, there were about 170 million cases of hepatitis C worldwide. An estimated 4 million Americans are infected, and about 12,000 die of the disease each year. The prevalence among prison inmates is alarmingly high, with over 40 percent infected in some communities.

Symptoms are similar to those of hepatitis B, but often less severe. People contract this virus mainly from shared hypodermic needles, contaminated body piercing and tattooing equipment, and (rarely) sexual contact. Before 1992, many people also were infected during blood transfusions, hemodialysis, or organ transplant surgeries.

Research efforts have focused on the 15 percent of hepatitis C patients who recover from the disease. A 2000 study showed that these patients' immune systems respond more effectively to the virus, eliminating each of its genetic variants. By contrast, in patients who later become chronic carriers, the genetic diversity of the virus increases dramatically during the first few months after infection.

There is no vaccine and no treatment for the acute form of hepatitis C. A drug called Rebetron (a combination of ribavirin and interferon), made by Schering-Plough, is used to treat the chronic form. Reports indicate that the drug costs about $18,000 per patient per year, and that the manufacturer has marketed it so aggressively as to become the target of a 2000 FDA investigation. Hepatitis C has achieved the dimensions of a bandwagon, with some journalists now claiming that 90 percent of Americans are infected. Available data suggest that such claims are exaggerated.

Lassa Fever. First recognized in 1969, this hemorrhagic fever occurs only in Africa, but like several other emerging diseases it has received some attention in the West due to the high case fatality rate (20–50 percent) and occasional outbreaks among laboratory workers and travelers returning from Africa. The agent is an arenavirus that occurs in various African rodent species, including the multimammate rat (*Mastomys natalensis*).

A related pathogen called the Machupo virus causes a hemorrhagic fever in South America that can spread by airborne transmission. In 1994, a person in Bolivia caught Machupo and transmitted it to six family members, all of whom died.

Until recently, there was no evidence that arenaviruses are associated with human disease in North America. In 2000, however, health officials in California reported three deaths from viral hemorrhagic fevers caused by arenaviruses found in native rodents. This new North American disease does not yet have a common name, and its mode of transmission is unclear.

Marburg Virus Disease. In 1967, 25 laboratory workers in Germany and Yugoslavia contracted this virus by contact with infected tissues of African green monkeys captured in Uganda. Seven of those workers died of a severe hemorrhagic fever. Sporadic cases later appeared in Zimbabwe, South Africa, and Kenya; Marburg also has spread by use of contaminated needles in a hospital and, in at least one case, by sexual contact. A recent outbreak in the Democratic Republic of the Congo involved 88 people, of whom 73 died. This outbreak was tentatively linked to unsanitary conditions in a Congolese gold mine.

The Marburg virus belongs to a newly recognized family of RNA viruses called filoviruses, which also includes the agent of Ebola hemorrhagic fever. Marburg is believed to occur only in Africa; as noted in the Ebola account, however, about 7 percent of people in Germany are seropositive for one or more filoviruses. It is not clear whether this fact is somehow related to the 1967 outbreak or to the presence of unknown filoviruses in Europe. As a result of the 1967 incident, the United States and many other countries now quarantine all imported monkeys for at least 31 days.

Meningitis (Viral). Many viruses can cause meningitis, including the echoviruses, the coxsackieviruses, and the agents of chickenpox, measles, mumps, and poliomyelitis. Unlike bacterial meningitis, viral meningitis is seldom fatal, although recovery may be slow.

Since most cases of viral meningitis in the United States result from enteroviruses (which occur in feces), adults who change diapers at home or in day care centers are at risk for this disease. As expected, people who wash their hands after changing diapers are less likely than others to contract viral meningitis. A 1999 study produced somewhat confusing results: women who

changed more than 90 diapers per month were at higher risk than women who changed fewer diapers; but men who changed more than 90 diapers per month were at *lower* risk than men who changed fewer diapers. Whether this finding reflects gender differences, societal roles, or faulty sampling, it is likely to provoke controversy.

Mononucleosis. Nearly everyone is exposed to the Epstein-Barr virus (EBV), the agent of mononucleosis. Exposure in early childhood rarely causes symptoms; in developed nations, however, exposure often does not occur until young adulthood, when illness is more likely to result. The main symptoms of "mono" are fatigue, fever, sore throat, and swollen lymph nodes, sometimes with an enlarged liver and spleen. The disease can last for several weeks or months, but is almost never fatal. It spreads from person to person by kissing or other contact that involves an exchange of saliva. Infected people continue to shed the virus in their saliva for as long as a year. No treatment other than rest is necessary. EBV is, however, one of several viruses recently identifed as a possible cause of multiple sclerosis.

Poliomyelitis (Polio or Infantile Paralysis). The agent of polio, a picornavirus, usually spreads by direct contact or occasionally in milk. Some sources indicate that polio is never waterborne, although the virus is found in water with fecal contamination; others state that water is often a vehicle. During the epidemics of the 1950s, the fear of public swimming pools was prevalent, whether justified or not. Regardless of the mode of transmission, the virus invades the body through the gastrointestinal tract and then destroys or damages motor nerve cells in the spinal cord.

The 1954 discovery of the Salk inactivated polio vaccine (IPV), followed by an enforced vaccination campaign, largely solved the problem for much of the world (Figure 5.5). In 1962, the Sabin oral polio vaccine (OPV) largely replaced the IPV, but both vaccines are still in use. As the OPV can occasionally cause paralytic polio (about one case for every 2.4 million vaccinations), the CDC now recommends the IPV for a child's first two doses, followed by two doses of OPV. Some doctors, however, have speculated that the OPV may cause paralysis in patients who already have an unrecognized enterovirus 71 infection.

The IPV in its modern form cannot cause polio, but it does not protect the community against polio as effectively as the OPV. The reason is that the body's immune system responds differently to the two vaccines. When people receive only the IPV and later swallow the polio virus, they will not contract polio, but the virus will pass through their bodies and emerge in a fully virulent form that may infect others. The OPV, by contrast, causes an immune response that will kill any ingested polio viruses.

Like many new products, the original Salk IPV released in 1954 suffered from quality control problems. The virus was supposed to be dead, but some batches were defective and still contained live virus. The hundreds of children who were crippled by that early vaccine, and the hun-

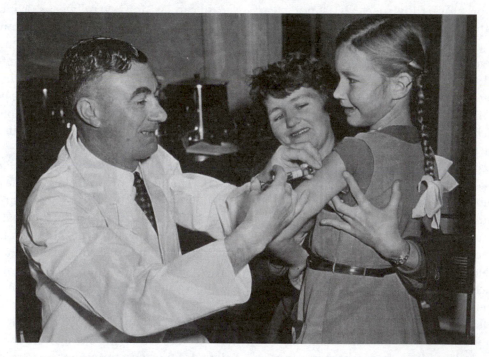

Figure 5.5. "Polio Pioneer" in Australia, 1954. The Salk and Sabin vaccines have rescued two generations of children from the disability and death caused by this greatly feared disease. (*Source*: U.S. National Library of Medicine.)

dreds of thousands who were not, were all heroes to whom the world owes its gratitude. Yet even after these problems were largely solved, many Americans remained suspicious of the vaccine, and to this day a few claim that polio would have disappeared faster without it. Despite these setbacks, and occasional small outbreaks from vaccine-derived strains, in 1994 WHO declared the Western Hemisphere free of "wild" polio. In all the world, fewer than 2000 people died of polio in 1999. About half of all cases now occur in India.

Although paralytic polio was known to the ancient Egyptians, the first large-scale epidemic on record took place in Sweden in 1887. Ironically, a polio outbreak is often most devastating when it strikes a developed nation with good hygiene and sanitation—such as the United States, where it arrived from Europe in about 1916. Under less tidy conditions, children tend to contract polio in infancy, when it rarely causes paralysis (despite its former name, "infantile paralysis"). In most epidemics, there are between 100 and 1000 inapparent or nonparalytic cases of polio for every one that ends in paralysis or death. The short-term effects of polio often are limited to an acute illness with fever, headache, and sometimes meningitis. But when an older child or adult gets the disease, the results tend to be worse. Finland, where a vaccination program had eliminated polio by 1964, had a small but unexpected outbreak of paralytic polio in 1984. Apparently, the IPV used in Finland at that time did not fully protect against one of the three polio serotypes.

Until recently, polio was little more than a memory and a source of vaccination controversy for most Americans. Then came the bad news: as many as one-quarter of all polio survivors, even those who were not initially paralyzed, develop muscular weakness and other complications decades later (Figure 5.6). Post-polio syndrome now affects hundreds of thousands of people who were born before the invention of the Salk vaccine. Here is a survivor's account:

The polio vaccine had not been invented when I was hospitalized with meningitis and a 106 fever in 1952. I remember seeing things crawling across the ceiling, dark and light, and a nice doctor with bushy eyebrows was talking to me, but I couldn't tell what he said.

When I left the hospital I was not paralyzed, just tired and weak. Nobody said "polio," just "meningitis," but my mother put away my tricycle for good. She built a big heated pool in the backyard, and I had to exercise in it. . . . So here I am, 40 years later, with post-polio syndrome.[12]

Rabies. This viral disease, also called hydrophobia, is virtually 100 percent fatal and untreatable once the virus reaches the brain. The symptoms in humans typically include headache, fever, agitation, dementia, and inability to swallow, followed by paralysis, convulsions, and death. Men with rabies sometimes have painful erections that last for days.

Antirabies serum injections (post-exposure prophylaxis or PEP) are effective, but they are not exactly a treatment; they are a preventive measure. After an infected animal bites a person (or the virus enters the body in some other way), the virus travels slowly from nerve endings in the skin at the

[12]2000 interview with polio survivor (name withheld).

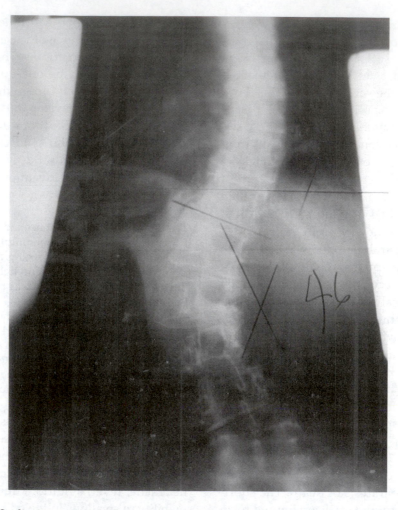

Figure 5.6. Scoliosis, a common late effect of childhood polio.

point of entry until it reaches the brain and causes rabies. The antirabies shots usually are effective during this incubation period, which lasts at least two weeks and sometimes as long as a year, depending on the point of entry.

The usual treatment after exposure consists of one injection of human rabies immunoglobulin followed by five doses of rabies vaccine over a four-week period. Persons at high risk for rabies, such as biologists who work with bats, may also be immunized before exposure. These injections are given in the arm and are now considered safe; as recently as the 1970s, however, rabies shots were an ordeal, consisting of 21 injections of horse serum in the abdomen. Reactions often were severe because of the foreign antigens in the horse serum and the number and locations of the shots.

There are at least six different rabies viruses in North America, each with a specific animal host. At one time, rabies was primarily a disease of dogs and other domesticated animals that contracted the disease by contact with wild animals. Now that most dogs are vaccinated, the pattern of the disease in the United States has changed, and most of the publicized human cases and exposures result from direct attacks by wild animals.

In 1999, for example, a rabid bobcat in Florida attacked seven people in two days before it was caught and killed. Other attacks by rabid bobcats were reported in New York State in 1997. Most human rabies cases in the United States, however, result from contact with bats. A 1999 study found rabies in 15 percent of a large sample of bats in Colorado, but the disease was present in 30 percent of bats that bit humans. For unknown reasons, just two bat species—the eastern pipistrelle (*Pipistrellus subflavus*) and the silver-haired bat (*Lasionycteris noctivagans*)—have caused about 75 percent of all bat-borne rabies cases in the United States in the past 20 years. Both are small bats with small teeth, and victims sometimes do not realize they have been bitten. In Mexico and Central America, vampire bats transmit rabies to cattle and other livestock.

Between 1980 and 1999, only 25 people in the United States contracted rabies, and in 22 cases the source was a bat. The others were two dogs and a skunk; in earlier years, raccoons also transmitted rabies. A 1999 study of rabies in Mexico showed that the majority of cases there result from skunk bites. In the early twentieth century, by contrast, about 100 Americans died of rabies each year, usually as a result of dog bites. Thus, routine rabies shots for dogs have saved many human lives. Worldwide, rabies accounts for about 40,000 deaths per year, and dogs are the source in 99 percent of cases.

In some parts of the United States, health officials have tried to control rabies by distributing baits that contain an oral rabies vaccine. Bats, of course, will not take such baits, but these programs may reduce the prevalence of rabies among coyotes and other animals that can transmit the disease to unvaccinated domestic dogs.

Two unusual incidents in 1996 and 1998 involved large numbers of people who drank unpasteurized milk from cows later found to be infected with rabies. Although there are no proven cases of rabies transmission by this route, caution was in order; thus, 18 persons received rabies shots in the first incident and 71 in the second.

In August 1999, the press reported an even more disturbing event: a black bear cub at an Iowa petting zoo died after displaying symptoms suggestive of rabies. When two subsequent tests at Iowa State University both confirmed the diagnosis, public health officials launched a vigorous campaign to contact all 400 people who had played with the animal, some of them tourists from as far away as Australia. At least 150 people received PEP; meanwhile, both the CDC and a second Iowa laboratory repeated the tests in September, but were unable to confirm that the bear had rabies. Apparently, only a few bears with rabies had ever been studied, and the test procedures were unreliable.

Roseola Infantum. This childhood disease, caused by human herpesvirus 6 (HHV-6), causes a sudden high fever and a rash on the body. Seizures may occur, but the illness lasts only a few days and complications are rare. The disease is important mainly because of its possible (but unproven) link to later development of multiple sclerosis.

Rotavirus. This virus may sometimes be foodborne, waterborne, or airborne, but researchers believe that most cases are transferred by direct contact between infected children. A 1999 study of foodborne diseases showed that rotavirus was foodborne in only 1 percent of cases. It is the most common cause of severe diarrhea among children in the United States, and is responsible for the hospitalization of 55,000 children in this country each year; about 40 times that number are infected. Worldwide, an estimated 600,000 children die of rotavirus infections each year. In adults, the infection tends to be much less serious.

Treatment of rotavirus, or any other severe diarrhea, consists of oral rehydration therapy (drinking to replace fluids and electrolytes). The FDA approved a vaccine in 1998, and more than 1 million American children received it. In 1999, however, doctors were advised to stop using the vaccine when at least 20 infants developed a life-threatening bowel obstruction after rotavirus immunization.

Rubella (German Measles). This is a mild viral disease that may cause a fever, rash, and swollen lymph nodes. Older patients sometimes have joint pain, but nearly half of all infected people have no noticeable symptoms. Once infected, a person has lifelong immunity to rubella.

The importance of rubella lies in the fact that, if the virus infects a woman in her first trimester of pregnancy, the results are likely to include birth defects or miscarriage. Thus, all women should request testing to make sure they are immune to rubella before becoming pregnant. In the United States alone, an estimated 20,000 children have been impaired by prenatal rubella infections. The disease spreads by direct contact or by airborne droplet transmission. Now that most children in the United States receive the combined measles-mumps-rubella (MMR) vaccine, rubella has become much less common.

Protozoan Diseases Transmitted by Other Contact

The agent of malaria, as discussed earlier, is a protozoan that has killed more human beings than any other pathogen in history. For all their virulence, however, protozoa have their limits. In simple terms, most of them need to stay wet. Most are transmitted only in water or food, or by intimate contact involving an insect vector or other exchange of body fluids. Thus, this section is brief.

Toxoplasmosis (see Chapter 3) and possibly other protozoan diseases can reach the fetus via the placenta, if the pregnant woman has a primary infection.

Trichomoniasis is a sexually transmitted disease, and amebiasis and giardiasis can be sexually transmitted under some circumstances, but are not transmissible by casual contact.

Fungal Diseases Transmitted by Other Contact

Alternaria Keratomycosis. Alternaria (see Chapter 6) is a fungus that infects tomatoes and other crop plants worldwide. In southern India, and probably elsewhere in the world, it sometimes also infects the cornea of the human eye. Agricultural workers appear to be at risk, but it is not clear if the infection is airborne or requires direct contact. The fungus contains a dark pigment, and one report describes the appearance of such an infection as "dramatic."

Ringworm or *Tinea*. This pathogen is not a worm, but a fungus that grows on the human skin and nails. Many different species of fungus are involved, most of them in the genera *Microspora*, *Trichophyton*, *Epidermophyton*, and *Candida*.

On the scalp, these fungi produce scaly patches with temporary loss of hair; school nurses sometimes confuse this condition with head lice. Ringworm of the body consists of ring-shaped crusted lesions that expand, leaving a clear area in the center. When the fungus colonizes the feet, it usually takes the form known as athlete's foot, with cracks or blisters between the toes. In a severe case of athlete's foot, an allergic reaction to the fungus products may also produce lesions on other parts of the body. Finally, ringworm of the fingernails or toenails causes thickening, discoloration, and brittleness of the nail.

People catch ringworm from other people or from various domestic animals, including dogs, cats, and cattle. Contaminated objects and surfaces frequently transmit the infection. All forms of ringworm respond fairly well to treatment with topical or oral fungicides, but the infection often returns.

Sporotrichosis. People who frequently handle thorny plants, sphagnum moss, or baled hay may contract this fungus (*Sporothrix schenckii*), which enters the skin through small cuts and causes small reddish bumps similar in appearance to insect bites. Later, these bumps resemble boils and finally become ulcerated. They are very slow to heal, but usually respond to treatment with iodides taken orally in droplet form. Outbreaks have occurred among nursery workers, gardeners, greenhouse workers, and children who play in hay. In rare cases, the infection may spread from the skin to other organs.

Multicellular Parasites Transmitted by Other Contact

This list might be considerably longer, but we have omitted certain parasites that seldom afflict humans in most of today's world.

Body Louse **(Pediculus humanus corporis)**. This parasite is less common in school children than the head louse, or at least less often reported. It is closely related to the head louse, described later in this chapter; the main difference is that the head louse lives on the head and the body louse lives on the body. The same medications work (or, more often, fail to work) on both. A third parasite, the crab louse, appears in the section on sexually transmitted diseases.

Body lice, unlike head lice, are not only annoying in themselves but also serve as vectors for several human diseases, including epidemic typhus, relapsing fever, and trench fever. By collecting body lice and subjecting them to DNA analysis, investigators have been able to diagnose and monitor these diseases in several countries where social conditions have led to their reemergence. People with long-standing infestations of body lice sometimes have enlarged lymph nodes and darkening of the skin, a condition known as vagabond's disease.

Chiggers. Several mite species have parasitic larvae called chiggers. They are very small, and their bites itch; as noted earlier in this chapter, mites also serve as vectors for scrub typhus. We mention chiggers here mainly because, in North America, they cause a fairly common syndrome that can easily be mistaken for a sexually transmitted infection. Since most victims are young boys, such a misdiagnosis might have grave consequences.

The condition is known in the medical literature as the summer penile syndrome. In other words, when boys play outdoors in summer they tend to accumulate chiggers, which often bite their genitals. The results typically include severe itching, difficulty in urination, and swelling due to a hypersensitivity reaction (see Chapter 7). Oral antihistamines and cold compresses typically relieve these symptoms.

Follicle Mite. This parasite (*Demodex folliculorum*) has attained minor cult status in recent years. Although it is a more or less normal inhabitant of human eyelash and eyebrow follicles, people in developed nations seem wary of colonization. In 2000, a popular New Age catalog portrayed a man whose nose resembled a large dill pickle, allegedly as a result of infestation with this mite. In the "after" photograph, after using the advertised product, he appeared normal and was smiling again. Some legitimate studies have linked the follicle mite to chronic blepharitis (pinkeye), rosacea, and other minor disorders.

Head Louse **(Pediculus humanus capitis).** Each year in the United States, head lice infest an estimated six to ten million children. The results can be catastrophic, but not for medical reasons. Unlike ticks and mosquitoes, head lice do not transmit disease, but families and school administrators sometimes react to their presence with hysteria.

Parents of children with head lice sometimes are visited by social workers and forced to sit through humiliating lectures on how to bathe themselves and wash their clothing. The parents then panic and call the family doctor, who recommends an over-the-counter medication that often fails to work (as explained below). In one tragic case, a parent who had been threatened with loss of his louse-infested child finally applied gasoline to the child's scalp, and a spark ignited the vapor. Often, lice are not even the real problem. To the untrained eye, ordinary dandruff may resemble louse eggs.

U.S. residents now spend as much as $100 million per year on over-the-counter head lice treatments, but the lice have become resistant. Studies have shown that American louse remedies are effective against head lice in Borneo, for example, but not on the domestic variety.

Probably the safest and most effective way to remove head lice is also the oldest and slowest. It requires a nonviolent but distracting videocassette—that part is new—plus a fine-toothed steel comb, a towel, some cotton balls, and a bottle of olive oil. While the child watches the movie, the parent goes through the child's hair a few strands at a time, rubbing the oil gently into the scalp and using the comb to remove the lice. The towel is to wipe up the mess. This process is the source of two English colloquialisms, "nit-picking" and "going over [something] with a fine-toothed comb."

Hookworm Disease. This parasite now occurs mainly in tropical countries and in the southeastern United States. Its name (*Necator americanus*) means literally "the American killer," but it rarely kills its host outright, although it may predispose to other infections. The larvae enter the body through bare skin, usually on the sole of the foot, and migrate to the lungs via the lymphatic and blood circulation. From there, they ascend the trachea to the throat. The person then swallows the larvae, which attach to the wall of the small intestine, grow to maturity, and lay eggs, which pass out in the feces to start another cycle.

Depending on the stage, hookworm disease may cause itching or infection on the foot or other point of entry; fever, cough, and pulmonary hemorrhage; nausea and diarrhea with weight loss; or heart failure and generalized edema. A heavy infestation of these worms, especially in children, may cause chronic anemia and developmental disabilities. Improved waste disposal has largely eliminated this disease in many areas. A public health program in Puerto Rico in the last century, for example, reduced the prevalence from 90 percent to about 15 percent. In 2000, the Gates Foundation awarded an $18 million grant to the Albert B. Sabin Vaccine Institute and Yale University for development of a hookworm vaccine.

Scabies Mite (**Sarcoptes scabiei**). This parasite burrows into the human skin, causing pimple-like lesions that itch intensely. It may infest various parts of the body, including the webs and sides of the fingers, the wrist, elbows, armpits, waist, thighs, genitalia, nipples, breasts, or lower buttocks. The mites spread from one person to another by direct contact (including sex) or by recently contaminated clothing or bedding. Skin lotions that contain insecticide are available as treatment and are usually applied to the entire body, except the head. It is also necessary to change and wash clothing and bedding to avoid reinfestation.

Enterobiasis. A generation or two ago, no one would have seriously entertained the notion that pinworms are a "biological hazard." Enterobiasis was a common parasitic infestation, especially in children, and that was the end of it. Even people who take baths can get pinworms; an estimated 15 percent of U.S. residents have them. Today, however, the very idea of (gasp) *worms* inhabiting our bodies is enough to send many Americans through the roof. This infestation, like follicle mites, may be more a psychological hazard than a biological one.

Pinworms have not yet been linked to any form of cancer, heart disease, or dementia. In rare cases, pinworms have caused appendicitis, which is also fairly common in people without pinworms. There may be some itching, especially when the worms crawl out at night to lay eggs, and so the groggy host scratches. The next time she bites her nails, she swallows the eggs again. People who find that the itching (or the entire concept) keeps them awake can ask the doctor to worm them.

REFERENCES AND RECOMMENDED READING

Aranda, M., and Lopez de Buen, L. "Rabies in Skunks from Mexico." *Journal of Wildlife Diseases*, July 1999, pp. 574–577.

"Bad to the Bone." *Discover*, October 1994, p. 11.

Baer, G.M. (Editor). 1991. *The Natural History of Rabies*. Boca Raton, FL: CRC Press.

Benini, Aldo A., and Bradford-Benini, Janet. 1995. *Ebola Strikes the Global Village: the Virus, the Media, the Organized Response*. San Luis Obispo: California Polytechnic State University.

Berkman, Alan, and Bakalar, Nicholas. 2000. *Hepatitis A to G: The Facts You Need to Know about All Forms of this Dangerous Disease*. New York: Warner Books.

Black, Kathryn. 1997. *In the Shadow of Polio: A Personal and Social History*. Cambridge, MA: Perseus Publishing.

Blackmore, D.K., and Schollum, L.M. "Risks of Contracting Leptospirosis on the Dairy Farm." *New Zealand Medical Journal*, September 1982, pp. 649–652.

Borchert, M., et al. "Filovirus Haemorrhagic Fever Outbreaks: Much Ado About Nothing?" *Tropical Medicine and International Health* 5(5), May 2000, pp. 318–324.

Brouqui, P., et al. "Chronic *Bartonella quintana* Bacteremia in Homeless Patients." *New England Journal of Medicine*, January 21, 1999, pp. 184–189.

Carithers, H.A., and Margileth, A.M. "Cat-Scratch Disease: Acute Encephalopathy and Other Neurologic Manifestations." *American Journal of Diseases of Children*, January 1991, pp. 98–101.

Dajer, Tony. "Taking It on the Jaw." *Discover*, October 1999, pp. 49–50.

Diamond, Jared. "A Pox upon Our Genes." *Natural History*, February 1990, p. 26 ff.

Diamond, Jared. "One-Way Plagues." *Wilson Quarterly*, Winter 1993, p. 146 ff.

Di Bisceglie, Adrian M., and Bacon, Bruce R. "The Unmet Challenges of Hepatitis C." *Scientific American*, October 1999, pp. 80–85.

Dolin, Raphael. "Entervirus 71—Emerging Infections and Emerging Questions." *New England Journal of Medicine*, September 23, 1999, pp. 984–985.

"Ebola Home Remedy." *Newsweek*, August 16, 1999, p. 4.

"Ebola Virus Infection in Imported Primates—Virginia, 1989." *Morbidity and Mortality Weekly Report*, December 8, 1989, p. 831 ff.

Fedarko, Kevin. "A Lousy, Nit-Picking Epidemic." *Time*, January 12, 1998.

"Fifty Visitors to Denver Zoo Ill with Salmonella from Lizards." *Washington Times*, March 4, 1996.

Finley, Don. 1998. *Mad Dogs: The New Rabies Plague*. Louise Lindsey Merrick Natural Environment Series, No. 26. College Station, TX: Texas A&M University Press.

Forton, F., and Seys, B. "Density of *Demodex folliculorum* in Rosacea." *British Journal of Dermatology*, Vol. 128, 1993, pp. 650–659.

Gould, Tony. 1997. *A Summer Plague: Polio and Its Survivors*. New Haven, CT: Yale University Press.

Halstead, Lauro. "Post Polio Syndrome." *Scientific American*, April 1998, pp. 42–47.

Haney, Daniel Q. "Breakthrough: Scientists Report First Effective Staph Vaccine." Associated Press, September 19, 2000.

Hirschhorn, R.B., and Hodge, R.R. "Identification of Risk Factors in Rat Bite Incidents Involving Humans." *Pediatrics*, September 1999, p. e35 ff.

Huang, C., et al. "Neurologic Complications in Children with Enterovirus 71 Infection." *New England Journal of Medicine*, September 23, 1999, pp. 936–942.

"Hyping Hepatitis C?" Reuters News Service, September 14, 2000.

"Iowa Bear Cub Places Zoo Visitors at Risk for Rabies." *Journal of the American Veterinary Medical Association*, November 1, 1999.

Kaplan, Colin. 1986. *Rabies: The Facts*. 2nd ed. New York: Oxford University Press.

Karvonen, M., et al. "Association Between Type 1 Diabetes and *Haemophila influenzae* Type B Vaccination: Birth Cohort Study." *British Medical Journal*, May 1, 1999, pp. 1169–1172.

Kavanaugh, John F. "Living by Appearance." *America*, February 5, 1994, pp. 38–39.

Krieger, Lisa. "Trench Fever of WW1 Flares

among the Homeless." *San Francisco Examiner*, December 29, 1997.

Lawren, Bill. "Armadillo Lepers." *Omni*, December 1984, p. 20.

Layton, C.T. "*Pasteurella multocida* Meningitis and Septic Arthritis Secondary to a Cat Bite." *Journal of Emergency Medicine*, May–June 1999, pp. 445–448.

Leirs, H., et al. "Search for the Ebola Virus Reservoir in Kikwit, Democratic Republic of the Congo." *Journal of Infectious Diseases*, February 1999, Suppl. 1, pp. S155–163.

Leroy, E.M., et al. "Human Asymptomatic Ebola Infection and Strong Inflammatory Response." *Lancet*, June 24, 2000, pp. 2210–2215.

Levy, Stuart B. "The Challenge of Antibiotic Resistance." *Scientific American*, March 1998, pp. 46–53.

Lies, Elaine. "Court Tells Japan to Compensate Leprosy Patients." Reuters News Service, May 11, 2001.

Littman, R.J., and Littman, M.L. "The Athenian Plague: Smallpox." *Proceedings of the American Philological Association*, Vol. 100, 1969, pp. 261–275.

"Lousy Kids Hard to Find in U.S., Doctors Say." Reuters News Service, September 14, 1999.

Lundsgaard, T. "Filovirus-Like Particles Detected in the Leafhopper *Psammotettix alienus*." *Virus Research*, April 1997, pp. 35–40.

Maldonado, A.E. "Hookworm Disease: Puerto Rico's Secret Killer." *Puerto Rican Health Science Journal*, September 1993, pp. 191–196.

"Mass Treatment of Humans Who Drank Unpasteurized Milk from Rabid Cows." *Morbidity and Mortality Weekly Report*, March 26, 1999, pp. 228–229.

"Measles Prevention: Recommendations of the Immunization Practices Advisory Committee (ACIP)." *Morbidity and Mortality Weekly Report Supplement*, December 29, 1989, pp. 1–18.

Melnick, J.L. "Enterovirus 71 Infections: A Varied Clinical Pattern Sometimes Mimicking Paralytic Poliomyelitis." *Review of Infectious Disease*, May–June 1984, Suppl. 2, pp. S387–390.

Melnick, J.L. "Current Status of Poliovirus Infections." *Clinical Microbiology Reviews*, July 1996, pp. 293–300.

"Meningitis Kills 10,000 in Africa." *New York Times* News Service, May 8, 1996.

Mohle-Boetani, J.C., et al. "Viral Meningitis in Child Care Center Staff and Parents: An Outbreak of Echovirus 30 Infections." *Public Health Report*, May–June 1999, pp. 249–256.

Monath, T.P. "Ecology of Marburg and Ebola Viruses: Speculations and Directions for Future Research." *Journal of Infectious Diseases*, February 1999, Suppl. 1, pp. S127–138.

"Most Bat Rabies Cases Tracked to Two Unusual Species." Associated Press, October 16, 1999.

Nass, Meryl. "Anthrax Epizootic in Zimbabwe, 1978–1980: Due to Deliberate Spread?" *Physicians for Social Responsibility Quarterly*, December 1992.

"New Virus Linked to Three California Deaths." Associated Press, August 4, 2000.

Olson, P.E., et al. "The Thucydides Syndrome: Ebola Deja Vu? [letter]." *Emerging Infectious Diseases*, April–June 1996.

Orent, Wendy. "Killer Pox in the Congo." *Discover*, October 1999, pp. 74–79.

Pan American Health Organization. 1999. *Measles Eradication: Field Guide* (Series TP-41). Washington, DC: Pan American Health Organization.

Pape, W.J., et al. "Risk for Rabies Transmission from Encounters with Bats, Colorado, 1977–1996." *Emerging Infectious Diseases*, May–June 1999, pp. 433–437.

Peters, Clarence J. "Biosafety and Emerging Infections: Key Issues in the Prevention and Control of Viral Hemorrhagic Fevers." Atlanta, GA: Proceedings of the 4th National Symposium on Biosafety, Atlanta, GA, January 1996.

Plagemann, Bentz. 1949. *My Place to Stand*. New York: Farrar, Straus.

"Rat-bite Fever, New Mexico 1996." *Morbidity and Mortality Weekly Report*, February 13, 1998, pp. 89–91.

Rogers, Naomi. 1958. *Dirt and Disease: Polio Before FDR*. New Brunswick, NJ: Rutgers University Press.

Roux, V., and Raoult, D. "Body Lice as Tools for Diagnosis and Surveillance of Reemerging

Diseases." *Journal of Clinical Microbiology*, March 1999, pp. 596–599.

Rupprecht, Charles E., et al. "The Ascension of Wildlife Rabies: A Cause for Public Health Concern or Intervention?" *Emerging Infectious Diseases* Volume 1, Number 4, October–December 1995, p. 107 ff.

Seppala, H., et al. "The Effect of Changes in the Consumption of Macrolide Antibiotics on Erythromycin Resistance in Group A Streptococci in Finland." *New England Journal of Medicine*, August 14, 1997, pp. 441–446.

Smith, G.A., et al. "The Summer Penile Syndrome: Seasonal Acute Hypersensitivity Reaction Caused by Chigger Bites on the Penis." *Pediatric Emergency Care*, April 1998, pp. 116–118.

Smith, Jane S. 1990. *Patenting the Sun: Polio and the Salk Vaccine*. New York: Morrow.

Sorensen, H.T., et al. "Diagnostic Problems with Meningococcal Disease in General Practice." *Journal of Clinical Epidemiology*, November 1992, pp. 1289–1293.

Sullivan, Nancy J., et al. "Development of a Preventive Vaccine for Ebola Virus Infection in Primates." *Nature*, November 30, 2000, pp. 605–609.

Thomas, Lewis. 1990. "On Disease." In *A Long Line of Cells*, pp. 169–177. New York: Viking Penguin.

Tobe, T.J., et al. "Hemolytic Uremic Syndrome Due to *Capnocytophaga canimorsus* Bacteremia After a Dog Bite." *American Journal of Kidney Diseases*, June 1999, p. e5.

"Update: Poliomyelitis Outbreak—Finland, 1984–1985." *Morbidity and Mortality Weekly Report*, February 14, 1986, pp. 82–86.

"U.S. Warns Hospitals About Antibiotic-Resistant Infection." Associated Press, January 6, 2000.

Vitek, Charles R., and Melinda Wharton. "Diphtheria in the Former Soviet Union: Reemergence of a Pandemic Disease." *Emerging Infectious Diseases*, October–December 1998, pp. 539–550.

Wacker, Bob. "Virus on Ice." *Health*, December 1989, pp. 48–51.

Webster, Robert G., and Granoff, Allan. 1995. *Encyclopedia of Virology Plus CD-ROM*. San Diego, CA: Academic Press.

OUTLOOK FOR THE TWENTY-FIRST CENTURY

Some of the most important diseases of the next decade are the ones described in this chapter, such as HIV and malaria.

For the most part, scientists now understand how HIV/AIDS is transmitted. Until an effective vaccine becomes available, individuals can do little more than avoid high-risk behavior and practice empathy while the world braces for the final numbers. In 2000, researchers at the University of California Los Angeles announced the development of a promising new AIDS vaccine, using a dead virus that has been turned inside out, in effect, thus enabling the immune system to detect hidden portions of the viral envelope. As noted earlier, human trials of another AIDS vaccine have already begun in England.

Group norms are at least as important as medicine in controlling any sexually transmitted disease, and a controversial movement in South Africa may help reduce the rate of HIV infection there. Andile Gumede and other Zulu women have recently revived the ancient custom of virginity testing, in which hundreds of young, unmarried Zulu girls gather to allow older women to determine if their hymens are intact. Some Westerners have criticized the practice as barbaric, while others note its similarity to the Western custom of an annual pelvic examination. The main difference is that the Zulu version inspires a sense of esprit de corps; each girl wants to pass and get her certificate.

Virginity testing is unreliable, and those who fail may be unfairly criticized, but a moment's embarrassment must be weighed against the disaster now facing Africa and the world. Men could share the burden by having their sons circumcised in infancy; studies in Africa have shown that circumcised heterosexual men rarely contract HIV. Even more radical solutions have been proposed. In 2001, President Daniel Arap Moi of Kenya asked all citizens to abstain from sexual relations for at least two years, and a Mexican official proposed a strict quarantine of AIDS patients.

One promising weapon against HIV is an economic boycott of the unaffordable drugs required to treat it. Brazil has achieved excellent results by manufacturing and distributing its own low-cost generic AIDS medications, thus forcing down the price of competing drugs sold by international corporations. In 2001, South Africa began a similar program.

For vectorborne diseases, the future is yet more hazy. Despite endless debate, no one really knows how global warming will influence the geographic and seasonal distribution of mosquitoes, sandflies, and other important disease vectors. Some researchers are certain that malaria will return to North America, while others insist it will not. Regardless of which viewpoint is correct, at least malaria is not some terrifying unknown. It was here before, and we know a great deal about the parasite and its life cycle. Pharmaceutical companies might work harder to develop effective antimalarial drugs if the millions of dying children were in the United States. Some advances have already occurred; in 1999, a German research team reported that the antibiotic fosmidomycin was effective against malaria, and in 2000, European scientists created a genetically modified *Anopheles* mosquito that produces antibodies to the malaria parasite.

REFERENCES AND RECOMMENDED READING

Buckley, Stephen. "Brazil a Model in Fight against AIDS." *Alta Vista*, September 17, 2000.

Kumate, J. "Infectious Diseases in the 21st Century." *Archives of Medical Research*, Vol. 28 No. 2, 1997, pp. 155–161.

McKenzie, John. "Malaria-Free Mosquitoes." ABCNews.com, July 19, 2000.

Szabo, R., and Short, R.V. "How Does Male Circumcision Protect against HIV Infection?" *British Medical Journal*, June 10, 2000, pp 1592–1594.

Wooten, James. "The Chastity Test." ABCNews.com, July 11, 2000.

THE GOOD OLD DAYS

Whenever today's environmental health problems threaten to overwhelm, we turn to the medical literature of past centuries, when human beings, disease vectors, and parasites lived together in peaceful harmony. The first example is an excerpt from a letter written by a man named William Barkley in Alabama, dated April 29, 1849 (original spelling preserved). The daughter's illness sounds like one of the vectorborne hemorrhagic fevers, but had it been yellow fever, the observer probably would have mentioned jaundice:

Our eldest daughter Anna Elizabeth took the newmonia on the 7 of March and 29 took to bleeding at the nose and an afful braking out, at first like messels then it appeared like brused blood under the skin and some blood under the arms, these got worse until the second of April when she expired about one hour and one half in the night and died pearfectly easy after being sick for 27 day and we have had a great deal of trouble for the loss.[13]

The same letter goes on to describe how, on the heels of this loss, a "Big Sow" destroyed most of the region's grain and fruit crops. The expression refers to a storm called a sou'wester, and does not imply that a pig trampled the fields, but one translation might be as good as the other. A disease, like a storm, was an inexplicable tragedy that left its survivors wondering who had sinned, who had left the gate open.

Overcrowded living quarters and unsanitary conditions have been the rule rather than the exception throughout much of human history. To understand how disease epidemics can arise under these circumstances, there is no example quite like a slave ship. Note, however, that the observer believed dysentery was transmitted by foul air rather than by contact or water:

The closeness of the place, and the heat of the climate, added to the number in the ship, being so crowded that each had scarcely room to turn himself, almost suffocated us. This produced copious perspiration, so that the air soon became unfit for respiration, from a variety of loathsome smells, and brought on a sickness [dysentery] among the slaves, of which many died. . . . This deplorable situation was again aggravated by the galling of the chains, now become insupportable; and the filth of necessary tubs, into which children often fell, and were nearly suffocated. The shrieks of the women, and the groans of the dying, rendered it a scene of horror almost inconceivable.[14]

FROM THE AUTHOR'S FILE CABINET

Every physician needs to exercise tact and good judgment, but this requirement is especially binding on those who treat sexually transmitted diseases (STDs).

In the early 1990s, during a routine OB/GYN checkup, a woman complained of a minor irritation and asked if it might be an allergy to her husband's latex condoms. The gynecologist, without performing any test, told her it was a chlamydia infection, and that both partners needed immediate treatment with Flagyl® (metronidazole)—an antibiotic normally reserved for highly resistant infections caused by protozoa or anaerobic bacteria. The reason for the prescription is not clear, as the drug of choice for chlamydia is (and was) an antibiotic with fewer potential side effects, usually tetracycline or erythromycin.

The patient, duly alarmed by what she believed was her first STD, filled the prescription and broke the news to her husband, expecting a rational response. After all, the same bacterium causes nonvenereal infections, such as pinkeye; she might have harbored it for years, or even caught it from him. Upon hearing this explanation, however, he hit the roof.

He went to the urology department of a world-renowned medical center and asked to be tested for chlamydia, explaining that his wife had been diagnosed with it. Although he spelled and pronounced the word correctly, things went wrong at that point. "There's no such thing," the urologist replied. "She probably means yeast."

[13]Frederick Smoot, "A Daughter Dies in Blue Pond" (<http://www.usgennet.org> 1997).
[14]From "The Interesting Narrative of the Life of Olaudah Equiano, or Gustavas Vassa, the African," in D. Mullane, *Crossing the Danger Water* (New York: Doubleday, 1993).

Bear in mind that chlamydia was already the most frequently reported STD in the United States, and that this doctor specialized in diseases of the urogenital tract. How could he not have heard of it? So the husband went home and demanded to know what his wife *really* had. What was she trying to conceal with her doubletalk? Was it syphilis? Or AIDS? Or both? She responded in kind, by recommending high-risk behavior with a donkey, and the war was on.

The next day, the husband called the gynecologist's office and confirmed the name of the microorganism, then called his urologist again. The urologist agreed to phone the gynecologist for instructions, and finally a laboratory test was done.

"My test was negative," the husband trumpeted to the heavens, "and yours was positive!"

"No," the wife insisted. "I never had a test." But this fact was lost in background noise, as both spouses packed their bags, consulted their attorneys, and inadvertently frightened the daylights out of their children.

By the time the feud ended, the wife had taken all of her Flagyl® (without adverse side effects) and should have been lily-pure. But only seconds into the reconciliation process, her original symptoms returned in full force. The problem was, in fact, a latex allergy.

CHAPTER 6

Crop and Livestock Pathogens and Pests

And there came out of the smoke locusts upon the earth; and unto them was given power, as the scorpions of the earth have power.
—Revelations 9:3

Books on biological hazards often refer to the Four Horsemen of the Apocalypse from the Book of Revelations: Famine, Pestilence, Destruction, and Death. People have known for a long time that famine—usually the result of crop failure—can be the first step in an all-too-familiar cascade. The weakened populace falls victim to disease epidemics, and then comes destruction—of the afflicted civilization itself, or of its neighbors and their coveted resources. As the Bible tells us, death follows after.

Now that the world's food supply has grown larger and foreign aid programs more effective, the power of this image has faded. Famines occur less often, and are no longer the cause of most epidemics; the third Horseman, Destruction, now tends to lead the parade. Destruction, whether in the form of a natural disaster or a war, is a major factor in spreading disease. (We will not add a fifth Horseman named Travel; tourism and immigration, to the epidemiologist, are surrogates for warfare.)

But Famine, the first Horseman, is never far away, and as the human population increases, we may see more of him. In 1997, the Population Council estimated that feeding the world adequately (by Western standards) in the year 2050 will require a 430 percent increase over today's level of food production. These facts underscore the urgent need for improved control of crop and livestock diseases.

CROSS-REFERENCE

This chapter discusses a few of the major pathogens and pests that afflict crop plants and livestock. Many diseases, however, occur in both humans and their domestic animals. Such diseases are called **zoonoses** (pronounced zo-o-NO-seez, singular zoonosis). Humans and plants also share at least a few diseases. Thus, references to some diseases appear in more than one chapter, and Table 6.1 provides a cross-reference.

Table 6.1
Cross-Reference: Other Biological Hazards Affecting Livestock and Crops

Disease	Chapter	Notes
Cryptosporidiosis	2	Mainly waterborne; humans and livestock
Giardiasis	2	Waterborne; humans and domestic animals
Leptospirosis	2	Contact, food, or water; humans and livestock
Tuberculosis	4	Airborne or contact; humans and livestock
Anthrax	3, 4, 5	Mainly contact; humans and livestock
Rabies	5	Contact; humans and livestock
Tularemia	5	Several modes; humans and wildlife
Poisonous plants	7	Ingested by range cattle, others
Turkey-X disease	7	Aflatoxin
Venomous organisms	7	May pose a risk to livestock
Predators	8	Bears, wolves, etc.

Some zoonoses, such as an obscure bacterial infection called seal finger, never really take off; either the disease is not highly communicable, or only a few people are exposed to it. Others, such as influenza (see Chapter 4) and plague (see Chapter 5), have caused the largest human disease epidemics in history. Still other animal pathogens find human beings unsatisfactory as hosts, but wreak havoc indirectly by destroying food supplies.

INTEGRATED PEST MANAGEMENT

Briefly, integrated pest management (IPM) combines a variety of methods to keep unwanted organisms at acceptable levels. This "unwanted" category includes not only pathogens and parasites of livestock and crops, but any plant or animal that turns up in numbers or locations that conflict with human interests. The methods of IPM include the conservation of existing natural enemies, such as mountain lions to control deer (and deer tick) populations; crop rotation and intercropping, to maintain existing biological control agents on a smaller scale and to reduce weed seedbanks; and the use of pest-resistant strains of plants and animals. IPM does not abandon more aggressive and sometimes risky methods such as pesticide application and genetic engineering, but it reduces the need for reliance on such methods.

DISEASES OF LIVESTOCK

Owing to the potential for massive economic losses in the livestock and farming industries, the U.S. Department of Agriculture (USDA) and other agencies have deployed legions of sacrificial chickens, suitcase-sniffing beagles, infertile flies, and other unlikely sentinels to ward off pestilence at our international borders and airports. If the chickens become sick or the dogs sit down, health officials investigate. At the first hint of invading screwworms or crop pests, the agencies release sterilized male insects to fire blanks into the gene pool. Few Americans are aware of the invaluable services that these animals provide, or of the ingenious efforts that have made their work possible.

Chapters 2–5 presented the majority of human pathogens and parasites that most readers are likely to encounter. If the ills of one species can fill four chapters, it is clear that a single chapter cannot begin to cover all the diseases of domestic animals. In the context of this book, hazards that affect livestock are secondary hazards, destroying resources rather than directly claiming human lives. Thus, the following paragraphs are limited to a few examples of livestock diseases and infestations. Table 6.2 provides examples of major outbreaks, and Tables 6.3 and 6.4 list livestock diseases that farmers are legally required to report. The reading material at the end of each main section,

and the resources in Chapters 11 and 12, provide more information.

Bacterial Diseases

Anthrax. This disease is a favorite topic at the start of the third millennium, as witness the fact that we have already discussed it in Chapters 3, 4, and 5. Despite its adaptability and audience appeal, however, anthrax is really a disease of cattle and other ruminants, which contract it by ingesting spores from soil or water. Outbreaks are more likely during a prolonged drought, when animals forage closer to the spore-laden soil and ponds begin to evaporate, causing the spores floating on the water to become more concentrated. Insect bites and contaminated feed also transmit the disease. Unlike ruminants, many carnivores are resistant to anthrax and often recover.

Infected animals may show respiratory distress, fever, loss of appetite, or other

Table 6.2
Examples of Major Outbreaks of Agricultural Diseases and Pests

Event	Date	Location	Deaths/Losses
Rinderpest	1600s	Europe	200 million cattle
Rinderpest	1890s	South Africa	90% of all cattle
Varroa Bee Mite	1980s	North America	95% of wild honeybees
Late Blight of Potato	1845–47	Ireland	Potato crop; 1 million people
Dutch Elm Disease	1930	North America	Millions of elm trees
Citrus Mycoplasma	1979	Florida	2 million trees
Avian influenza	1983–84	Northeastern U.S.	17 million chickens
Newcastle Disease	1971–74	Southern California	12 million chickens
Classical Swine Fever	1997	The Netherlands	6 million pigs
Foot-and-Mouth Disease	2001	England	4 million cattle

Note: Losses in the 2001 FMD epidemic represent animals slaughtered to prevent further spread.
Sources: Smithcors and Smithcors (1997); United States Animal Health Association; Office International des Epizootie.

Table 6.3
List A Reportable Animal Diseases, 2000

Disease	Species Affected
Foot-and-Mouth Disease	Cattle
Vesicular Stomatitis	Cattle
Swine Vesicular Disease	Swine
Rinderpest	Cattle
Peste des Petits Ruminants	Goats; also sheep and other small ruminants
Contagious Bovine Pleuropneumonia	Cattle
Lumpy Skin Disease	Cattle
Rift Valley Fever	Cattle, sheep, and goats; also humans
Bluetongue	Sheep and other ruminants
Sheep Pox and Goat Pox	Sheep and goats
African Horse Sickness	Horses
African Swine Fever	Swine
Classical Swine Fever (Hog Cholera)	Swine
Highly Pathogenic Avian Influenza	Domestic fowl and other birds
Newcastle Disease	Domestic fowl and other birds

Source: Office International des Epizootie.

signs. Frequently, however, anthrax in a ruminant presents as sudden death of an animal that appeared normal a few hours earlier. (If this sounds less complicated than anthrax in humans, the most likely reason is that the cow cannot describe its symptoms.) Some Biblical scholars believe that the fifth Egyptian plague in the Book of Exodus was anthrax, based on the reported high mortality and the fact that the sixth plague presented as boils on the Egyptian people.

Treatment with penicillin or oxytetracycline usually is effective if started early enough. An anthrax vaccine also is available to protect livestock in endemic areas.

Avian Cholera or *Fowl Cholera*. The same bacterium that causes this disease (*Pasteurella multocida*) also tends to occur on dogs' teeth (see Chapter 5). It affects all birds, especially turkeys, often causing a rapidly fatal septicemia. The birds may die without any obvious signs of illness, or there may be fever, loss of appetite, diarrhea, and a mucous discharge from the mouth. Necropsy findings often include pneumonia, hemorrhages, and necrotic areas in the liver and spleen. Birds that survive may develop a chronic form of fowl cholera, with local infections of the feet, eyes, lungs, or other parts.

Both live and killed vaccines are available and are the most effective way to protect poultry. Waterfowl and other wild birds serve as a natural reservoir for the disease, and mass die-offs occur on a regular basis, often associated with cold weather and high population densities during migration.

Brucellosis. This is primarily a disease of livestock, but humans also contract it on

Table 6.4
List B Reportable Animal Diseases, 2000

Disease	Species Affected
Anthrax	Cattle, sheep, goats, horses, swine; also humans
Aujeszky's Disease (Pseudorabies)	Swine and other livestock
Echinococcosis/Hydatidosis	Dogs, cattle, sheep, horses, swine; also humans
Leptospirosis	Cattle, horses, swine; also humans
Rabies	All mammals including humans
Paratuberculosis (Johne's disease)	Cattle and other ruminants
Heartwater (Cowdriosis)	Cattle and other ruminants
New World and Old World Screwworm	All mammals including humans
Bovine Brucellosis	Cattle
Bovine Genital Campylobacteriosis	Cattle
Bovine Tuberculosis	Cattle
Enzootic Bovine Leukosis	Cattle
Infectious Bovine Rhinotracheitis/ Infectious Pustular Vulvovaginitis	Cattle
Trichomonosis	Cattle
Bovine Anaplasmosis	Cattle
Bovine Babesiosis	Cattle
Bovine Cysticercosis	Cattle
Dermatophilosis	Cattle
Theileriosis	Cattle
Haemorrhagic Septicaemia	Cattle
Bovine Spongiform Encephalopathy	Cattle; also linked to CJD in humans
Ovine Epididymitis (*Brucella ovis*)	Sheep and goats
Caprine and ovine brucellosis (excluding *Brucella ovis*)	Sheep and goats
Contagious Agalactia	Sheep and goats
Caprine Arthritis/Encephalitis	Sheep and goats
Maedi-Visna	Sheep and goats
Contagious Caprine Pleuropneumonia	Sheep and goats
Enzootic Abortion of Ewes/Chlamydiosis	Sheep and goats
Contagious Equine Metritis	Horses
Dourine	Horses
Equine Encephalomyelitis (E and W)	Horses; also humans
Equine Infectious Anemia	Horses
Equine Influenza	Horses
Equine Piroplasmosis	Horses
Equine Rhinopneumonitis	Horses
Glanders	Horses
Horse Pox	Horses
Equine Viral Arteritis	Horses
Horse Mange	Horses

(continued)

Table 6.4   (Continued)

Disease	Species Affected
Venezuelan Equine Encephalomyelitis	Horses
Epizootic Lymphangitis	Horses
Japanese Encephalitis	Horses
Atrophic Rhinitis of Swine	Swine
Porcine Brucellosis	Swine
Trichinellosis	Swine
Enterovirus Encephalomyelitis	Swine
Transmissible gastroenteritis	Swine
Infectious Bursal Disease	Domestic fowl, other birds
Marek's Disease	Domestic fowl, other birds
Avian Mycoplasmosis (*M. gallisepticum*)	Domestic fowl, other birds
Avian Chlamydiosis	Domestic fowl, other birds
Fowl Typhoid and Pullorum Disease	Domestic fowl, other birds
Avian Infectious Bronchitis	Domestic fowl, other birds
Avian Infectious Laryngotracheitis	Domestic fowl, other birds
Avian Tuberculosis	Domestic fowl, other birds
Duck Virus Hepatitis	Domestic fowl, other birds
Duck Virus Enteritis	Domestic fowl, other birds
Fowl Cholera	Domestic fowl, other birds
Salmonella enteritidis and *S. typhimurium*	Domestic fowl, other birds
Myxomatosis	Rabbits
Tularemia	Rabbits; also humans
Rabbit Haemorrhagic Disease	Rabbits
Acariosis of Bees	Honeybees
American Foulbrood	Honeybees
European Foulbrood	Honeybees
Nosemosis of Bees	Honeybees
Varroosis	Honeybees

Source: Office International des Epizootie.

occasion, by working with livestock or laboratory cultures or by eating contaminated cheese or drinking unpasteurized milk.

The agents are the bacteria *Brucella abortus*, which causes bovine (cow) and human brucellosis; *B. suis*, which can cause porcine (pig) or human brucellosis; and *B. melitensis*, which can cause caprine (goat), ovine (sheep), bovine, or human brucellosis. Related species are *Brucella ovis* in sheep and *B. canis* in dogs. All these bacteria exist in various serotypes, and the nomenclature may change. Camels, buffalo, and many other mammals are susceptible to brucellosis; the buffalo herd in Yellowstone Park is believed to carry this disease, and management is a controversial issue because of the animals' endangered status and cultural importance to Native Americans.

Brucellosis often causes cows to abort, and may also cause inflammation of the testicles in bulls. If the cow's mammary glands are infected, the milk will be contaminated. Other symptoms of the disease may include infertility and fluid-filled cysts in the joints. The symptoms in sheep, goats, and pigs are similar. Vaccines are available to prevent brucellosis in livestock. The disease in humans is more serious but usually not fatal, starting with a high, intermittent fever and often causing meningitis, pneumonia, inflammation of the sacroiliac joints, or other complications.

Contagious Bovine Pleuropneumonia. The agent of this disease is the bacterium *Mycoplasma mycoides*, which causes fever, loss of appetite, and respiratory illness in cattle. Humans do not catch this disease, and the only susceptible wild mammal appears to be the American buffalo. Vaccines have been used for nearly a century in an effort to control CBPP, but most have been ineffective. One mild strain is satisfactory as a vaccine and is often given in combination with a rinderpest vaccine.

Glanders. The agent of this highly contagious, often fatal disease is the bacterium *Burkholderia* (or *Pseudomonas*) *mallei*. It causes nodules in the lungs of horses, mules, and donkeys. Humans who work with these animals or their products can easily contract the disease, but actual human cases have been rare, although 95 percent fatal. In 2000, an Army researcher working on a glanders vaccine contracted the disease, but reportedly survived with antibiotic treatment. Cattle, sheep, and pigs are resistant to glanders. A closely related bacterium, *Pseudomonas pseudomallei*, causes the human disease melioidosis (see Chapter 2).

Glanders, like leprosy, is a disease that people have recognized and hated since antiquity. Today, most developed nations, including the United States, have eliminated glanders. It still persists in some Eastern European, African, and Asian countries, including China, Mongolia, and Myanmar. U.S. federal regulations prohibit the import of any horse that has not tested negative for glanders.

Heartwater. This tickborne rickettsial disease of cattle and other ruminants derives its name from the autopsy findings, which usually include fluid buildup in the sac surrounding the heart and in the lungs. Heartwater is often fatal within a week after the first appearance of symptoms, which usually include high fever with convulsions and abnormal behavior; the disease may easily be mistaken for rabies, tetanus, meningitis, or poisoning. It also occurs in a milder form in endemic areas. The disease apparently originated in South Africa and later spread to the Caribbean, where it now occurs on several islands.

The disease is not present in the United States, but the white-tailed deer is highly susceptible to the infection and could serve as a reservoir if it were accidentally introduced. In 1999, scientists in Florida found the heartwater pathogen in ticks found on tortoises imported from Africa.

Johne's Disease or *Paratuberculosis*. This infection is present in about 20 percent of all cattle herds in the United States, where it costs the cattle industry an estimated $200 million per year by causing diarrhea and weight loss. The agent, *Mycobacterium avium paratuberculosis* (MAP), was discussed in Chapter 3 as the possible agent of Crohn's disease in humans. Johne's disease also affects sheep, goats, deer, elk, and bison. It is presently incurable and hard to eradicate, as the agent can survive for years in soil, water, and manure. In some cases, this bacterium may even survive pasteurization of milk.

Leptospirosis. An account of this disease appears in Chapter 2, as it also affects humans in significant numbers. Susceptible livestock species include cattle, sheep, horses, and swine. The effects of leptospirosis may include meningitis, jaundice, infertility, abortion, and/or a decrease in milk production; many animals become chronic carriers of the disease. Commercial vaccines based on whole cell products are available, and experimental vaccines based on cellular extracts have been tested.

Pneumonic Pasteurellosis or *Shipping Fever*. The agent of this disease, a bacterium called *Pasteurella haemolytica*, causes greater economic losses to the beef cattle industry than all other pathogens combined. Most of the deaths occur in weaned beef calves soon after they arrive at the feedlot.

Shipping fever is not always contagious in the usual sense. The bacteria that cause this disease are normally present in the lungs and do not pose a threat to healthy cattle. When the animal undergoes environmental stress, however, the associated physiological changes cause these bacteria to multiply rapidly and change their surface antigens. This biotype switch enables the bacteria to colonize the upper respiratory tract, and the infected animal then releases them as an aerosol that can infect the rest of the herd. (Of course, if the rest of the calves are equally stressed, this step may be unnecessary.) Meanwhile, the bacteria release an exotoxin that attacks leukocytes, and the death of these cells releases chemicals that cause necrosis of the surrounding lung tissue. The animals often develop pneumonia and heart failure.

Reducing the incidence of this disease may involve better management of calves to reduce stress associated with shipping and processing, as well as the development of effective vaccines.

Viral Diseases

African Swine Fever (ASF). This acute infectious disease of pigs causes a high fever with hemorrhages in the skin and various internal organs. The fatality rate sometimes approaches 100 percent, and the virus can survive for months in fresh or salted meat products. As of 2001, only one African nation, the Ivory Coast, had succeeded in eradicating ASF. This victory required a public awareness campaign, import restrictions, and the slaughter of infected pigs. The United Nations Food and Agriculture Organization (FAO) has established programs in several African countries to aid in control of this disease.

The ASF virus is similar to the poxviruses. Without laboratory tests, this disease is hard to distinguish from classical swine fever or hog cholera. At present, no ASF vaccine is available.

Avian Influenza. This disease can infect chickens, turkeys, and other poultry as well as wild birds. There are many different strains, including an extremely infectious and deadly form called HPAI (highly pathogenic avian influenza). Birds often die suddenly, sometimes after showing signs such as coughing, diarrhea, or nasal discharge. Migratory ducks are the natural reservoir, and most strains are not directly transmissible to humans (see Chapter 4). In Hong

Kong in 1997, however, at least 18 people contracted an influenza strain called H5N1 directly from chickens, and six of the victims died. Poultry workers should use face masks and other safety equipment, both to protect themselves and to avoid spreading influenza from one farm to another. Birds cannot legally be imported to the United States without testing negative for this disease.

Borna Disease. This neurological disease occurs not only in horses, cattle, and sheep, but also in rabbits, ostriches, and primates. Although Borna is not yet a recognized zoonosis, recent evidence suggests that the virus can infect people, possibly causing schizophrenia and other neuropsychiatric disorders.

In horses, the disease takes the form of viral encephalomyelitis. The animals typically lose coordination, show abnormal yawning and chewing movements, and tend to lean against objects. Once symptoms appear, the case fatality rate may be 95 percent in horses and 50 percent in sheep; however, many cases are clinically inapparent. Animals apparently acquire the virus from contaminated food and water or by contact with infective secretions of other animals. The virus enters the central nervous system through nerve endings in the nose and throat. The disease apparently results from the host's cell-mediated immune response, not from the virus itself.

Classical Swine Fever or *Hog Cholera*. Although eradicated from the United States in 1978, this highly contagious viral disease of swine causes frequent outbreaks in other countries. In its acute form, the disease causes a high fever and death within two weeks. Chronic and clinically inapparent cases also occur. Contaminated food or objects can transmit the disease; birds, flies, and human beings can also transfer the virus from one pig to another, but do not become infected.

Europe has had three major outbreaks of this disease since 1990. The latest, in 1997, resulted in the deaths of nearly six million pigs in the Netherlands alone. At present, the only treatment is to slaughter the infected animals and quarantine the affected area.

Equine Infectious Anemia. This highly contagious and often fatal disease affects horses, donkeys, and related animals. It has a worldwide distribution and was first recognized in the United States in 1888. The virus first attacks the immune system and then the red blood cells. Horses that survive the acute phase develop a chronic illness with fever, small hemorrhages in the mucous membranes, loss of weight, and anemia.

The agent is a type of retrovirus called a lentivirus, similar in many respects to HIV. It is unique among known retroviruses, however, in that it is vectorborne. Horseflies, deerflies, and other large biting insects can transmit the disease. The virus shows antigenic drift, or the ability to change its form in such a way that existing antibodies do not recognize it. U.S. Federal regulations prohibit the import of any horse that has not tested negative for this disease. There is no vaccine or treatment at present. A live attenuated virus is available, but many researchers are concerned about the possibility of infecting healthy horses.

Foot-and-Mouth Disease (FMD or Hoof-and-Mouth Disease). This is a highly contagious disease of cattle, pigs, and sheep. It

Crop and Livestock Pathogens and Pests

causes fever with lesions on the mouth, teats, and feet. Animals catch the disease by contact with infected animals or contaminated objects and surfaces, by ingestion of contaminated feed or water, or by airborne transmission. Infected bulls also have transmitted the virus in their semen. Most animals recover but are often weakened, and severe economic losses can result from reduced production of meat and milk. Vaccines available as of 2001 are helpful, but not entirely effective. Several other livestock diseases can cause similar symptoms, and owners should promptly report any suspicious illness to animal disease control officials.

The last outbreak in the United States occurred in 1929, but the disease remains widespread in Africa, South America, Asia, and parts of eastern Europe. Recent large FMD outbreaks have occurred in Iraq and in the Community of Independent States, which lack the infrastructure needed for an effective vaccination program. In 2001, Great Britain also had an outbreak, with 2030 confirmed cases in livestock. About four million animals were killed as a control measure; a more innovative response was the use of a mathematical model to determine the relative efficacy of vaccination vs. culling to stop epidemics. A few people also contracted the disease, but all recovered. (At a news conference, Prime Minister Tony Blair described how a farm worker contracted FMD when a rotting cow carcass exploded.)

Hendra Virus or *Equine Morbillivirus*. This recently identified virus affects both horses and humans (see Chapter 4) and is often fatal. The virus is closely related to the agents of measles, canine distemper, and rinderpest. The only known outbreak occurred in Australia in 1994, and the natural host has not yet been identified. Symptoms include a high fever, labored breathing, and a nasal discharge. Autopsy shows fluid and blood in the lungs. Horses appear to contract the disease from contact with secretions of an infected animal. There is no evidence that this disease can spread from one person to another, but it is hard to generalize from only three known human cases.

Lumpy Skin Disease. The agent of this disease is a poxvirus that causes fever, ulcerating nodules on the skin and mucous membranes, swollen lymph nodes, and death in as many as 20 percent of cases. Lumpy skin disease apparently infects only cattle, although sheep and goats have similar diseases. The virus is not transmissible to humans.

The virus appears to be vectorborne, and its range has expanded rapidly in the past century. It appeared in Zambia in 1929, spread to Botswana in 1943, and finally reached South Africa, where it infected over eight million cattle and caused great economic loss. In 1957 it reached Kenya in the form of a sheep pox epidemic. The disease was in the Sudan by 1970 and in Nigeria by 1974, and by the mid-1980s it affected much of central Africa. In 1988 it spread to Egypt, and isolated outbreaks have occurred in Israel and Bahrain.

Attenuated strains of the virus have been used successfully as vaccines; strains derived from sheep and goats are also effective in cattle and vice versa.

Maedi-Visna. This retrovirus causes two different diseases in sheep: a chronic form of pneumonia called maedi, first described in Iceland in 1947, and a progressive inflammation of the brain and spinal cord called visna. The disease spreads slowly through a flock, probably by direct contact, and has an incubation period of at least two years. Clinical illness may last several months and is always fatal. Maedi-visna now occurs in North America, Africa, Asia, and Europe, as well as in Iceland. There is no known treatment or cure.

Newcastle Disease. Also called exotic Newcastle disease, this is one of the most highly contagious and virulent diseases of poultry. Many birds die without showing clinical signs, and the fatality rate is nearly 100 percent in unvaccinated flocks. Symptoms include respiratory distress, diarrhea, paralysis, and swelling of the eyes and neck. The agent is an airborne virus that also spreads by direct or indirect contact; even persons who vaccinate flocks may inadvertently spread the disease between birds in the process. The vaccine is available for administration either as an aerosol (in a tightly closed building) or in drinking water.

Although Newcastle has not occurred in domestic poultry in the United States since 1974, it is still prevalent in other countries. Parrots may carry the disease without showing symptoms, and there is a risk that smuggled parrots and other pet birds from South America may reintroduce this disease to the United States. The USDA is so concerned about this possibility that it advises poultry farmers not to hire employees who own pet birds.

In 1997 and 1998, wildlife officials reported that Newcastle disease had killed several thousand double-crested cormorants at southern California's Salton Sea. Earlier mass die-offs of wild birds east of the Rockies had also resulted from Newcastle outbreaks, which pose a continual threat to the poultry industry.

Pseudorabies. The agent of this highly contagious disease of swine and other livestock is a herpesvirus that spreads by contact and affects the central nervous system. It has been present in the United States for over 150 years, and it now costs the pork industry over $30 million each year in lost animals and vaccination costs. Despite an effective eradication program, nearly two million swine in this country remained infected as of 1998, more than half of them in Indiana and Iowa. Recently, some producers have stopped vaccinating their herds in order to cut costs, and the result could be a serious resurgence of pseudorabies. USDA programs are in place to prevent this outcome.

Pseudorabies has two forms, neurotropic and pneumotropic. The first form causes the pig to behave in an uncoordinated fashion, often with severe itching and convulsions. The second appears as an upper respiratory infection with nasal irritation and pneumonia, sometimes in combination with depression or other neurological signs. Both forms may cause fetal death and abortion. Some pigs become chronic carriers of pseudorabies and can infect others. Cattle, sheep, and other animals that catch pseudorabies usually die within a few days.

Rabies. Chapter 5 describes this important disease of livestock and humans.

Rift Valley Fever. The agent of this vectorborne hemorrhagic fever is a bunyavirus that can infect humans or livestock. Cattle, sheep, and other ruminants develop a high fever and enlarged lymph nodes, often with vomiting and diarrhea; the actual cause of death appears to be liver damage.

The death rate in sheep can be as high as 100 percent, and pregnant sheep often abort. Cattle are less susceptible than sheep, with death rates usually on the order of 10 percent. Symptoms in cattle may include salivation and reduced milk production. In humans, the disease may resemble influenza, sometimes with complications such as liver or eye damage or encephalitis.

Outbreaks of this disease in livestock often are associated with above-average rainfall that favors a high mosquito population. Human outbreaks have resulted from mosquito bites and also from laboratory accidents. Both live and attenuated vaccines are available for livestock, and there is also an experimental vaccine for humans, although it is not widely available. In 2000, an outbreak of Rift Valley fever in Saudi Arabia and Yemen killed over 200 people.

Rinderpest. This deadly cattle plague is caused by a virus that is closely related to the agent of measles. A major outbreak in east Africa in 1982–1984 not only devastated local economies, with total losses estimated at U.S. $500 million, but also threatened wildlife in Serengeti National Park. Thus, in 1997, the FAO began a major campaign of vaccination and surveillance, with the ambitious goal of eradicating rinderpest from the world by 2010.

Vesicular Stomatitis. This reemerging viral disease of cattle, horses, and swine occurs only in North, Central, and South America. It is often confused with foot-and-mouth disease, as both cause painful lesions on the tongue, lips, nostrils, teats, and feet. Most animals infected with vesicular stomatitis do not become ill, but can still transmit the disease. About 10 percent of animals in a herd are likely to show symptoms; the disease is not fatal, but the animals lose weight, produce less milk, and may refuse to nurse. Economic losses can be severe for dairy farmers and moderate for beef producers. Transmission usually results from contact with contaminated objects and surfaces, but insect vectors also may be involved. Many wild animals are susceptible and may serve as a reservoir for the disease. People who handle livestock also can contract vesicular stomatitis in a mild flu-like form, usually without the lesions. A vaccine for cattle is available, but its effectiveness is in question.

Protozoal Diseases

Babesiosis. Several tickborne protozoans in the genus *Babesia* cause severe illness in livestock and occasionally in humans (see Chapter 5). The agents of cattle babesiosis are *Babesia divergens*, *B. bovis*, *B. bigemina*, and possibly other related species. The vectors are ticks (*Ixodes* and others), and the disease occurs in the Americas, Africa, Asia, Europe, and Australia. It is not clear whether any of these same protozoans also infect humans, but a related species found in mice (*Babesia microti*) has caused human babesiosis in the United States. Another form of babesiosis found in horses is described later in this chapter as equine piroplasmosis.

Babesiosis is similar to malaria in that both pathogens are protozoa that multiply inside red blood cells. In cattle, the main symptoms are a high fever, anemia, a lack of coordination, and general circulatory shock. Animals that recover have lifelong immunity. An effective live vaccine is available.

Blackhead Disease of Turkeys. At present, no treatment is available for this common and serious disease, caused by the protozoan *Histomonas meleagridis*. Turkeys ingest it while scratching in contaminated soil. The parasite cannot survive long outside a host, but can live in the common earthworm or in eggs of a harmless parasite of birds called the cecal worm. The eggs may remain viable for a long time. A medication for this disease was pulled from the market because of possible health risks to humans. Chickens can be carriers, but usually do not get sick. A feed additive is available to help prevent infection, but the additive is toxic to waterfowl if released into the environment. Symptoms are loss of appetite with wasting of the breast muscle, and damage to the intestine and liver.

Coccidiosis. The agents of this disease are protozoa (*Eimeria*, *Isospora*, and others) that occur in cattle, sheep, swine, dogs, chickens, turtles, and many other animals. Related protozoans also cause three diseases shared with humans: cyclosporiasis, cryptosporidiosis, and toxoplasmosis (see Chapters 2 and 3). The main symptom in most animals is diarrhea, and the life cycle is similar to that previously described for the human coccidioses. Cattle may ingest the protozoa in water or when grazing near the roots of plants. Anticoccidial medications are available for most livestock and poultry.

Dourine. This often-fatal disease results from infestation with a flagellated protozoan (*Trypanosoma equiperdum*) that occurs in horses, donkeys, and related animals. It is the only known trypanosome that is sexually transmitted rather than vectorborne, and the only one that is mainly a tissue parasite and rarely invades the blood. U.S. federal regulations prohibit the import of any horse that has not tested negative for this disease; control requires slaughtering infected animals.

A related parasite of cattle (*Trypanosoma theileri*) also is called dourine; studies have shown that up to 70 percent of cattle in some herds are infected without evidence of disease.

Equine Piroplasmosis. This tickborne disease is a form of babesiosis that results from infection with either of two agents, *Babesia equi* or *B. caballi*. It occurs mainly in Central and South America, Africa, and the Middle East. The case fatality rate is as high as 20 percent. U.S. federal regulations prohibit the import of any horse that has not tested negative for this disease. The last major outbreak in the United States was in Florida in 1961.

Surra. The agent of this disease, *Trypanosoma evansi*, can infest many different mammals including cattle, sheep, pigs, horses, camels, elephants, dogs, and deer. Symptoms vary widely from one species to another. The acute form of the disease causes intermittent fever, emaciation, swelling of the legs, and death in horses, camels, and llamas. In cattle, sheep, and pigs, the disease may be clinically inapparent. The two main vectors of this pathogen are *Tabanas* horseflies and (in the New World) vampire bats. No vaccine is available.

Fungal Diseases

Cryptococcosis. This is also a disease of human beings (see Chapter 4). Cattle may contract cryptococcosis by inhaling the spores, by eating contaminated feed, or by contact with contaminated milking equipment. As in humans, infection is most likely

159

to occur near accumulations of dried bird droppings. The disease, however, takes a different form in cattle than in humans, appearing as a primary infection of the mammary glands. Our best advice is to keep the barn clean.

Histoplasmosis. Again, this disease also affects humans (see Chapter 4). It causes a mild respiratory illness in cattle that inhale the spores, a common occurrence in barns with large accumulations of pigeon or starling droppings. The disease is less severe in cattle than in humans.

Multicellular Parasites

Livestock, like the rest of creation, can harbor numerous worms and other parasites. As some of these appear in earlier chapters as human parasites, the following discussion is limited to a few relatively interesting examples.

Screwworm (**Cochliomyia hominivorax**). The New World screwworm is the larva (maggot or immature stage) of a large tropical fly that lays its eggs in the open wounds of cattle and other livestock, as well as wild mammals and occasionally humans (see Chapter 4). The eggs hatch, and the larvae feed on the flesh surrounding the wound. When full-grown, the larvae drop to the ground, where they form protective cases and later hatch into adult flies.

The United States has been free of screwworm since 1966, except for a 1976 outbreak in Texas that cost over $375 million to control. The reintroduction of this insect could cost the livestock industry an estimated $750 million in production losses each year.

USDA eradicated the screwworm from the southwestern and southeastern states in the 1950s and 1960s by releasing laboratory-raised sterile male screwflies to mate with females. In 1972, the United States and Mexico formed a joint commission to eliminate the screwworm from Mexico, an effort that succeeded in 1991; two outbreaks in Mexico in 1992 and 1993 were successfully contained. The next goal is to push the fly-free zone southward to the border of Colombia.

Infection or toxicity resulting from a heavy screwworm infestation, if not treated, can kill an animal in a few weeks. In some cases, a single wound contains as many as 3000 larvae. Treatment of an infested animal involves removing the larvae from wounds with tweezers and applying organophosphate insecticides.

Tracheal* and *Varroa Mites of Honeybee. Prophecy is easy to identify after the fact. In 1975, the author of a bestselling cookbook wrote:

Although most grains are wind-pollinated, few of us realize how large and often unexpected a role insect life plays in pollination, and how insecticides can destroy this vital link in the food chain. The current abundance of fruit and vegetables in America can be traced in large part to the importation of the honeybee. . . . Today, guarding against losing helpful insects is as important as destroying insect enemies.[1]

A few years later, the premonition came true, but in an unexpected way. It was not the much-maligned pesticides that killed the honeybees after all, but two of God's own creatures. The first varroa and tracheal mites arrived on bees imported from

[1]Irma S. Rombauer and M.R. Becker, *The Joy of Cooking* (New York: Bobbs-Merrill, 1975).

Europe in the mid-1980s, and within ten years had destroyed 95 percent of all wild honeybees in North America. (Honeybees were foreign to North America in the first place, but we have no record of what native bees their importation might have displaced.)

The varroa mite (Figure 6.1) attaches itself to the top of the bee's head, and the smaller tracheal mite invades the bee's equivalent of a windpipe. In only 15 years since their arrival, these bee mites have become resistant to the pesticides beekeepers use to control them. The scarcity of wild honeybees has seriously affected over 90 bee-pollinated fruit and vegetable crops, as well as the honey industry itself. Early efforts to control the mite focused on massive use of pesticides, which, of course, selected for resistant strains of mites. To combat these strains, the industry hopes to introduce Russian honeybees, which are better able to withstand the mites than their American cousins.

***Vampire Bat* (Desmodus rotundus).** A mosquito does not draw enough blood to weaken an animal, so we usually call it a

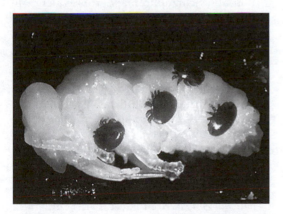

Figure 6.1. Varroa Bee Mite (*Varroa jacobsoni*). (*Source*: Texas A&M University.)

disease vector rather than a parasite. The vampire bat, however, qualifies as both. In parts of South America, as many as 20 vampires may feed on one cow in a day. The bite can transmit various diseases, including rabies and surra. At least 100,000 cattle in Latin America die each year from rabies transmitted by this bat (which also bites humans). Vampire bats do not occur in the United States at present.

Prion Diseases

A prion is an infectious particle that is smaller than a virus and composed entirely of protein. It is difficult to kill, as it is not alive in the first place. Prions cause disease in humans and in domesticated cattle, sheep, mink, dogs, and cats, as well as in wild deer, elk, and other mammals. Chapter 3 discusses bovine spongiform encephalopathy (BSE) and scrapie, and their apparent relationship to human Creutzfeldt-Jakob disease.

***Bovine Spongiform Encephalopathy (BSE)* or *Mad Cow Disease*.** As explained earlier, the origin of this disease is controversial, but alternative theories are unproven at present, so we will stick to the party line. First diagnosed in Great Britain in 1986, BSE is a prion disease that has substantially impacted the cattle industry in several European countries. To date, there have been no confirmed cases of BSE in the United States, and strict programs are in place to keep it out, including a ban on the import of ruminants from Europe.

Symptoms of BSE include changes in behavior or temperament, lack of coordination, and loss of body weight. The infected cow develops symptoms after an incubation period of two to eight years and dies within a few weeks or months. No test is currently available to detect the disease in a living animal; the diagnosis is made by post-mortem examination of brain tissue, which appears spongy when viewed under a microscope. Mice can be inoculated with material taken from cows believed to be infected, but detection of the agent by that method can take up to two years.

Scrapie. This neurological disease of sheep apparently originated in the British Isles or in western Europe and now occurs throughout the world, except in Australia and New Zealand. The first known case of scrapie in the United States was in Michigan in 1947. Since then, the disease has appeared in nearly 1000 flocks in this country.

Infected sheep display changes in behavior, such as lack of coordination, hopping, swaying, or a tendency to bite themselves and rub against objects. If startled, an infected sheep may fall down or have convulsions. Scrapie is 100 percent fatal within a few months, but several other diseases and toxins can cause similar clinical signs in sheep. A genetic mutation in some sheep protects them from scrapie by prolonging the incubation period; these individuals tend to die of natural causes before they have time to contract the disease.

REFERENCES AND RECOMMENDED READING

Alvord, Valerie. "Illegal Import of Exotic Birds Is Growing." *San Diego Union-Tribune*, October 11, 1999.

Beran, George W., and Steele, James H. (Editors). 1994. *Handbook of Zoonoses, Section A: Bacterial, Rickettsial, Chlamydial, and Mycotic.* 2nd ed. Boca Raton, FL: CRC Press.

Beran, George W., and Steele, James H. (Editors). 1994. *Handbook of Zoonoses, Section B: Viral.* 2nd ed. Boca Raton, FL: CRC Press.

"Cholera Kills 4,000 Birds at Migratory Stopover." Associated Press, January 6, 1999.

Cockrum, E. Lendell. 1997. *Rabies, Lyme Disease, Hanta Virus, and Other Animal-Borne Human Diseases in the United States and Canada.* Cambridge, MA: Fisher Books.

Cravens, R. "Epidemiology and Pathogenesis of Pneumonic Pasteurellosis and a Statistical Analysis of Vaccine Trials." *Pfizer Technical Bulletin*, July 1996.

Diamond, Jared. 1992. "The Arrow of Disease." *Discover*, October 1992, pp. 64–73.

Ferguson, N.M., et al. "The Foot-and-Mouth Epidemic in Great Britain: Pattern of Spread and Impact of Interventions." *Science*, May 11, 2001, pp. 1155–1160.

"Foot-and-Mouth Disease Outbreak in Great Britain." Richmond, VA: United States Animal Health Association, National Animal Health Emergency Management System, February 2001.

Garvin, Glenn. "Vampire Bats Have Nicaragua under Siege." Knight Ridder News Service, December 17, 1999.

Hungerford, Tom G. 1991. *Diseases of Livestock.* 9th ed. New York: McGraw-Hill.

"Imported Bees Enlisted for War." Reuters News Service, August 13, 1999.

Iwahashi, K., et al. "Borna Disease Virus Infection and Schizophrenia: Seroprevalence in Schizophrenia Patients." *Canadian Journal of Psychiatry*, March 1998, p. 197.

Liess, B. (Editor). 1988. *Classical Swine Fever and Related Viral Infections.* Developments in Veterinary Virology series. Zoetermeer, The Netherlands: Martinus Nijhoff.

Morrison, Douglas (Editor). 1998. *Prions and Brain Diseases in Animals and Humans.* New York: Plenum Press.

Office International des Epizooties. 1997. *Diagnostic Manual for Aquatic Animal Diseases.* 2nd ed. Paris: OIE.

Office International des Epizooties. 2000. *International Animal Health Code.* Paris: OIE.

Olsen, Glenn H., and Orosz, Susan E. 2000. *Manual of Avian Medicine.* St. Louis: Mosby.

Pasteur, Louis. 1969. *Correspondence of Pasteur and Thuillier Concerning Anthrax and Swine Fever Vaccinations*. Translated and edited by Robert M. Frank and Denise Wrotnowska. University, AL: University of Alabama Press.

"Researcher on Army Vaccine Infected with Rare Bacterial Disease." Associated Press, May 15, 2000.

Roberts, Ronald J. 1997. *Handbook of Trout and Salmon Diseases*. 3rd ed. Cambridge, MA: Fishing News Books.

Sainsbury, David. 1998. *Animal Health: Health, Disease, and Welfare of Farm Animals*. Malden, MA: Blackwell Science.

Smithcors, J.F., and Smithcors, A. 1997. *Five Centuries of Veterinary Medicine*. Pullman, WA: Washington State University Press.

Spence, Cinty. "Varroa Bee Mite, Now Resistant to Miticide, Again Threatens Honeybees." News Release, University of Florida, March 11, 1998.

Studdert, M.J. (Editor). 1996. *Virus Infections of Equines*. New York: Elsevier.

Swartz, T.A., et al. (Editors). 1981. *Rift Valley Fever*. New York: S. Karger Publ.

United Nations Food and Agriculture Organization. 1988. *Rice in Indonesia: Status after Three Crop Seasons*. Jakarta: FAO.

U.S. Department of Agriculture. 1976. *Ticks of Veterinary Importance*. Washington, DC: U.S. Government Printing Office.

U.S. Department of Agriculture. 1989. *Rift Valley Fever: A Mosquito-Borne Exotic Disease of Sheep, Cattle, and Humans*. Washington, DC: U.S. Government Printing Office.

DISEASES OF CROPS

There are so many different plant crops and associated diseases that the following paragraphs can present only a small sample. For more information on plant diseases or their control, readers should contact their local Cooperative Extension Service or Integrated Pest Management project, or consult the references at the end of this section and in Chapter 12.

Bacterial Diseases

Bacterial Leaf Spot (BLS). The pathogen is a bacterium (*Xanthomonas campestris*) that infects the leaves and stems of various plants, including citrus fruits, peppers, cucumbers, and lettuce. Related bacteria also affect stone fruits and other crops. The spots first appear on the underside of leaves (or on outer leaves in lettuce), gradually turning black and becoming larger until the leaves drop off. Spots also appear on fruit, where they resemble blisters that may extend into the interior of the fruit. The disease is transmitted by seed and by infected transplants.

Bacterial Wilt. This disease, caused by the bacterium *Ralsonia* (or *Pseudomonas*) *solanacearum*, is one of the most important bacterial plant diseases in the world. It is particularly devastating in the tropics, where it affects tomato, potato, banana, eggplant, ginger, and other crops. The wide host range, latency in nonhost plants, resistance to control measures, and problems in identification have made this disease hard to eradicate. Researchers in Australia are developing a molecular identification system for use in the field, and are also studying the genetic interaction between the bacterium and its plant host, to determine how the bacterium can switch from virulence to avirulence.

Citrus Canker. This highly contagious disease, caused by the bacterium *Xanthomonas axonopodis* var. *citri*, may be the world's most serious disease of citrus crops. Lesions appear on the fruit, leaves, and twigs of infected plants, resulting in damaged fruit, loss of leaves, and sometimes the destruction of entire crops. The disease first appeared in the United States in 1910; it was eradicated in this country by 1933, but not before it destroyed some 20 million citrus trees in the Gulf Coast states. Sporadic outbreaks have occurred more recently in Florida but were quickly contained by quarantine measures and the removal of infected trees. Wind, flooding, overhead irrigation, insects, birds, and humans all may spread citrus canker.

Pierce's Disease of Grape and *Variegated Chlorosis of Citrus*. An insect called the glassy-winged sharpshooter is the vector for a bacterium called *Xyella fastidiosa*, which infects grapevines and citrus trees in South America. In the early 1990s, the insect arrived in southern California, but growers expressed minimal concern because California had no citrus pathogen that it could vector. But a different strain of *Xylella fastidiosa*—one that does not infect citrus trees—was already present in northern California, where it had infected grapevines for many years with the help of a different vector, the blue-green sharpshooter. The two expatriates found each other, and in 1998 the duo began attacking vineyards in southern California. If the bacterial strain that infects citrus later arrives from Brazil, it will find its vector well established in the United States, and the cost to the citrus industry could be enormous.

At present, the most effective control measure is a soil-applied insecticide that kills the insect vectors. Releasing a parasitic wasp to destroy sharpshooter eggs is another possibility, but such biological control measures require extensive study to make sure they do not backfire.

Viral Diseases

Cassava Mosaic Virus. Like other mosaic viruses, this pathogen causes mottled coloring and malformation of leaves, resulting in necrotic lesions and reduced crop yields. Cassava is an important food crop in Africa, and devastating epidemics have recently occurred in Uganda and Kenya; the same virus also affects tobacco and datura plants. Heat treatment can produce virus-free plants, but vector control also is necessary. The vectors for this disease are whiteflies, tiny insects in the order Homoptera, which also includes the aphids, scale insects, and other important plant pests. The Consortium for International Crop Protection has recently begun a program to develop strains of cassava that are resistant to this virus and its vector.

Tobacco and Tomato Mosaic Viruses (Tobamoviruses). These viruses affect a wide range of plant species, including not only tobacco and tomatoes but also peppers, eggplant, potato, and several other crops and ornamental plants. The symptoms vary depending on the strain of plant and virus, but usually include a yellow and dark-green mottled pattern on the leaves with some leaf malformation, such as narrowing of the leaves in cool weather or a fern-like appearance. The overall result is stunting of the plant and reduction of yield.

The virus is transmitted by mechanical inoculation, grafting, contact between plants, and especially by seed, as the virus is found on the seed coat. Workers who handle tobacco products can even transmit the virus from their hands to live plants. No insects or nematodes appear to act as vectors. The virus often occurs on fresh market tomatoes, but is harmless to humans. Control methods include spraying plants and washing hands with milk; inoculating plants with a weak strain of the virus; treating seeds with heat to kill the virus (at temperatures low enough to avoid killing the seeds); and sterilizing equipment and structures.

The tobamoviruses, first reported on tobacco in 1899 and on tomato plants in 1909, were among the first plant viruses ever discovered. These viruses are very stable and can survive for many years in plant debris or on contaminated clothing. In 1999, scientists reported that this virus (and possibly others) can survive for hundreds or even thousands of years in Arctic ice. When climate change melts this ice and releases viruses back into the atmosphere, they could again infect hosts if the viral protein coats have survived intact. Some scientists believe this phenomenon may partly explain the emergence or reemergence of "new" disease epidemics.

Tomato Spotted Wilt. Despite its name, this viral disease affects not only tomatoes but several other important crops such as peanuts, onions, lettuce, and peppers. The symptoms include yellowing of leaves, dead spots on leaves and shoots, ring-shaped markings on fruit (if any), and general stunting of the plant. The virus was unknown before 1985, but now has a worldwide distribution.

The vectors for this virus include several species of tiny insects called thrips. The pathogen has a somewhat unusual structure for a plant virus, and the fact that it is not lethal to thrips has led some investigators to suggest that it might have originated as an insect virus. When immature thrips feed on an infected plant, they acquire the virus and keep it for the rest of their lives. Grafting and mechanical inoculation also can infect plants. The peanut industry in Georgia alone lost an estimated $40 million to this virus in 1997.

Insecticides can control thrips populations, but no treatment is available to kill the virus itself. Some varieties of certain crops are resistant to the virus, including several peanut varieties recently developed at the University of Florida. Some resistant tobacco varieties also are available, thanks to research funding by that industry. For most crops, the main control measures are to remove the infected plants and to avoid planting susceptible crops next to each other.

Tristeza Virus. This virus of citrus trees causes yellowing and loss of foliage. The tree may die within three to four months following infection, or may survive for several years in poor condition, typically producing small fruit. Tristeza is one of the most economically important plant diseases worldwide. It originated in South America and spread to other continents on imported trees and fruit; by the early 1990s it had destroyed over 100 million citrus trees, not only in its homeland but also in Florida and some European countries. At present, citrus growers in Florida lose about 15 percent of their trees to this disease each year.

The vectors of tristeza are the melon aphid (*Aphis gossipyii*) and other aphids. Grafting on sour orange rootstocks also can transmit the disease, which affects oranges, grapefruit, lemon, and other citrus trees. The only control measures are to destroy infected trees and to use virus-free budwood and rootstock. Preimmunization strategies and quarantine restrictions also have been effective in limiting the spread of the disease in some areas.

Algal Diseases

Algal Leaf Spot. The agent of this plant disease is the single-celled alga *Cephaleuros virescens*. It can infect citrus, apple, pecan, macadamia, cocoa, and fig trees, as well as many other plants of economic importance, such as oak, orchids, and various ornamental shrubs. It usually affects the leaves, causing discolored, circular spots with a netlike surface and wavy or feathered margin. The alga may also cause girdling lesions on twigs, providing an opportunity for fungal infection.

Recommended control practices include removal of spotted and fallen leaves, pruning of overhanging trees to reduce humidity, and applying a time-honored fungicide called Bordeaux mixture—which also works on algae—according to label directions and EPA guidelines (or the equivalent in other countries).

Fungal Diseases

In general, the most important diseases affecting crop plants are those that result from fungal infections. The following paragraphs describe a few representative fungal diseases.

Alternaria Rot. Fungi in the genus *Alternaria* affect a variety of crops including citrus, tomato, pistachio, figs, carrots, and ornamental plants. These fungi also cause asthma and can infect the cornea of the human eye (see Chapters 7 and 5, respectively).

Alternaria citri, for example, is commercially important on orange and lemon crops, causing the fruits to change color prematurely and develop dark spots at one end that extend into the core. Infection also affects seedlings, causing lesions followed by leaf drop. On carrots, the related fungus *Alternaria radicina* starts in the carrot crown at the point of leaf attachment, where a weakened black area develops that causes leaves to break off; the same fungus also can cause a leaf blight. The fungus is seedborne and also survives in plant debris and in the soil. Rain or irrigation during warm weather encourages its growth. Seeds can be soaked in hot water to kill the fungus, and crop rotation may prevent the buildup of the fungus in the soil.

Apple Scab. The agent of this disease is a fungus (*Venturia inaequalis*) that survives in dead leaves on the ground. During spring rains, the fungus releases its spores to infect young leaves and fruits; established infections on trees also release spores. The disease causes dark spots on leaves and fruits that later resemble scabs. For effective timing of fungicide application, growers must predict outbreaks on the basis of temperature and moisture conditions. Tables are available for this purpose.

Dutch Elm Disease. Most history students have heard of this wilt disease, which originated in Asia and later spread to Europe, finally reaching North America in about 1930 on a shipment of contaminated wooden crates or logs. A second accidental introduction occurred in Canada in 1944, and from there it spread to England in the 1960s. The disease has destroyed millions of elm trees (*Ulmus*) in North America, continental Europe, and England, causing losses of billions of dollars in valuable wood in addition to major aesthetic damage. As recently as the late 1990s, new outbreaks were reported.

The agents are two related fungi (*Ophiostoma ulmi* and *O. novo-ulmi*) that block the vascular system of the tree, causing wilting of shoots and yellowing of the leaves, followed by rapid defoliation. The tree may die within weeks following infection, or more slowly over a period of years. Both native North American and European bark beetles serve as vectors for the fungus, which also spreads on root grafts and contaminated pruning tools. Control of the disease requires the removal and disposal of dead wood combined with insecticide

spraying and fungicide injection. Various experimental methods are being tested.

Late Blight of Potato **(Phytopthora infestans).** This fungus (Figure 6.2) caused the Irish Famine of 1845–1847, killing an estimated one million people who depended almost entirely on the potato crop for food. More than 150 years later, late blight is still the most important pest of potato plants. The world's potato farmers now spend $1.6 billion each year controlling this fungus, and pesticide-resistant strains have recently appeared. The fungus grows very quickly in favorable weather, producing a full cycle of infection, lesion development,

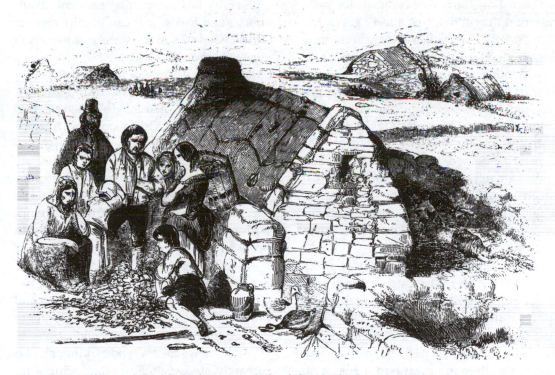

Figure 6.2. Effects of late blight fungus in Ireland during the famine of 1847. This fungus destroyed the Irish potato crop and caused a famine that killed an estimated one million people and forced another million to emigrate. (*Source*: Heraldic Artists Ltd.)

167

spore formation and dispersal, and new infection all in as little as five days.

Even opponents of biotechnology may have breathed a covert sigh of relief in 1994 when Purdue University scientists announced the development of a genetically modified potato with a built-in fungicide. As of 2001, however, such potatoes are not yet commercially available. Plant breeders using conventional methods have developed several partly resistant strains, such as the Elba potato. Promising new hybrids include AWN86514–2, developed in 1998 at the University of Idaho, and New York 121, which Cornell University announced in 2000. Trials of new fungicides also are in progress.

Peach Leaf Curl. This is one of the most common fungal diseases affecting peaches and related crops such as plums, nectarines, and almonds, particularly in areas with wet, cold winters. It causes discolored and deformed leaves, reddish lesions on fruit, and reduced yield; severely infected trees often lose branches. The agent (*Taphrina deformans*) infects leaves in the bud, and once they are infected there is no treatment. Spores are released from the surfaces of diseased leaves to infect other buds. Fortunately, growers can control peach leaf curl by applying fungicides in late winter before budding.

Wheat Rust. The term "rust" refers to a number of different parasitic fungi that infest crops, typically forming orange-red spots on the plants. Until the 1920s, wheat rust cost farmers millions of dollars every year. The disease was well known in ancient times; the Romans even had a rust god, named Robigus, and a festival called Robigalia in his honor.

When a devastating epidemic struck in 1916, Canadian farmers threatened to go on strike unless the government funded research to find a solution. That same year, Dr. Margaret Newton, a Canadian geneticist and plant pathologist, began a study of wheat rust fungi (*Puccinia graminis* and related species) and made it possible to breed rust-resistant grains that have benefited agriculture worldwide. Outbreaks still occur, however, and in regions where the fungal spores survive the winter, local rust epidemics typically reduce wheat yields by 2–10 percent. Fungicide, if required, must be applied early enough in the season to avoid leaving a residue in the grain. The Department of Plant Pathology at Kansas State University has a computer program available, called Rusty, that can predict rust severity based on soil moisture, rust inoculum survival, and other factors.

This fungus is one of many plant pathogens that also affect human health. In 1924, doctors studying asthma described the first case associated with a specific fungus, which turned out to be wheat rust. Unfortunately, Dr. Newton and other rust researchers were among those whose lungs were damaged beyond repair by years of exposure to the fungus. Scientists who work with spores now wear filtration masks to protect themselves.

At one time, biological warfare researchers in the former Soviet Union and elsewhere reportedly stockpiled wheat rust and other pathogens as potential weapons to destroy the food crops of enemy nations. In 1998, the news media reported that similar research is now aimed at deploying a related fungal strain against opium poppy crops in southern Europe and Asia. If this is true, one hopes that the plan includes suitable precautions to prevent the spread of the agent beyond its intended targets.

In the nineteenth century, farmers in England largely eliminated a wild plant called barberry (*Berberis*), which served as an intermediate host for the wheat rust fungus. In the process, they nearly drove the barberry carpet moth (*Pareulype berberata*) to extinction, as it requires the barberry plant for food; a recovery plan is now in progress. Biological control measures, although preferable to pesticide use, often involve such tradeoffs.

In 1970, American agronomist Dr. Norman Borlaug received the Nobel Peace Prize for his contributions to the development of high-yield, rust-resistant wheat strains and his efforts to introduce this crop to developing nations around the world.

Witches' Broom. This fungus (*Crinipellis perniciosa*) takes the form of a mushroom rather than a mold, and in recent years it has destroyed a significant part of the cocoa bean crop in Brazil. Between 1990 and 2000, the witches' broom and two other fungi destroyed an estimated 3 million tons of cocoa beans in South America. In some parts of Brazil, the yield has been reduced by more than 75 percent. Worldwide panic regarding a possible chocolate shortage has prompted aggressive research programs by USDA and other agencies.

One of the most promising control methods is to spray infected trees with a mixture of several strains of another fungus, called *Trichoderma virens*, which attacks the witches' broom. This method reduced the infection by about one-third in recent field trials. Efforts also are in progress to develop fungus-resistant cultivars of the cacao tree.

Multicellular Parasites

Many nematodes, arthropods, and other invertebrates attack agricultural crops, but there is a somewhat fuzzy line between microscopic plant parasites and the usually larger "pests," which follow this section.

As nematodes are the most numerous organisms on earth, we cannot begin to do them justice here, but two examples may suffice. Both of the following nematode species are subject to federal quarantine regulations.

Burrowing Nematode. This species (*Radopholus citrophilus* or *R. similis*) is a tiny endoparasitic worm that tunnels through the roots of citrus crops, causing a disease known as spreading decline that rapidly destroys infested groves. Related nematodes affect bananas and other crops. At present, the burrowing nematode occurs only in Florida.

Golden Nematode. These microscopic South American worms (*Globodera rostochiensis* and *G. pallida*) attack potato roots and have drastically affected potato yields in Europe. The species does not occur in the United States, but past introductions have occurred, and agricultural inspectors are concerned that it might be imported accidentally in soil. For that reason (and others), it is illegal to import potted plants into the United States.

PREDATORS, PESTS, AND WEEDS

Pest is an imprecise expression that usually means a small (but not microscopic) animal that damages crop plants or their stored products. A vampire bat clinging to the leg of a cow is doing about the same

169

thing that aphids do to plants, but most sources call the bat a parasite and the aphid a pest. An elephant that tramples a field in Africa is not exactly a pest; it is more like a competitor, but no specific term applies to this situation. A coyote that eats chickens is not a pest either, but an example of a **predator**. A **weed** is a plant that most people want removed from its present location, either because it competes with crop plants or because it has some other unwanted characteristic.

Many of the most serious pests and weeds in the United States are not native to this continent, but were accidentally imported from somewhere else. According to a recent estimate, non-native insect pests alone cost the U.S. economy over $19 billion each year. Some regions of the world also have non-native predators and nuisance animals that people have introduced to new areas for one reason or another, such as the mongoose (*Herpestes auropunctatus*) in Hawaii, the brown tree snake (*Boiga irregularis*) in Guam, and the black bear (*Ursus americanus*) in southern California.

Predators

Chapter 8 discusses several predators in the context of human depredations, but these animals are far more likely to attack domestic animals than humans, and livestock predation takes a heavy economic toll. The largest predators, such as the big cats, grizzly bears, and crocodiles, can kill prey of all sizes from cattle on down. Smaller livestock and poultry are also subject to predation by smaller animals, such as weasels and snakes.

The USDA estimates that predator damage costs the U.S. economy over $60 million each year, including $40 million in losses to cattle producers and over $20 million to the sheep and goat industry. Although this may sound like a lot of money, it is pocket change compared with the billions lost to pathogens and parasites. More than half the total cost of predation in the United States is attributable to one species, the coyote (*Canis latrans*), which kills hundreds of thousands of sheep and calves every year. Some other livestock predators in the United States are mountain lions (*Felis concolor*), bobcats (*Lynx rufus*), foxes (mainly *Vulpes fulva*), and bears (*Ursus horribilis* and *U. americanus*).

The USDA Wildlife Services Division has developed a device called the Electronic Guard that uses sound and light to frighten predators. The agency reports that this space-age scarecrow has been successful in keeping bears out of vineyards, deer out of cornfields, and birds out of fish farms. None of these situations quite meets the usual definition of livestock predation, however, and it is not clear whether the device would discourage mountain lions, for example, from taking sheep.

A second high-tech option, effective mainly against coyotes, is to equip sheep and goats with protective collars that contain a poison called Compound 1080. The device theoretically explodes in the predator's mouth, causing an environmentally safe and theoretically painless death. This method is controversial, for reasons that should be apparent. The M-44 cyanide ejector is another aggressive and risky way to manage predators. Livestock owners have the right to protect their investment, but safer and more effective methods would be desirable.

The traditional livestock-guarding dogs used for centuries in Europe can be highly effective if properly trained and managed. Some sheep and cattle ranchers have virtually eliminated coyote and mountain lion predation by using these large dogs, but it is important to warn human visitors. A few ranchers have successfully used llamas to guard sheep.

Crop, Cargo, and Warehouse Pests

Army Worm. Among the worst insect pests worldwide are caterpillars called army worms, the larvae of several species of owlet moths or cutworms (family Noctuidae) that lay their eggs on the leaves of various crop plants. The name refers to their habit of marching through a field in large numbers, causing widespread destruction, and then moving on.

These caterpillars have emerged in recent years as major pests of canola in Canada, corn in Pennsylvania, hay in South Carolina, and sorghum in Africa. Army worms are related to several other important crop pests, including the pink bollworm, which appears later in this chapter. Some common army worms in North America are the true army worm (*Cirphis unipuncta*), which occurs worldwide and mainly attacks grains and grasses; the beet armyworm (*Spodoptera exigua*), which attacks not only beets but also cotton, cereal, citrus, tomatoes, and other crops in Europe and the western United States; and the western army cutworm (*Chorizagrotis agrestis*), of which one author wrote in 1926: "They commonly appear in small, though occasionally in enor-mous numbers, and travel in armies, devastating everything green in their path, including native grasses and weeds, truck, forage, and cereal crops, cotton, forest, and fruit trees."[2]

Biological controls for this species include a parasitic wasp and several predators, such as spiders and damsel bugs. When the percentage of nonparasitized army worms falls below a certain level, insecticide spraying may be necessary.

Asian Long-Horned Beetle (**Anoplophora glabripennis**, *Figure 6.3*). Perhaps the only good thing about this insect is its Chinese name, which translates into English as "the shiny-shouldered starry-heaven beetle." It hitchhiked to the United States on wooden crates from China in 1998, and no known pesticide can kill it. Scientists, mindful of the song about the old woman who swallowed a fly, are properly reluctant to import Chinese predators as biological controls. Until a better solution is found, the only way to deal with the problem is to cut down all infested trees. Thus far, the beetle has turned up only in cities such as New York and Chicago—but if it becomes established in North American forests, the price tag could be on the order of $138 billion.

Boll Weevil (**Anthonomus grandis**). Although the cotton plant produces fiber and oil rather than food, its economic importance is great, and cotton pests represent a legitimate hazard. For over 100 years since its arrival from Mexico, the boll weevil has been the most important U.S. cotton pest, with total losses estimated at $14 billion.

The USDA's boll weevil program monitors all fields planted with cotton by placing traps

---

[2]E.O. Essig, *Insects of Western North America* (New York: Macmillan, 1926).

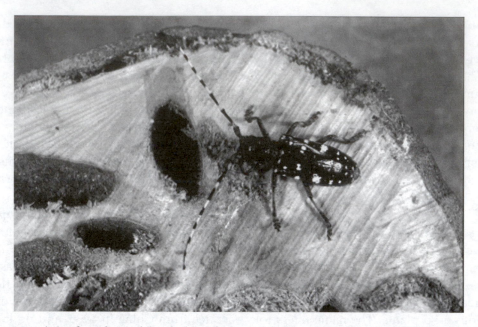

Figure 6.3. Asian long-horned Beetle (*Anoplophora glabripennis*). (*Source*: Cornell University.)

baited with a pheromone that attracts weevils and kills them using an insecticide. This method is more effective than visual detection alone in identifying low levels of weevil infestation; by killing some weevils, it also serves as a control measure. As of 2000, this program had eradicated the boll weevil in Virginia, North and South Carolina, Georgia, Florida, southern Alabama, California, and Arizona. The insect remains a serious problem in several other states.

In 1995, Texas cotton growers demonstrated the complexity of species interactions by spraying large amounts of the insecticide malathion over a wide area, with the intention of killing boll weevils and protecting the cotton crop. With the weevils out of the way, the result was a massive outbreak of their competitors, such as beet armyworms, cotton aphids, and sweet potato whiteflies. All are secondary cotton pests, and they proceeded to destroy more cotton than the boll weevil alone could have done.

Brown Planthopper (**Nilapanuata lugens**)**.** In the 1970s, Java joined the list of nations where pesticides have caused unexpected problems. In an effort to reduce its dependence on foreign rice imports, the government launched a "green revolution" program with high-yield rice strains, irrigation, and extensive pesticide and fertilizer use. Such programs often are successful if combined with integrated pest management (IPM) principles, such as multiple cropping and rotation; in this case, however, the outcome was poor.

The pesticides killed predators that normally kept the brown planthopper in check, and thus the insects multiplied, destroying over two million hectares of rice in less than two years. In 1986, when this pest threatened 70 percent of Java's rice harvest, the government established new agricultural policies that included IPM and reduced pesticide use. This program was successful, and the rice crop survived. As in all such success stories to date, however, farmers could only reduce but not eliminate the use of pesticides.

Locust Bird (Quelea quelea). Like the vampire bat in the parasite section (above), this animal may seem out of place here, simply because it has bones. But in its native Africa, the locust bird or red-billed quelea qualifies as a true agricultural pest and is treated as such.

A quelea colony can number in the tens of thousands, and a flying flock resembles a column of smoke. Although the individual birds are small, they are so numerous that rural people in Zimbabwe use them as food, sometimes gathering more than a ton of baby queleas per day during the nesting season. But that food comes at the expense of the nation's economy; the bird is so destructive to winter cereal crops that farmers are reluctant to plant them, sometimes resorting to food aid instead. Others switch to growing maize, which the quelea cannot eat, but the maize crop needs more water to grow and often fails in dry years. Foreigners who do not understand the problem make it worse, by demanding that the little birds be allowed to live in peace. Africans need the protein in one form or another, whether as the cereal they planted or the birds that consumed it.

The usual method of controlling queleas (other than eating them) is to spray fields with high levels of organophosphate pesticides. In 1995, Senegal and Mauritania began a joint spraying program to combat the quelea in the Senegal River Valley. Although driven by necessity, such plans have obvious disadvantages that call for safer and more environmentally responsible alternatives. IPM measures include lethal control combined with other methods such as crop management, better forecasting of outbreaks, exclusion netting, and variations on the traditional scarecrow.

Locust. There are many different species of locusts, but the one we usually mean is the desert locust of Biblical fame, *Schistocerca gregaria*. The second part of its name, *gregaria*, tells the story. These insects aggregate at times in immense swarms, and billions may descend on a field, destroying the entire crop within hours. Without pesticides, a country such as Tunisia would lose an estimated 40 percent of its wheat and barley crops to locusts.

FAO and other organizations have developed computer models to predict locust outbreaks, based on weather and vegetation data from satellite images and on historical trends in locust population dynamics. Ground surveillance programs by national crop protection services and the military also are effective in finding locust bands and swarms. Anticipating these outbreaks can help greatly in planning effective control operations. Technology and communications have come a long way since Moses confronted the Pharaoh Ramses with a similar challenge; but forecasting is an inexact science without divine aid, and locust plagues continue.

An interesting alternative to pesticides, practiced in much of French-speaking West and North Africa, is to serve the locusts for dinner as *crevettes du Sahara* ("shrimp of the desert"). The sheer biomass of locusts, if harvested on a large scale, could help solve the problem of protein shortage in Africa. Both control strategies cannot be used at the same time, however, and more efficient harvesting methods would be needed to make a significant dent in the problem.

Mediterranean Fruit Fly **(Ceratitis capitata).** The Medfly, called Moscamed in Spanish-speaking countries, is one of the world's most destructive agricultural pests. The female fly lays its eggs under the skin of more than 250 varieties of fruit; the larvae hatch and feed, causing extensive damage.

Despite its name, this insect is nothing like the tiny *Drosophila* fruit flies used in laboratory experiments, nor is it native to the Mediterranean region. The Mediterranean fruit fly originated in Africa and has spread through most tropical and subtropical regions of the world. It is nearly as large as a common housefly, with dark blue eyes and a yellow abdomen with silver crossbands. The wings have a blotched pattern of yellow, brown, and black.

The Medfly became established in Hawaii in 1910. Outbreaks have occurred in Florida, California, and several Mexican states, but aggressive campaigns of trapping, spraying, and sterile Medfly release have been largely successful, despite legitimate public concern about the human health effects of organophosphate pesticides. If the Medfly ever becomes established in the continental United States, the annual losses to the fruit industry could exceed $1.5 billion.

Pink Bollworm. This caterpillar, considered the world's most destructive cotton pest, is the larva of a small moth (*Pectinophora gossypiella*) that lays its eggs on young cotton bolls. When the larvae hatch, they bore into the cotton bolls and eat the seeds, then drop to the ground to complete their life cycles. The same insect can also live on the okra plant.

The species originated in Asia and arrived in the United States before 1917, probably in a shipment of cotton seed from Mexico. It is reported to cause cotton losses of 20 percent or higher in countries where it is well established, such as Brazil and China. In the United States, the pink bollworm presently occurs in Oklahoma, Texas, New Mexico, Arizona, and parts of several other southern states. A program of releasing sterile bollworm moths has helped to limit its spread. Scientists at the University of California are trying to improve upon this technique by introducing a lethal gene into the pink bollworm population.

Rats and Other Rodents. Two rodent species, the Norway rat (*Rattus norvegicus*) and the house mouse (*Mus musculus*), cause significant damage to stored grain and other agricultural products each year worldwide. Although one rat eats only about 25 pounds of food per year, and one mouse only about two pounds, the early maturation and high reproductive rates of these animals make the total losses staggering. According to a 1999 study, rats alone destroy about $19 billion worth of stored grain and other products in the United States each year. Rats and mice also transmit several human and livestock diseases (see Chapters 2–5) and contaminate more food than they actually eat.

Various poisons and mechanical barriers can reduce the problem; predictably, however, rats in Great Britain and other areas have become resistant to warfarin and other common rodenticides.

Weeds

Every year, the U.S. Department of Agriculture publishes the Federal Noxious Weed List on its Web site <http://www.aphis.usda.gov/ppq/weeds/>. There were nearly 100 plant species on the 1999 list. It is not entirely clear how a weed qualifies for this list, as some of the most highly publicized plant pests appear not to be on it.

The prickly yellow star thistle (*Centaurea solstitialis*), for example, is a Mediterranean weed that arrived in California at about the same time as the Gold Rush. By 1965, it occupied an estimated one million acres in the state; at latest count it had expanded to 20 million acres, thanks to El Niño rains and zealous hay-spreading operations by the highway department. Beekeepers like the thistle because it blooms late in the year, but taken as a whole it is a highly unpopular plant with many drawbacks. Its long tap root, high fecundity, and chemical arsenal enable it to outcompete more desirable native plants. In large quantities, it is poisonous to livestock, and it also has sharp spines that stick people's feet and discourage cattle from grazing. Goats will eat it, however, and fire will burn it. More aggressive measures, such as herbicide use and biological controls, may have long-term environmental consequences of their own.

One unusual weed that definitely made the federal list is American witchweed

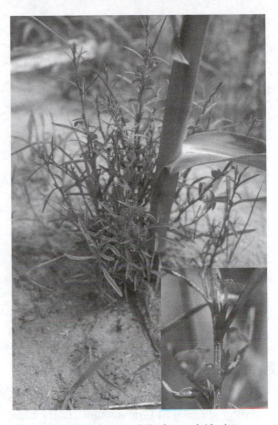

Figure 6.4. American Witchweed (*Striga asiatica*). (*Source*: Dr. Daniel L. Nickrent, Southern Illinois University, Carbondale.)

(*Striga asiatica*, Figure 6.4), a parasitic plant of African or Asian origin that arrived in the United States sometime before 1955. It is not only a weed in the usual sense, but also a parasite that extracts nutrients from the root systems of sorghum, sugar cane, rice, corn, and certain wild grasses. The USDA Animal and Plant Health Inspection Service currently offers a $25 reward to anyone who finds and reports this weed. It is about a foot tall, and its flowers are red or pink.

REFERENCES AND RECOMMENDED READING

Abrams, Isabel S. "Alien Invaders." *Current Health*, March 1992, pp. 18–20.

Allen, R. 1997. *The Grain-Eating Birds of Sub-Saharan Africa*. Kent, UK: University of Greenwich.

Becker, Hank. "Potential Chocolate Shortage May be Foiled by Beneficial Fungi." *Agricultural Research Service News*, October 25, 1999.

Benbrook, Charles M. 1997. *Pest Management at the Crossroads*. Annapolis Junction, MD: Professional Mailing and Distribution Services.

Bryant, Kris. "The Barking Anatolian Army." *Mother Earth News*, April–May 1994, p. 10.

Burton, Robin. "Unwelcome Hitchhikers." *Oceans*, July–August 1985, pp. 32–35.

Carlile, W.R. 1995. *Control of Crop Diseases*. 2nd ed. New York: Cambridge University Press.

Cooke, Martin. "The West's Secret Weapon to Win the Opium War." *Sunday Times* (UK), June 28, 1998.

"Cornell Develops Potato Resistant to Late Blight and Other Diseases." News Release, Cornell University, February 8, 2000.

Davis, John J., and Satterthwait, A.F. "Life-History Studies of *Cirphis unipuncta*, the True Army Worm." *Journal of Agricultural Research*, August 21, 1916, pp. 799–812.

Day, Peter R. (Editor). 1977. *Conference on the Genetic Basis of Epidemics in Agriculture, New York, 1976*. Annals of the New York Academy of Sciences, Vol. 287. New York: New York Academy of Sciences.

Elliott, C., and Craig, A. "Quelea: Integrated Pest Management vs. Lethal Control." In Adams, N.J., and Slotow, R.H. (Editors). Proceedings of the 22nd International Ornithological Congress, Durban. *Ostrich*, Vol. 69, 1998.

Fry, William E., and Goodwin, Stephen B. "Resurgence of the Irish Potato Famine Fungus." *BioScience*, June 1997.

Gibson, R.W., et al. "Unusually Severe Symptoms Are a Characteristic of the Current Epidemic of Mosaic Virus Disease of Cassava in Uganda." *Annals of Applied Biology*, Vol. 131, 1996, pp. 259–271.

Goto, Masao. 1992. *Fundamentals of Bacterial Plant Pathology*. San Diego: Academic Press.

Gowans, Jill. "Feathered Locust Plague." *The Sunday Tribune*, Durban, August 17, 1998.

Gray, Peter. 1995. *The Irish Famine*. New York: Harry N. Abrams.

Hayward, A.C., and Hartman, G.L. 1994. *Bacterial Wilt: The Disease and Its Causative Agent, Pseudomonas solonacearum*. Wallingford, UK: CAB.

Liu, D., et al. "Osmotin Overexpression in Potato Delays Development of Disease Symptoms." *Proceedings of the National Academy of Sciences*, Vol. 91, 1994, p. 1888 ff.

MacKenzie, Debora. "Run, Radish, Run." *New Scientist*, December 18, 1999.

Maramorosch, Karl, and McKelvey, John J., Jr. 1985. *Subviral Pathogens of Plants and Animals: Viroids and Prions*. Orlando, FL: Academic Press.

Pimentel, David, et al. "Environmental and Economic Costs Associated with Non-indigenous Species in the United States." Report presented at the annual meeting of the American Association for the Advancement of Science, Anaheim, CA, January 24, 1999.

Pottinger, Matt. "China Scientist Battles Beetle that Bugs Us." Reuters News Service, October 27, 1998.

Rahn, Dan. "The Trouble with Thrips." *University of Georgia Research Reporter*, Summer 1999, pp. 25–31.

Somerville, Alexander. 1995. *Letters from Ireland during the Famine of 1847*. Dublin: Irish Academic Press.

Spake, Amanda. "Robbing Fruit of Its Vine." *U.S. News and World Report*, June 26, 2000.

"Star Thistle Ranges Far, Spreading Its Misery." Associated Press, January 20, 1999.

Sutic, D.D., Ford, R.E., and Tosic, M.T. (Editors). 1999. *Handbook of Plant Virus Diseases*. Boca Raton, FL: CRC Press.

Thurston, H. David. "Plant Disease Management Practices of Traditional Farmers." *Plant Disease*, Vol. 74, 1990, pp. 96–102.

"U.S. Releases Wasps to Kill Plant-Sucking Bugs." Reuters News Service, September 20, 1999.

Walker, Matt. "Back from the Dead." *New Scientist*, September 4, 1999.

Wood, Marcia. "Potato Offers Resistance to Late Blight Disease." *Agricultural Research Service News*, December 17, 1998.

Wrobel, M., and Creber, G. (Editors) 1998. *Elsevier's Dictionary of Fungi and Fungal Plant Diseases*. New York: Elsevier.

Zalon, Frank, and Fry, William. 1992. *Food Crop Pests and the Environment: The Need and Potential for Integrated Pest Management*. St. Paul, MN: American Phytopathological Society.

OUTLOOK FOR THE TWENTY-FIRST CENTURY

Genetic engineering may confer resistance on more crop plants and domestic animals, but this process carries its own risks (and costs), and may not be widely available in Third World nations where it is most needed. Improved pesticides are another solution; some of the most dangerous (and effective) pesticides such as DDT have been eliminated from the agronomist's arsenal, but the controversy and public health risks associated with pesticide use will continue. The organophosphate pesticides now used to control the Medfly, BSE, and mosquito vectors have serious potential human health effects, and unless safer alternatives become available, the choice is a difficult one. Our species' dependence on a few food crops presents the risk of widespread famine in the event of a resistant disease outbreak or bioterrorism.

THE GOOD OLD DAYS

Insecticides and fungicides have caused incalculable harm to environmental health and quality—and yet their inventors might be forgiven, if anyone still living could remember the days when farmers had to get along without them. In 1997, Nobel Laureate and agronomist Norman Borlaug stated the issue as follows:

Without high-yield agriculture, either millions would have starved or increases in food output would have been realized through drastic expansion of acres under cultivation—losses of pristine land a hundred times greater than all losses to urban and suburban expansion . . .

If they [U.S. environmentalists] lived just one month amid the misery of the developing world, as I have for fifty years, they'd be crying out for tractors and fertilizer and irrigation canals, and be outraged that fashionable elitists back home were trying to deny them these things.[3]

Many agronomists believe that, without pesticides and artificial fertilizers—or equally controversial processes, such as genetic engineering—crop yields and shelf life would once again be so unpredictable that farmers could not feed today's enormous and ever-growing human population.

In 1845, something as simple as a fungicide might have saved a million lives in Ireland and averted one of the greatest human migrations in history. But there were no fungicides then; a wise farmer planned for failure and avoided dependence on a single crop. The Irish and those who governed them had forgotten that lesson, and are unlikely to forget it again. The Potato Famine has been the subject of several recent books and television documentaries, but like the Holocaust, it is a story that demands retelling:

[3]G. Easterbrook, "Forgotten Benefactor of Humanity" (*Atlantic Monthly*, January 1997).

In this black year of '47 in which the potato crop failed a third time—a total failure this time—in which far more than half a million died of famine and of plague begotten by famine, and far more than a quarter million fled the country, Larcom (the Government Commissioner) estimated at forty-five million pounds the value of the food-crops produced. The greater portion of these crops crossed the channel—sold to satisfy the landlord and tax gatherer. Travellers were often appalled when they came upon some lonely village by the western coast, with the people all skeletons on their own hearths. . . .

. . . We saw sights that will never wholly leave the eyes that beheld them, cowering wretches almost naked in the savage weather, prowling in turnip fields, and endeavouring to grub up roots which had been left, but running to hide as the mailcoach rolled by: groups and families, sitting or wandering on the highroad, with failing steps, and dim, patient eyes, gazing hopelessly into infinite darkness and despair; parties of tall, brawny men, once the flower of Meath and Galway, stalking by with a fierce but vacant scowl: as if they realised that all this ought not to be, but knew not whom to blame, saw none whom they could rend in their wrath.[4]

REFERENCES AND RECOMMENDED READING

Maher, T. M. "How and Why Journalists Avoid the Population-Environment Connection." *Population and Environment*, March 1997.

FROM THE AUTHOR'S FILE CABINET

Many round organisms have confusingly similar names, all derived from the Greek word *kokkos* ("berry"). A spherical bacterium is called a coccus (plural, cocci), giving us names such as *Streptococcus* ("string of berries") and *Deinococcus* ("terrifying berry"). But *Echinococcus* ("spiny berry") is a tapeworm, not a bacterium. *Coccus* also refers to a scale insect; *Coccidioides* ("similar to a berry") is a fungus; and the Coccidia ("little berries") are protozoa, the topic of this anecdote.

As noted earlier, victims of intestinal coccidiosis tend to lose weight, owing to the nature of the parasite and its life cycle. Human victims usually eat more to compensate for lost nutrients, or simply take in their belts by a notch or two. Wild animals and their domesticated relatives, however, cannot afford these luxuries, and have evolved nutrient-conserving strategies that will never catch on with humans. One of these is coprophagy, or the consumption of one's own feces.

In some animals, such as rabbits, coprophagy is a normal phase of digestion. It is similar to cud chewing by a cow, in that the animal extracts more nutrients from the same food by eating it twice. Other species resort to this behavior when food is scarce, or when a disease interferes with absorption. Some human groups have practiced it on occasion. In the eighteenth century, for example, Native Americans in Baja California had a civilized form of coprophagy: during the season when cactuses were fruiting, they ate the fruit and excreted the undigested seeds. Later in the year, when no fruit was available, they gathered their dried feces and dissolved them in water to extract the seeds; then they ground and cooked the seeds, and ate them again. Whatever the missionaries might have thought of this custom, it was a highly practical alternative to starvation. Even today, a few diehard connoisseurs prac-

[4]Seumas Macmanus, *The Story of the Irish Race* (Old Greenwich, CT: Devin-Adair, 1921).

tice coprophagy by drinking *kopi luwak* —the world's most expensive coffee at U.S. $300 per pound, brewed from beans that have been eaten and then excreted by a small Indonesian marsupial.

Precedent notwithstanding, dog owners frequently react in horror when their beloved pets begin eating their own feces. Some dogs acquire this habit for unknown reasons, but in others, it can be a symptom of coccidiosis. In the 1970s, the author's roommate bought a four-month-old German Shepherd puppy from a reputable, high-priced kennel. It was a very nice dog, but every pet has its drawbacks. Although housebroken, it had uncontrollable diarrhea 20–30 times in every 24 hours. It would discharge a pool of this material onto the carpet, immediately eat most of it, then walk through the remainder and leap onto the nearest human's lap, whining and licking her face to be let out. We were fond of dogs, but not to this extent.

The kennel assured the frantic owner that this behavior was normal, as all their dogs did the same thing. Finally, the owner consulted a veterinarian and learned that the puppy had a heavy infestation of coccidia. Treatment stopped the objectionable behavior for a few days; but either the treatment was not entirely effective, or the puppy became reinfected from contaminated household objects, and the problem soon returned. Eventually, the kennel took back the puppy, saying how sorry they were that things hadn't worked out. Most kennel owners nowadays are better-informed and can recognize obvious signs of disease.

REFERENCES AND RECOMMENDED READING

Soave, O., and Brand, C. D. "Coprophagy in Animals." *Cornell Veterinarian*, Vol. 81, 1991, pp. 357–364.

CHAPTER 7

Venoms, Toxins, and Allergens

> But just as Teddy was stooping, something wriggled a little in the dust, and a tiny voice said: "Be careful. I am Death!"
> —Rudyard Kipling, *The Jungle Book* (1894)

The science of poisons, unlike the science of pathogens, has been around for a long time. Poisons of biological origin, called **toxins**, form the main subject matter of this chapter.

The benefits of toxins are many. They can paralyze game animals, kill enemy soldiers, knock beetles off the cucumbers, summon visions of gods or pink elephants, and (in small doses) serve as powerful medicines. The associated risks also are great, as evidenced by the present worldwide epidemic of substance abuse, medical quackery, and less visible phenomena, such as the economic clout of the pharmaceutical, pesticide, and defense industries.

Allergens are similar to toxins in that they are chemicals (usually proteins) that cause harmful effects. The main difference is that a toxin harms everyone, in a somewhat predictable, dose-dependent fashion, whereas an allergen affects only sensitized individuals. Some allergens, such as the resin of plants in the genus *Toxicodendron*, are so universally disliked that people regard them as poisons, and have given the plants such names as poison oak and poison ivy. (In fact, however, only about 80 percent of the human population is allergic to *Toxicodendron*.)

It is possible to become sensitized to a chemical that is also a toxin. Bee venom, for example, always causes at least minor pain, and several hundred bee stings might kill anyone; but a sensitized (allergic) person can die from a single sting.

CROSS-REFERENCE

As some biological hazards involve more than one mode of action, toxins and related topics appear at several locations in this book. It is conventional to refer to staphylococcal food poisoning as a foodborne disease, for example (see Chapter 3), although the actual cause of the illness is the bacterial toxin. Also, certain predators (such as the Komodo dragon, Chapter 8) use bacterial colonies and decomposition products in their mouths as a sort of venom equivalent. For the reader's convenience, Table 7.1 provides a cross-reference to related topics found in other chapters. For consistency with earlier chapters, Table 7.2 lists a few examples of "outbreaks" of related phenomena. Table 7.3 puts the subject matter of this chapter in perspective; venomous animals attract a great deal of attention, but in reality they claim few victims.

MORE DEFINITIONS

A **venomous** animal is one that injects a toxin when it bites or stings you. Such an animal keeps its toxin (called venom) in a specific gland or other body part. By contrast, a **poisonous** animal (or plant) is one whose tissues are toxic if you ingest or contact them. A standard measure of toxicity is the LD_{50}, meaning the dose of a chemical needed to kill 50 percent of exposed subjects of a given species.

There are many venomous snakes, but no known poisonous snakes; rattlesnake meat is delicious, if the chef recognizes the problem and discards the head end. (The media often refer incorrectly to "poisonous snakes," and even the U.S. Navy has published a book entitled *Poisonous Snakes of the World*.) In birds and amphibians, the situation is reversed; both groups include poisonous species, but no known venomous ones in the strict sense. A few mammal species are venomous, and certain organs of some mammals are poisonous. Finally, among the fishes and arthropods, there are many examples of both venomous and poisonous species.

A third category of intoxication results when an organism, such as a fungus, releases toxic chemicals into its environment for one reason or another. These toxins often contaminate water or become concentrated in foods that are not toxic in themselves.

Table 7.1
Cross-Reference: Biological Toxins in Other Chapters

Disease	Chapter	Notes
Cholera	2	Cholera toxin
Food poisoning	3	Bacterial toxins in food
Aspergillosis	4	More on aflatoxin
Diphtheria	4	Diphtherotoxin
Chiggers	5	Hypersensitivity reaction mimics disease
Strep Group A	5	"Flesh-eating bacteria" produce a toxin
Tetanus	5	Tetanus toxin
"Ptomaine"	8	Bacteria and toxins on the Komodo dragon's teeth
Biological Warfare	9	Potential role of biological toxins

Table 7.2
Examples of "Outbreaks" of Envenomations and Poisonings

Agent or Event	Date	Location	Est. Cases	Est. Deaths
Lepidopterism	1984	Venezuela (on ship)	34	0
Ergotism	A.D. 857	Europe	NR	Thousands
Ergotism?	1374	Aix-la-Chapelle, France	Hundreds	NR
Ergotism	1692	Salem, MA	NR	20+
Trichothecenes	1944	Russia	Thousands	10%
Pfiesteria	1997	Atlantic Coast	NR	1 bil. fish
Irukandji (jellyfish)	1996	Northern Australia	62	0
Blue-green algae	1970	Australia	150+	0
Death cap mushroom	1997	California	9	0
Gyromitra mushroom	1957	Poland	132	19
Jimson weed (*Datura*)	1990	Tanzania	10+	0

Sources: Dinehart et al. (1985); Little and Mulcahy (1998); Kendrick (1992); Rwiza (1991); *Morbidity and Mortality Weekly Report*, various.

VENOMOUS ANIMALS

Venomous Mammals

There are at least three solid examples of venomous mammals, plus borderline cases, as discussed below.

***Duck-billed Platypus* (Ornithorhynchus anatinus).** Males of this primitive, egg-laying Australian mammal have spurs on their hind legs, which they can use to inject a potent venom. Humans who have been spurred report that the chief symptom is intense pain. In small mammals, the venom can be lethal.

Shrews. Since ancient times, naturalists have claimed that shrews were venomous and that their bite could kill. Some of those same naturalists, however, claimed that shrews were evil and could cause paralysis by running over a person's leg. Most biologists dismissed the whole idea as superstition, until recent studies confirmed the

Table 7.3
Estimated Human Mortality Caused by Venomous Animals

Organism	Deaths per Year, U.S.	Deaths per Year, World
Spiders	3	200
Scorpions	0	5,000
Snakes	6	10,000
Bees	50	NR

Sources: Reptile Gardens, Rapid City, SD; Amdur et al. (1991); U.S. National Center for Health Statistics, Vital Statistics of the United States, 1992.

presence of a venom in the saliva of the North American short-tailed shrews (genus *Blarina*) and the European water shrews (genus *Neomys*). The venom probably serves the purpose of immobilizing the shrew's insect prey, and is not considered harmful to humans. Like snake venoms, it may not even be injected with every bite. Some victims, however, have reported severe reactions:

The burning sensation, first observed, predominated in the immediate vicinity of the wounds, but was now greatly intensified, accompanied by shooting pains, radiating in all directions from the punctures but more especially running along the arm, and in half an hour, they had reached as high as the elbow. All this time, the parts in the immediate vicinity of the wounds, were swelling, and around the punctures the flesh had become whitish. . . . [the pains] did not entirely disappear until the total abatement of the swelling, which occurred in about a fortnight.[1]

A more recent report, on a shrew Web site, describes the short-tailed shrew's bite in less dramatic terms: "The bite was painful, but more odd feeling than severe. . . I do recall that my finger was a bit numb for a few hours afterward."[2] The amount of venom injected, the age or condition of the animal, or individual reactions might account for the difference.

Solenodon. Few readers will ever encounter a solenodon. There are only two living species, one in Cuba (*Solenodon cubanus*) and the other in the Dominican Republic and Haiti (*Solenodon paradoxus*), and both are presently listed as endangered. They resemble large shrews with long noses, and they have submaxillary glands that produce a toxic saliva.

Skunks **and** *Others*. Skunks are famous for smelling bad, but the animal itself is not the problem. With its musk gland removed, a skunk makes a charming pet, or an excellent if rather small roast. When threatened, however, skunks can use the gland to squirt a glandular secretion into the eyes of a predator. This chemical spray causes painful burning and temporary blindness, and is clearly an effective defense. It is not exactly a venom, but along those lines.

"Venomous" Birds

No known bird injects or actively deploys a venom, but seabirds called fulmars (*Fulmarus glacialis* and related species) do something similar: they spit a bad-smelling oil from their stomachs to repel invaders from their nests, accurately striking targets up to five feet away. The name fulmar, in fact, is derived from two Norse words meaning "foul gull."

The oil is not poisonous, and people in some North Atlantic countries burn it as lamp oil and regard fulmars as a delicacy. When oil squirted by a fulmar comes in contact with other marine birds, however, it can mat their feathers and cause them to drown. Thus, it can be as lethal as any toxin, in a behavioral sense, when used against the predators that the fulmar normally encounters. The oil has also repelled cats and other

[1]C. J. Maynard, "Singular Effects Produced by the Bite of a Short-Tailed Shrew, *Blarina brevicauda*" (*Contributions to Science*, Vol. 1, 1889, pp. 57–59).
[2]"Shrew Culture, Myths, Stories and Poisonous Facts," <http://members.vienna.at/shrew/cult-poison.html>.

animals, but its level of effectiveness is unknown. Comparable behavior occurs in a few other bird species.

Venomous Reptiles

Nearly all the world's venomous reptiles are snakes. There are two venomous lizard species, both in the New World, and no known venomous turtles or crocodilians. The only living reptile not in one of these groups is the tuatara of New Zealand, which is not venomous either. (Despite *Jurassic Park*, scientists have no idea if any dinosaurs were venomous or not.)

The fear of snakes is widespread, even in places where snakes are common. In 1999, a man successfully robbed a convenience store in Oklahoma by carrying a harmless snake and telling the clerk it was a copperhead. As discussed below, many snakes are dangerous, but injury and disfigurement are more likely outcomes than death. Some journalists have exaggerated the risk of snakebite—as do pharmaceutical companies that sell high-priced antivenoms. Conservationists, by contrast, tend to downplay the risk of snakebite in an effort to discourage the needless slaughter of reptiles. The truth, as usual, lies somewhere in between.

Every year in about May, rural newspapers around the country publish two general types of rattlesnake stories. One type announces that rattlers are emerging from their dens in unusually high numbers, and that people need to be careful; the other type claims that rattlers are not dangerous. Both statements are false. Nothing can appear in unusually high numbers every year, and rattlers most certainly are dangerous.

No more than ten people in North America die from snakebites in a typical year, but many more are injured. Some sources claim that 8000 U.S. residents suffer venomous snakebites every year, but this number is misleading. Many people (including many doctors) cannot identify a venomous snake; even if the snake is venomous, many bites are "dry," with no venom injected. In Asia and Africa, however, snakes take a far higher toll. No accurate global statistics are available, but some sources estimate that more than 10,000 people worldwide die from snakebites each year and that another 100,000 are severely injured, either by the venom itself or by the infections that so often follow snakebites. A book published in 1896 states that 21,538 people died of snakebites in India alone in 1894.

Crotalid Snakes (Rattlesnakes, Pit Vipers). Snakes in this group are the only venomous reptiles that most U.S. residents will ever encounter. Most are easy to identify by the familiar "rattle" on the end of the tail. The snake will not always sound a warning; the young ones cannot, as their rattle has only one button. East of the Rockies, there are two crotalids without rattles: the copperhead (*Agkistrodon contortix*) and the cottonmouth (*Agkistrodon piscivorus*). The best way to avoid being bitten is simply to avoid touching or approaching any snakes.

If a rattler is on your property and you have children or outdoor pets, have a qualified person remove it. In 2000, a two-year-old Florida boy died from a rattlesnake bite in his own yard. Entrepreneurs in some cities have set up shop as "critter gitters" who will relocate unwanted animals for a fee. You can also call the biology department of

185

a local college and ask for help. If the snake is in a place where you absolutely must kill it, just whack it on the neck with a long stick. There is no need for a gun or axe; even large snakes are fragile and easy to kill. Be aware, however, that some rattlesnake species—including the timber rattler (*Crotalus horridus*) of the eastern United States, the ridge-nosed rattlesnake (*Crotalus willardi*) in New Mexico, and the red rattlesnake (*Crotalus ruber*) in southern California—are protected under federal or state laws. Unless the snake is an immediate and genuine threat, killing it may be illegal.

Rattlesnakes bite only when they perceive a threat, but they make mistakes like everyone else. If a person walks past a rattler concealed in the bushes, it might strike, regardless of the victim's intentions. (Possibly for that reason, the rattlesnake motif on an early American colonial flag did not catch on as a national symbol.)

Some rattlesnake species are more likely to bite than others, and some produce a more dangerous venom than others, or a larger quantity of venom. All rattler venoms contain enzymes that digest protein; some species also produce neurotoxins. The copperhead, for example, is not very dangerous unless the victim has an allergic reaction, but the western diamondback rattlesnake (*Crotalus atrox*, Figure 7.1) is widely regarded as perhaps the most dangerous snake in the world. Between those two extremes, rattlesnakes cover the full hazard spectrum. The Mojave rattlesnake (*Crotalus*

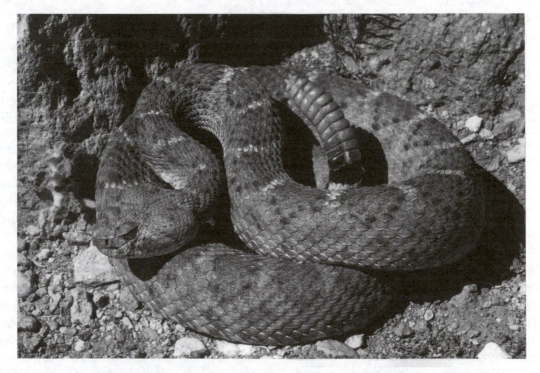

Figure 7.1. Western Diamondback Rattlesnake (*Crotalus atrox*). (*Source*: David L. Hardy, Sr., M.D.)

scutulatus) has one of the world's most dangerous venoms, but is somewhat less inclined to bite than the diamondback.

Although rattlesnake bites rarely are fatal to healthy adults, untreated bites can cause severe injuries. By "severe," we mean tissue necrosis with major scarring or loss of a toe or finger, often with prolonged disability or permanent weakness of a damaged muscle (Figure 7.2). Life-threatening anaphylaxis (a severe allergic reaction) may occur in some victims. Again, people can avoid these outcomes by leaving snakes alone. Many rattlesnake bites involve victims who were drunk and showing off (see the File Cabinet section at the end of this chapter).

The public's fear of rattlenakes may express itself in various ways. Every year, the news media cover the "rattlesnake round-up" that has become a Texas tradition. Although this fear of snakes may be partly instinctual, example also plays a role. In 1974, a youth leader confronted a rattlesnake on a hiking trail in California; with a half-dozen children looking on, he killed the small animal with an axe while shouting about Satan. Many gopher snakes and other harmless species also are killed every year by people who think they are doing society a service. With these predators out of the way, rodent populations increase, damaging stored food and spreading disease (see Chapter 6).

Many "snakebites" do not even involve snakes. Herpetologist Lawrence Klauber told the story of a hunter who stuck himself

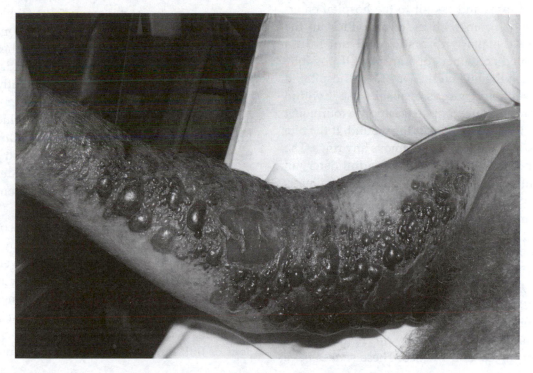

Figure 7.2. Injury caused by a rattlesnake bite. (*Source*: David L. Hardy, Sr., M.D.)

on a barbed-wire fence, thought it was a rattler, and promptly suffered a heart attack. In 2000, a southern California resident reached into his woodpile, felt a sting, and concluded that it was the bite of an unseen timber rattler (a species not found in California). He then drove to a hospital, where he demanded and received antivenom. Several days later, he developed a slight fever and flu-like symptoms, so he returned to the doctor and demanded treatment for serum sickness. Some Native American tribes believed that a person who dreamed of a rattlesnake bite should receive the same treatment as the victim of a real bite; today's potent treatments, however, are best reserved for the truly bitten.

To avoid such misunderstandings, always kill the snake (see above) for identification purposes and take it to the hospital emergency room with the victim. Pick up the dead snake with a stick and put it in a sealed container for transport. If possible, wash the bite on the way to the hospital. If a suction device is available, use it within three minutes, but do *not* apply a tourniquet or ice, and do *not* cut the wound. If the bite is on a hand, quickly remove any rings. The doctor will most likely administer an antivenom, which may cause severe illness, but at least it will prevent further tissue damage. (Ideally, the victim will have medical insurance, as the antivenom alone for treating one snakebite may cost $5,000-$15,000.)

Elapid Snakes (Coral Snakes, Cobras, Others). The only elapids in North America are coral snakes: *Micrurus fulvius* in the southeast and *Micrurus euryxanthus* in the southwest and Mexico. These snakes have small teeth and seldom bite humans, but if the snake gets a grip, envenomation occurs in 75 percent of cases. The venom is neurotoxic, and severe symptoms (including respiratory paralysis) may appear up to 12 hours after the bite. Drooping eyelids often are an early symptom. Antivenom treatment is effective.

Most coral snake bites result when someone picks up a coral snake, thinking it is a harmless scarlet kingsnake (*Lampropeltis triangulum*), which has similar bands of color in a different sequence. The jingle bears repeating: "Red and yellow kills a fellow." In other words, if the red and yellow (or white) bands are next to each other, the snake is a coral snake.

Some of the world's most dangerous snakes are elapids, including the first six snakes on the "most venomous" list (Table 7.4). All produce powerful neurotoxins, but may be less inclined to bite than some other venomous snakes; note that the elapids, other than cobras, figure less prominently on the "most dangerous" list (Table 7.5). One person who survived a bite by the blue krait (*Bungarus caeruleus*), an elapid, claims to have seen "beautiful texture and tapestry and colors."[3] Despite the worldwide demand for mind-altering drugs, krait venom is unlikely to emerge as a favorite.

The elapids also include the sea snakes of Australia's Great Barrier Reef, which have potent venom but rarely bite humans even when handled. Most sea snake bites occur on fishing boats, as the snakes sometimes become entangled in nets. An antivenom is available. According to one report, 95 percent of folk remedies are effective against

[3]Bill Haast, owner of a venom laboratory in Florida, quoted in *Outside Magazine*, July 1997.

Table 7.4
The Ten Most Venomous Snakes in the World

Not all authorities are in agreement, and four other snakes are tied for tenth place: the African mamba (*Dendroaspis*, three species) and the Mojave rattler (*Crotalus mohavensis*).

Species	Geographic Range	Notes
1. Inland Taipan (*Oxyuranus microlepidotus*)	Australia	The most toxic venom of any snake, delivered in large doses (enough in one bite to kill over 100 people).
2. Australian Brown Snake (*Pseudonaja textilis*)	Australia	Highly potent venom.
3. Malayan Krait (*Bungarus candidus*)	SE Asia and Indonesia	50% of bites are reported fatal even with antivenin treatment.
4. Taipan (*Oxyuranus scutellatus*)	Australia	The venom in one bite will kill up to 12,000 guinea pigs.
5. Tiger Snake (*Notechis scutatus*)	Australia	Highly venomous and also aggressive (see Table 7.5).
6. Beaked Sea Snake (*Enhydrina schistosa*)	Arabian Sea to Coral Sea	Highly potent venom.
7. Saw-Scaled Viper (*Echis carinatus*)	Middle East, Asia	Venom is 5 times as toxic as that of the cobra; also aggressive (Table 7.5).
8. Coral Snake (*Micrurus fulvius*)	North America	Highly potent venom, but the snake is small and rarely bites.
9. Boomslang (*Dispholidus typus*)	Africa	The most venomous rear-fanged snake in the world.
10. Death Adder (*Acanthophis antarcticus*)	Australia, New Guinea	Can deliver enough venom in one bite to kill about 18 people.

Source: Reptile Gardens, Rapid City, SD.

sea snake bites—a fairly good indication that the victim was not in danger.

Viperid Snakes (Old World Vipers). Some of the most dangerous Old World snakes belong to this group. Representatives include the European viper (*Vipera berus*) and asp viper (*Vipera aspis*), the only venomous snakes found in northern Europe; Russell's viper (*Vipera russelli*) of India and Southeast Asia, considered the world's most dangerous viperid (Table 7.5); the horned sand viper or asp (*Cerastes cornuta*), which resembles the unrelated North American sidewinder; and the saw-scaled viper (*Echis carinatus*), said to cause many fatalities in northern Africa and India. The name "asp" refers to several different snakes, and it is not clear which (if any) of these species Cleopatra used to commit suicide, but the odds-on favorite is the Egyptian cobra (*Naja haje*)—actually an elapid, and not a viperid at all.

Colubrid Snakes (Mostly Harmless). All native North American snakes, other than the pit vipers and coral snakes, are colubrids and are harmless. They have teeth, of course, and can bite if you pick them up. Their teeth are not clean, and the wound

Table 7.5
The Most Dangerous Snakes in the World

Criteria for inclusion in this table include the snake's reported tendency to bite and its probability of coming in contact with humans, as well as the potency of its venom. Note that only two snakes appear on both lists.

Region	Species	Notes
North America	Western Diamondback Rattlesnake (*Crotalus atrox*)	Common near populated areas; aggressive when cornered; large dose of highly potent venom.
Asia	Indian Cobra (*Naja naja*)	May kill more people in India than any other snake.
	Russell's Viper (*Vipera russelli*)	One of the most dangerous snakes in China and southeast Asia.
Africa	Saw-Scaled Viper (*Echis carinatus*)	Potent venom; aggressive.
	Egyptian Cobra (*Naja haje*)	Cleopatra's asp?
	Puff Adder (*Bitis arietans*)	Many fatalities in Africa.
Australia	Tiger Snake (*Notechis scutatus*)	Kills more people each year than any other Australian snake.
Europe	European Viper (*Vipera berus*)	The only dangerous snake found in most of Europe.

Source: Reptile Gardens, Rapid City, SD.

may become infected unless you wash it promptly with soap and water. People who have not had a recent tetanus booster should also see a doctor, but there is no point in killing the snake.

Reptile collectors, zookeepers, herpetologists, and residents of Africa and Asia may encounter some highly dangerous Old World colubrids, such as the African boomslang (*Dispholidus typus*), the African twig snake (*Thelotornis kirtlandi*), and the Asian red-necked keelback (*Rhabdophis subminiata*). In all these snakes, the venom apparently works by first inducing massive blood clotting that exhausts the body's supply of clotting proteins, followed in a day or two by multiple hemorrhages and death. There are two mildly venomous colubrids in California, but their venom poses no risk to humans: the night snake (*Hypsiglena torquata*) and the lyre snake (*Trimorphodon biscutatus*).

Venomous Lizards. Only two lizards in the world are venomous, and both occur in North America: the Gila monster (*Heloderma suspectum*) of the southwestern United States and Sonora, Mexico and the Mexican beaded lizard (*Heloderma horridum*) of western Mexico and southern Guatemala. These large lizards are slow-moving and can attack only if you handle them. The venom contains a mixture of substances, including serotonin (a neurotransmitter), several enzymes, and a chemical similar to the hormone secretin. Although Gila monster venom is seldom fatal to humans, the bite is painful and messy, as the lizard hangs on and chews, often flipping itself upside down in the process. When you pull it away, its teeth break off in the wound, adding to the problem by causing infection. The venom can also cause a drop in blood pressure, rapid heartbeat, nausea, and difficulty in breathing. No commercial antivenom is available.

"Venomous" Amphibians

Although many amphibians have potent toxins in their skin, these animals are poisonous rather than venomous. Many fishermen believe that the hellbender (*Cryptobranchus alleganiensis*) is venomous, but in fact it is harmless. Another large salamander, the conger-eel (*Amphiuma means*), has a nasty bite that may become infected, but there is no actual venom.

Some reports indicate that the cane toad (*Bufo marinus*) can use its parotid glands to squirt its skin toxin as far as a meter in the direction of an enemy's eyes. If so, then this large toad qualifies as both venomous and poisonous. Cane toads are native to Central and South America, but have been introduced to many locations worldwide, including Hawaii and Australia, where they have caused great damage to native wildlife.

Venomous Fishes

At latest count, there are more than 200 venomous species of marine fishes, and this book cannot begin to do them justice.

Some of the most important examples are in the stingray family (Scorpaenidae). These fish deliver their venom using their tails, which are equipped with spines and venom-secreting cells. The venom causes severe pain and also affects the human cardiovascular system. A large dose is dangerous, but very few of the estimated 750 annual stings are lethal. Treatment involves prompt removal of any stingray tissue from the wound, followed by irrigation with salt water and immersion in a hot bath. Larger wounds may require sutures, and a tetanus booster is advisable.

Venomous Arthropods

Insects. The best-known North American examples are bees, wasps, and the imported red fire ant. These insects and their relatives cause more deaths in the United States than all other venomous animals combined. One sting can kill a person who has been sensitized by previous exposures; even someone who is not allergic can die if stung at least 100 times.

Africanized killer bees (*Apis mellifera scutella*) were accidentally released in Brazil in 1956 and began expanding their range northward at the rate of 200–300 miles per year, arriving in Texas in 1991. In the 40 years following their release, killer bees killed an estimated 1000 people and injured thousands more. These bees produce less honey than their European counterparts, and are more likely to sting people; on the plus side, they are resistant to bee mites (see Chapter 6). Their individual stings are no more dangerous than those of the familiar honeybee, but hundreds or even thousands of killer bees may sting the same person.

Venoms, Toxins, and Allergens

Wasps receive less publicity than bees, but their stings also can be lethal. In 1998, a two-year-old Florida boy died after a swarm of yellowjackets stung him more than 200 times. In 2641 B.C., the Egyptian pharaoh Menes reportedly died of anaphylaxis after a wasp sting.

The red fire ant (*Solenopsis invicta*) arrived in the southern United States from Brazil before 1940 and has recently extended its range to southern California. Since its arrival, its stings have killed more than 80 people and injured many others. In areas that the ant has colonized, parents must warn young children never to play outdoors without shoes, babies cannot crawl on the ground in their own yards, and bedridden elderly people—particularly those in nursing homes—may be swarmed and stung repeatedly. In one publicized case, an 87-year-old Florida woman was stung 1625 times before anyone noticed the problem. The ants also attack livestock and damage crops, and have even caused electrical blackouts by nesting in traffic lights and junction boxes. Agricultural officials have tried releasing parasitic flies as a biological control measure, but with little success thus far.

Several less famous insects also cause frequent envenomations. In Texas, a caterpillar popularly known as the puss or asp—not a snake, but the larva of the moth *Megalopyge opercularis*—is responsible for about 100 reported injuries each year. Its sting causes an intense, radiating pain, often with a skin rash, swelling, itching, or other symptoms. The larvae of several other U.S. moth species, notably the io moth (*Automeris io*) and the brown-tailed moth (*Euproctis chrysorrhea*), cause similar injuries.

Several aquatic insects in the order Heteroptera deserve mention, as people seldom expect to find a venomous, biting insect in the water. Some of the giant water bugs (Belostomatidae) can cause a serious wound by injecting proteolytic enzymes, much as a rattlesnake does. A few tropical species are over 4 inches long, but their North American cousins, such as the toe biter (*Lethocerus americanus*), are about half that size. The water scorpions (Nepidae), the backswimmers (Notonectidae), and even the small creeping water bugs (Naucoridae), also can deliver a painful bite. In Africa, related insects may serve as vectors for the agent of Buruli ulcer (Chapter 2).

Spiders. Journalists often claim that the black widow and brown recluse spiders are the only venomous spiders in the United States. Strictly speaking, nearly all spiders in the world are venomous; the catch is that most have mouthparts too small to inject their venom into humans, or else the venom is not harmful to large animals such as ourselves. An estimated 200 human deaths per year worldwide result from spider bites. In 1997, the American Association of Poison Control Centers received reports of more than 13,000 spider bites, none of them fatal.

The female black widow spider (*Latrodectus mactans* and related species) causes most reported spider bite injuries in North America. The death rate for untreated bites is said to be about 5 percent, but an effective antivenom is available. The usual symptoms are muscle cramps, sweating, weakness, and rapid pulse. In one reported case, a 13-year-old boy was bitten in bed and required emergency room treatment twice during the next four days, but finally recovered after antivenom treatment. More typical cases, however, do not require any treatment, and most do not find their way into the medical literature. The symptoms in the mildest cases range from a tiny pinprick sensation with no aftermath to a brief flu-like illness.

The brown recluse spider (*Loxosceles reclusa*, Figure 7.3) and related violin spiders have become famous in recent years, largely as the result of a Utah woman's severe injury in 1986. The story appeared in *Reader's Digest*, *Good Housekeeping*, and other widely read magazines; although tragic, the case was not typical. A 1999 study of 149 brown recluse bites showed that only 40 percent caused any tissue necrosis, and 43 percent of those healed within two weeks. Only one person in that study had more extensive necrosis that required hospitalization. Brown recluse bites (or allergic reactions to

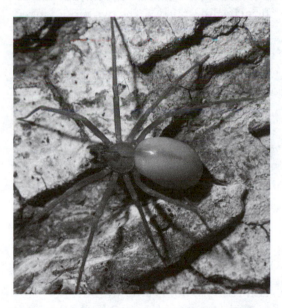

Figure 7.3. Brown recluse spider (*Loxosceles reclusa*). (*Source*: Dr. John A. Jackman, Texas A&M University.)

them) have caused circulatory collapse and gangrene on occasion, but such outcomes are rare. Various skin diseases, such as cutaneous anthrax, skin cancers, and herpes lesions, sometimes are mistaken for recluse spider bites.

The large tarantula spiders (of various species) also can inject a venom, but for most people the bite is no more serious than a bee sting. An Italian dance called the tarantella is said to resemble (or cure) a person who is jumping up and down with pain after a tarantula bite. As in the case of a bee sting, however, repeated exposures can lead to sensitization. Also, the body hairs of pet tarantulas can cause severe irritation of the skin, eyes, and respiratory tract.

The Sydney funnel web spider of Australia (*Atrax robustus*) and related species are another famous group of arachnids, partly because of the motion picture *Crocodile Dundee*—and an exaggerated *Reader's Digest* article that made such statements as "the funnel-web will attack anything that crosses its path." In reality, about 30–40 bites occur each year in eastern and southern Australia, of which three or four require antivenom treatment. Between 1927 and 1980, this spider caused a total of 13 human deaths in Australia. It is probably the most dangerous spider in the world, but spiders in general are not among humanity's greatest problems.

Ticks. These small eight-legged arthropods figure prominently in Chapters 5 and 6, as they are vectors for several important human and livestock diseases. Certain ticks, however, also produce a neurotoxic protein that causes paralysis. (Other ticks cause a similar reaction due to allergy rather than a true toxicosis. The bites of some ticks also cause skin ulcers, but it is not clear if a toxin or a bacterial infection is responsible.)

The tick paralysis victim usually is a young child, and the tick often is concealed by hair at the back of the child's head. After about six days, when the tick is engorged, the child develops a flaccid paralysis that starts with the feet and moves upward. At one time, this syndrome was commonly mistaken for polio. Unless the problem is quickly identified and the tick removed, respiratory failure follows, with death in as many as 12 percent of cases.

Tick paralysis is less common and less severe in adults than in children. In one such case, an adult experienced muscular weakness, purple spots (possibly allergic purpura), and a general sick feeling, but recovered within a few hours after an engorged tick was found and removed from the pubic area. Tick paralysis is fairly common in domestic animals as well as in humans. An antiserum is available for treating dogs with tick paralysis, and research is in progress to develop a vaccine for veterinary use.

Scorpions. Some of the world's most venomous scorpions live in Mexico, where an estimated 200,000 people are stung every year and at least 300 die. One of the most dangerous species is the bark scorpion (*Centruroides exilicauda*, Figure 7.4), which also occurs in southern Arizona. No scorpion-related deaths have been reported in Arizona since 1968, however, and the lethality of this species may be somewhat exaggerated in the literature.

In northern Africa and the Middle East, several deadly species of scorpions kill either several thousand people each year or almost none, depending on who is count-

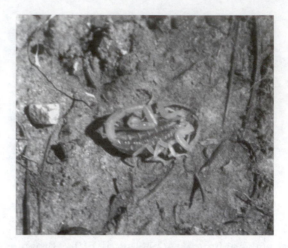

Figure 7.4. Arizona Bark Scorpion (*Centruroides exilicauda*). (Photo by David B. Richman, New Mexico State University.)

ing. If such deaths occur, they may be among people who do not seek medical treatment, and thus are not included in official health statistics. The two most dangerous species in that region are the death stalker (*Leiurus quinquestriatus*) and the fat-tailed scorpion (*Androctonus crassicauda*). In India, the red scorpion (*Buthus tamalus*) is reported to cause some deaths.

A scorpion stings by flicking its curved tail, which has a venom apparatus at the tip. Even the sting of a nonlethal scorpion is unpleasant, causing pain, swelling, discoloration, and sometimes anaphylaxis. Lethal scorpion stings typically cause a sharper pain followed by numbness, drowsiness, itching, slurred speech, and muscle spasms, sometimes with nausea and vomiting. Victims may die from respiratory or circulatory failure 24–48 hours after the bite.

Antivenoms are available for the most dangerous species. It is important to avoid most of the first aid measures recommended in older books; do not apply ice or a tourniquet, and do not give the person morphine or codeine. A recent unexpected finding is that insulin—the same hormone used to treat diabetes—may be the most effective treatment for severe scorpion envenomations. Another unexpected finding, reported in November 2001, is that some people in Pakistan grind scorpion stings and smoke them as an low-cost alternative to heroin.

Centipedes. Despite their reputation, most centipedes are not particularly dangerous. Their bite is painful, and may cause a swelling that lasts several weeks. If the bite becomes infected, it requires medical attention like any other animal bite. A few of the largest tropical species, however, are quite venomous. The 12-inch giant centipede (*Scolopendra gigantea*) of South America, for example, eats mice and can easily send a human to the hospital. It is greatly in demand as a pet, of course, and captive-bred adults typically sell for U.S. $70–$80 as of 2001.

Other Venomous Invertebrates

Jellyfish and *Corals*. Every year, an estimated 130 million people spend their vacations enjoying warm tropical or subtropical waters that hold more than 300 species of jellyfish. Some of these, notably the Australian sea wasp or box jellyfish (*Chironex fleckeri*), the irukandji (*Carukia barnesi*), and the Portuguese man-of-war (*Physalia physalis* and related species), can kill a human being. Many other jellyfishes are not deadly but can inflict a severe burn. Despite these facts, few people are seriously injured. For most minor jellyfish injuries, home rem-

edies will suffice, such as vinegar, meat tenderizer, or a paste of baking soda and water.

The basketball-sized Australian sea wasp, with its 15 feet of stinging tentacles, is considered the world's most dangerous jellyfish. A standard local precaution against its sting is to wear pantyhose while swimming. A sea wasp antivenom also is available, and efforts are currently in progress to develop antivenoms for irukandji syndrome and other jellyfish poisonings. Israeli scientists have developed a protective cream with chemical ingredients similar to those that protect certain fishes from the stings of sea anemones (a sedentary stage in the life of a jellyfish). The cream may prove useful in preventing jellyfish injuries, particularly if combined with a sun block for convenient one-step application.

Some corals also can cause serious injury. One of the most famous is the so-called death seaweed of Hana (*limu-make-o-Hana*), which is not a seaweed but a soft coral, with the scientific name *Palythoa toxica*. This coral and its relatives produce a highly unusual poison called palytoxin. Besides being (arguably) the most toxic organic substance ever discovered, it also has the longest chain of carbon atoms found in any natural product. At one time, the Hawaiians used it to poison their spear points; the coral grew only in one closely guarded tide pool. Filefishes that feed on these corals may also become poisonous.

Starfishes and *Sea Urchins*. Animals in this group have caused few (if any) fatalities, but their spines can inflict painful injuries. The crown-of-thorns starfish (*Acanthaster planci*), for example, not only destroys coral reefs but can also injure humans, causing severe pain, swelling, and skin irritation.

Mollusks. The most famous venomous mollusks are the cone snails (*Conus* sp.) found in all tropical and subtropical oceans, and the blue-ringed octopus (*Hapalochlaena maculosa*) of Australia. (Shellfish poisoning is a separate issue that appears later in the chapter.)

In a recent motion picture, a character states that cone toxin travels through the body faster than the speed of light, or some such rot. In fact, it is a potent but fairly ordinary nerve toxin. All the cone snails (400–500 species) use toxins to subdue their prey, but only the larger fish-eating cones can harm humans. A few fatal cases are in the literature, the first dated 1915:

[A native of New Caledonia] unhappily took a good-sized shellfish (*Conus textile*) and put it in his basket. He immediately felt a painful sensation running up his right arm to the shoulder. He went home. The pain increased until he writhed in agony. The body swelled to an enormous size, and by daylight he was a corpse.[4]

Another detailed description dates from 1936, and we include it mainly because it describes a different cone species (*Conus geographicus*) and entirely different symptoms. A 1982 study concluded, in fact, that this is the most dangerous of all the cones, although the other description might sound worse:

Local symptoms of slight numbness started almost at once. There was no pain at any time. Ten minutes afterwards there was a feeling of stiffness about the lips. At twenty minutes the sight became blurred with diplopia; at thirty minutes the legs were paralysed; and at sixty minutes unconsciousness appeared and deepened into coma. . . . Death took place five hours after the patient was stung.[5]

The blue-ringed octopus of Australia might qualify as the world's most dangerous mollusk if it bit people more often. Like the puffer fish and *Taricha* newts described later in this chapter, it produces a highly toxic chemical known as tetrodotoxin. (Some sources call it maculotoxin instead, after the scientific name of the octopus, but the two toxins are chemically the same.) Unlike the puffer fish and newts, the octopus injects this toxin as a venom, rather than simply storing it in body tissues as a poison.

In a widely reported case in 1954, an Australian diver found an octopus about six inches long and played with it for several minutes, then tossed it to his friend. The octopus crawled across the friend's back and dropped into the water. Although this man never reported a sting or other warning sign, his mouth soon became dry, and the other diver noticed a puncture wound. An hour or two later, the victim was dead. Laboratory studies have confirmed the lethality of this octopus.

REFERENCES AND RECOMMENDED READING

Amdur, Mary O., et al. (Editors). 1991. *Casarett and Doull's Toxocology*. 5th ed. New York: McGraw-Hill.

Bahuaud, J., et al. "Les Piqures par Cones Venimeux Observées en Nouvelle-Caledonie et ses Dependances [The stings of venomous

---

[4]H. Flecker, "Cone Shell Mollusc Poisoning, with Report of a Fatal Case" (*Medical Journal of Australia*, April 4, 1936, pp. 464–466).
[5]Ibid.

cones observed in New Caledonia and Dependencies]." *Medicina Tropical*, March–April 1982, pp. 197–202.

Boone, Cary. "Snake Bites Man." *Idyllwild* [CA] *Town Crier*, September 29, 2000.

Brodie, E. 1986. *Venomous Animals: A Golden Guide*. New York: Golden Books.

Cacy, J., and Mold, J.W. "The Clinical Characteristics of Brown Recluse Spider Bites Treated by Family Physicians." *Journal of Family Practice*, July 1999, pp. 536–542.

Chippaux, J.P. "Snake-Bites: Appraisal of the Global Situation." *Bulletin of the World Health Organisation* Vol. 76, 1998, pp. 515–524.

Coniff, Richard. "The Ten Most Venomous Animals." *International Wildlife*, March–April 1888, p. 18 ff.

Davis, Calvin L. 1979. *Insects, Allergy and Disease: Allergic and Toxic Responses to Arthropods*. Oshawa, Ont: C.L. Davis.

Dehesa-Davila, M., and Possani, L.D. "Scorpionism and Serotherapy in Mexico." *Toxicon*, September 1994, pp. 1015–1018.

Dittrich, Ken, et al. "Scorpion Sting Syndrome: A Ten Year Experience." *Saudi Medicine*, March 1995, pp. 148–155.

Dufton, M.J. "Venomous Mammals." *Pharmacology and Therapeutics*, Vol. 53, 1992, pp. 199–215.

Dumbacher, J.P., and Pruett-Jones, S. "Avian Chemical Defense." Chapter 4 in Nolan, V., Jr., and Ketterson, E.D. (Editors). *Current Ornithology*, Vol. 13. New York: Plenum Press, pp. 137–174.

Ernst, Carl H. 1999. Venomous Reptiles of North America. Washington, DC: Smithsonian Institution Press.

"Experts Fear Phorid Flies Fail in Quest to Fell Fire Ants." Associated Press, June 8, 2000.

Foster, Steven, and Caras, Roger. 1998. *Venomous Animals and Poisonous Plants: North America North of Mexico* (Peterson's Field Guide). Boston: Houghton Mifflin.

Haas, Danielle. "Jellyfish Protection: New Cream Protects against Sting." Reuters News Service, August 21, 2000.

Halstead, Bruce W. 1988. *Poisonous and Venomous Marine Animals of the World*. 2nd ed. Princeton, NJ: Darwin Press.

Henkel, John. "For Goodness Snakes! Treating and Preventing Venomous Bites." *FDA Consumer Magazine*, November 1995.

Hinde, Julia. "The Stinging Seas." *New Scientist*, November 27, 1999.

Huntley, A. "Lethocerus americanus, the 'Toe Biter'." *Dermatology Online Journal*, October 1998, p. 6.

Jahn, Ed. "UCSD Doctors Use a New Serum on Woman Bitten by Rattlesnake." *San Diego Union-Tribune*, September 16, 1993.

Keegan, Hugh L. 1980. *Scorpions of Medical Importance*. Jackson: University Press of Mississippi.

Kemp, E.D. "Bites and Stings of the Arthropod Kind." *Postgraduate Medicine*, June 1998, p. 88 ff.

Kemper, Steve. "Something Just Bit You?" *Smithsonian Magazine*, September 1999.

Keyler, D.E., and Vandervoort, J.T. "Copperhead Envenomations: Clinical Profiles of Three Different Subspecies." *Veterinary and Human Toxicology*, June 1999, pp. 149–152.

Kitchens, C.S., and Van Mierop, L.H. "Envenomation by the Eastern Coral Snake (*Micrurus fulvius fulvius*): A Study of 39 Victims." *Journal of the American Medical Association*, September 25, 1987, pp. 1615–1618.

Klauber, L.M. 1956. *Rattlesnakes: Their Habits, Life Histories, and Influence on Mankind*. Berkeley: University of California Press.

Lee, Douglas. "Black Mamba!" *International Wildlife*, November–December 1996, p. 48 ff.

Little, M., and Mulcahy, R.F., "A Year's Experience of Irukandji Envenomation in Far North Queensland" (*Medical Journal of Australia*, 1998, Vol. 169, pp. 638–641).

Maguire, Tony. "Meanest Spider Alive." *Reader's Digest*, April 1994, p. 41 ff.

"Man Uses Snake to Rob Convenience Store." Associated Press, December 14, 1999.

Martin, I.G. "Venom of the Short-Tailed Shrew (*Blarina brevicauda*) as an insect immobilizing agent." *Journal of Mammalogy*, Vol. 62, 1981, pp. 189–192.

Masina, S., and Broady, K.W. "Tick Paralysis: Development of a Vaccine." *International Journal of Parasitology*, April 1999, pp. 535–541.

Master, Edwin J. "Loxoscelism." *New England Journal of Medicine*, August 6, 1998, p. 379.

Mathew, J.L., and Gera, T. "Ophitoxaemia (Venomous Snakebite)." *International Journal of Medicine*, June 22, 2000 (online at <www.priory.com>).

Meier, J., and White, J. (editors). 1995. *Handbook of Clinical Toxicology of Animal Venoms and Poisons*. Boca Raton, FL: CRC Press.

Miller, Thomas A. "Latrodectism." *American Family Physician*, January 1992, p. 181 ff.

Minton, Sherman A., Jr. 1974. *Venom Diseases*. Springfield, IL: Thomas.

Moore, R.E., and Scheuer, P.J. "Palytoxin: A New Marine Toxin from a Coelenterate." *Science*, April 30, 1971, pp. 495–498.

Murthy, K.R., and Hase, N.K. "Scorpion Envenoming and the Role of Insulin." *Toxicon*, September 1994, pp. 1041–1044.

Nielsen, G.R., and MacCollom, G.B. "Problem Insects in Swimming Areas." University of Vermont Extension Publication EL54, 1997.

Nordt, S.P. "Anaphylactoid Reaction to Rattlesnake Envenomation." *Veterinary and Human Toxicology*, February 2000, p. 12.

O'Malley, G.F., et al. "Successful Treatment of Latrodectism with Antivenin after 90 Hours." *New England Journal of Medicine*, February 25, 1999.

Pournelle, G.H. "Classification, Biology, and Description of the Venom Apparatus of Insectivores of the Genera *Solenodon, Neomys*, and *Blarina*." In Pournelle, G.H. (Editor). 1967. *Venomous Animals and Their Venoms*, pp. 31–42. New York: Academic Press.

Rhoades, Robert B. 1977. *Medical Aspects of the Imported Fire Ant*. Gainesville, FL: University Presses of Florida.

Rubio, M., and Brown, W. S. 1998. *Rattlesnake: Portrait of a Predator*. Washington, DC: Smithsonian Institution Press.

Russell, F.E., and Dart, R.C. "Toxic Effects of Animal Toxins." In Amdur, Mary O., et al. (Editors). 1991. *Casarett and Doull's Toxocology*. 5th ed. New York: McGraw-Hill.

Schrader, Esther. "Fire Ants Take the Fun Out of the Backyard." *Los Angeles Times*, December 5, 1998.

Senior, Kathryn. "Taking the Bite Out of Snake Venoms." *Lancet*, June 5, 1999, p. 1946 ff.

Shiflett, D. "Men O'War." *National Review*, November 13, 2001.

Skinner, K.M. "Oil-Spitting in Fulmars: An Example of Chemical Defense in Birds?" Chemical Ecology, Colorado State University, Spring 1998.

"Snake-Bite Crisis: Not Enough Antidote for Poisonous Bites." Associated Press, August 7, 2000.

Sugiarto, J.R., et al. "Clinical Profile of Snakebite Patients Admitted at RITM July 1995–July 2000." Paper presented at 11th European Congress of Clinical Microbiology and Infectious Diseases, Istanbul, Turkey, April 3, 2001.

Sutherland, S.K. "New First-Aid Measures for Envenomation, with Special Reference to Bites by the Sydney Funnel-Web Spider (*Atrax robustus*)." *Medical Journal of Australia*, April 19, 1980, pp. 378–379.

Texas A&M University. Imported Fire Ant Web site, <http://fireant.tamu.edu>

Trempe, Suzanne. "Along Came a Spider." *Good Housekeeping*, April 1993, p. 54 ff.

Vetter, R.S., Visscher, P.K., and Camazine, S. "Mass Envenomations by Honey Bees and Wasps." *Western Journal of Medicine*, April 1999, pp. 223–227.

Visscher, P.K., Vetter, R.S., and Camazine, S. "Removing Bee Stings." *Lancet*, August 3, 1996, pp. 301–302.

Wood, William. "New Components in Defensive Secretion of the Striped Skunk, *Mephitis mephitis*." *Journal of Chemical Ecology*, Vol. 16, 1990, pp. 2057–2065.

ORGANISMS THAT RELEASE TOXINS

Various plants, fungi, protozoa, algae, and bacteria release toxins with effects ranging from memory loss to rapid death. People may acquire these toxins by passive contact with the organism, by drinking contaminated water, or by eating animals that previously fed on the toxic organisms. Some plants also inject a toxin; we cannot call such plants "venomous," as their immediate role is passive, but the sequence of events is similar.

A less obvious form of toxin, produced by some fungi and microorganisms, causes damage to the DNA in living cells. The effects of such chemicals, called mutagens, may appear months or years later in the form of cancer or a defective fetus, depending on the circumstances. Cancer-causing mutagens, known as carcinogens, may be responsible for about one-third of all cancers in the United States. A mutagen that causes birth defects is called a teratogen.

Insects that Release Toxins

When most people think of toxin-releasing organisms, moths do not immediately come to mind. Yet many people are injured every year by clouds of tiny barbed spines released into the air by several moth species, particularly in South America and Mexico. The spines are covered with toxic secretions from the moth's glands and are constantly shed. When inhaled by humans, the barbs cause respiratory injuries, sometimes resulting in large outbreaks of a condition called lepidopterism (moths and butterflies are in the insect order Lepidoptera). Symptoms include throat pain, coughing, and sneezing that typically last several days. Inhalation of airborne spines from caterpillars causes dermatitis and/or rhinitis in an estimated 500,000 people each year.

Plants that Release Toxins

The most familiar example of a toxin-injecting plant is the nettle (*Urtica dioica* and related species). Unlike poison ivy and other plants that rely on an allergic reaction, nettle affects everyone. Its leaves are armed with hollow stinging hairs that inject a mixture of histamine, acetylcholine, and serotonin into the skin. All these chemicals are normally present in the human body, but elsewhere and in their proper amounts. Histamine is a chemical that the body releases in response to allergies, and it acts as a constrictor of bronchial smooth muscle (which explains why we take antihistamine drugs for asthma); but some fungi and plants, such as ergot and nettles, grow their own histamine. Similarly, acetylcholine and serotonin are neurotransmitters in the human body, but many other organisms also produce them.

Nettles contain no actual toxins, and the young leaves make a nutritious vegetable when boiled. Just be sure to identify the plants correctly, and wear gloves to pick and wash them.

Fungi that Release Toxins

Aflatoxin. Several different fungi produce this mycotoxin, which takes its name from its most common source, *Aspergillus flavus.* These fungi grow as molds on stored foods such as corn, rice, and peanuts, especially in developing nations where high temperature and humidity levels may encourage toxin formation. A 1987 article predicted that aflatoxin and other mycotoxin contamination of food might be eliminated from the world by the year 2000, but this did not come to pass.

Aflatoxin is a powerful carcinogen that attacks the liver, causing primary liver cancer; it has been linked to several other diseases, including Reye's syndrome in children. Like many chemicals that act as carcinogens, it can also cause defects in the developing fetus. In 1960, more than 100,000 turkeys in England died of a previously unknown disease that the press called "Turkey-X disease." An investigation showed that the turkeys had eaten peanut meal contaminated with *Aspergillus flavus*, and the actual cause of death was liver damage from aflatoxin.

Ergotism. A fungus called *Claviceps purpurea* that grows on rye plants in damp weather can release powerful alkaloids. These chemicals have profoundly influenced human history, from the outbreaks of "dancing mania" in Medieval Europe and the later Salem witch trials, to the Haight-Ashbury phenomenon of the 1960s and the eventual discovery of effective drugs to treat migraine headaches—quite a track record for a smelly black mold.

In the ninth century, a strange plague afflicted Europe, and recent scholars have interpreted the recorded symptoms as those of ergotism. In some victims, this malady caused bizarre hallucinations with a sense of flying, followed by convulsions and death. In others, however, it produced gangrene with a burning pain in the legs. The *Annales Xantenses* describes an outbreak in A.D. 857 as follows: "A great plague of swollen blisters consumed the people by a loathsome rot so that their limbs were loosened and fell off before death."[6]

In the 1930s, an American chemist identified the nucleus of ergot as a chemical now called lysergic acid. While handling one of its derivatives, called LSD-25, the chemist became aware of strange sensations and pretty colors, and the rest of the story is well known. The same research, however, identified several ergot derivatives that have proven useful in the treatment of migraine headaches. Ergot is a vasoconstrictor, which explains why some people in A.D. 857 lost their legs; in high doses, the drug cut off the peripheral circulation, and necrosis set in. But the same action, in controlled doses, can counteract the vasodilation that contributes to migraine. One interesting theory attributes postpartum psychosis to the medical use of ergot derivatives before and during childbirth.

Stachybotrys. In the past few years, this black mold has evolved into a story too strange to evaluate. The fungus itself really exists, often growing on damp paper in basements. Some good researchers are working on it, but its effects remain controversial. In 1995, when a number of infants in Detroit and other cities had pulmonary hemorrhages, the Centers for Disease Control and Prevention (CDC) investigated the outbreak and identified *Stachybotrys* as the cause. At that time, experts stated that it was fairly easy to remove the mold using a bleach solution.

In 2000, however, the CDC reexamined the mold data and retracted its conclusions, citing "serious shortcomings" in the original investigation. During the five-year interim, the mold had grown beyond its original confines and acquired a following and a nickname ("stacky"). Anecdotal reports now claimed that *Stachybotrys* could cause memory loss and many other symptoms in adults as well as children, and that it was nearly impossible to remove from buildings. In the late 1990s, several families in Arizona

---

[6]George Barger, *Ergot and Ergotism* (London: Gurney & Jackson, 1931).

and other states reported outbreaks of *Stachybotrys* in their homes. One such family became the subjects of one of the oddest television documentaries ever filmed. Here is a sample from an AP news release: "[The subject] and her family fled their Scottsdale home more than a year ago when a garden of fluorescent mushrooms and molds were found growing in the walls of their 5,000-square-foot home."[7]

It is not clear how we got here from the black mold *Stachybotrys*, but no matter; many fungi grow in buildings, and some of the most ordinary ones are fluorescent. This sounds strange mainly because few people study fungi or go crawling around inside their walls. As discussed elsewhere in this chapter, fungi do cause allergic reactions; in interviews, however, these family members reported health problems ranging from headaches and fatigue to seizures and liver disease. One man's boss stated that the fungus had turned his employee into a "nincompoop" (his word, not ours).

Finally, on the advice of consultants, at least one of these families had their beautiful house and all its contents demolished, even china and glassware that might seem easy to clean. Either this family and others have lived through an astounding tragedy, or perhaps there is some other explanation. And on that note, we will proceed to the next topic.

Trichothecenes. Several fungi, including the aforementioned *Stachybotrys*, *Trichoderma* (see Chapter 6), and a common mold called *Fusarium*, produce a group of toxic chemicals known as trichothecenes. In Russia in 1944, a large outbreak of human tox-icity resulted when wartime conditions made it necessary for farmers to leave their grain crops in the field all winter. The dampness promoted the growth of trichothecene-producing molds, and more than 10 percent of the people who ate the grain died, with symptoms that included vomiting, diarrhea, and hemorrhaging. Lower levels of exposure to trichothecenes apparently can also suppress the immune system. A review of the recent medical literature fails to establish any link between trichothecenes and memory loss, personality changes, seizures, or other neurological problems reported in the media.

Protozoa, Algae, and Bacteria that Release Toxins

Although these three categories of organisms are not closely related, the names sometimes are used interchangeably. Dinoflagellates are protozoa, but the media often call them algae when reporting on the latest red tide menace. Cyanobacteria are bacteria, but they are often known as blue-green algae. Finally, some "real" algae also release toxins.

Protozoa. Dinoflagellates are protozoa, but some of them contain chlorophyll and make food by photosynthesis as plants do. Most of the so-called red tides, highly publicized in recent years for killing wildlife and humans, result from blooms of dinoflagellates. Such blooms have become more frequent, probably as a result of nutrients from sewage runoff in coastal areas.

One of the most famous of these dinoflagellates is pfiesteria (*Pfiesteria piscicida*),

[7]"Moldy Homes Making Arizonans Ill," Associated Press, December 14, 1999.

hailed in the press as the "Cell from Hell." Like some other marine toxins, it can affect behavior and memory in humans, but there are no confirmed reports of poisonings from eating contaminated fish; all reported cases were in fishermen or others who handled contaminated water. The fish themselves develop bleeding sores and often die, typically in huge numbers. One outbreak in the late 1990s killed an estimated one billion fish off the Atlantic coast.[8]

The most common red tide organisms are dinoflagellates such as *Gymnodinium breve*, *Gonyaulax catanella*, and related species, which produce several toxic chemicals including saxitoxin. Mussels, clams, and other shellfish that ingest these organisms become highly poisonous to humans; the resulting condition is called paralytic shellfish poisoning, although the shellfish themselves are not the source of the toxin. Saxitoxin blocks action potentials in nerves and muscles, causing paralysis and sometimes death. During widespread red tide events, these toxins can also become airborne, causing irritation to people's eyes and throats. Another dinoflagellate, *Gambierdiscus toxicus*, causes a form of fish poisoning called ciguatera. Symptoms in humans include nausea, itching, dizziness, and weakness, often with a sensation of loose teeth in the lower jaw. Some patients with this syndrome have been treated for depression.

Algae. Diatoms are single-celled algae that live in fresh and salt water worldwide. They resemble miniature canoes or jewels when viewed through a microscope. Some of them, unfortunately, release a toxin called domoic acid, which attacks the brain. When people or wildlife ingest the toxin by eating fish or shellfish that have fed on diatoms, a syndrome called amnesic shellfish poisoning may result. Besides causing loss of memory, domoic acid in sufficient doses can also cause vomiting, diarrhea, and death. Nearly 400 California sea lions died in 1998 after feeding on anchovies that had eaten diatoms. Sea lions that survived the incident showed abnormal behavior such as head waving and scratching.

Bacteria. Chapter 3 describes several bacteria that multiply in food and release toxins, causing illness ranging from mild nausea to circulatory collapse and death. Another type of bacteria, however—cyanobacteria, confusingly called blue-green algae—release toxins directly into the natural bodies of water where they live. Some of the cyanobacteria often involved in human and animal poisonings are *Microcystis*, *Cylindrospermopsis*, and *Anabaena*. Most of them have no popular names, and the public seems largely unaware of them.

In one case, a group of British Army recruits were practicing eskimo rolls in kayaks in a lake when they encountered a toxic bloom of *Microcystis*. Two soldiers developed acute pneumonia, and the rest suffered vomiting, diarrhea, sore eyes, and blisters in their mouths. In the 1970s, another cyanobacterium found its way into a public water system in Australia and poisoned at least 150 people, many of whom were hospitalized with liver and kidney damage. Animals also are affected; in 2000, a hunter's Labrador retriever died after

[8]For more information, see J.R. Callahan, *Recent Advances and Issues in Environmental Science* (Phoenix, AZ: Oryx Press, 2000).

drinking cyanobacteria-contaminated water from a lake in Idaho.

REFERENCES AND RECOMMENDED READING

"Algae's Role Confirmed in Dog's Death." Associated Press, January 6, 2000.

Anderson, Donald M. "Red Tides." *Scientific American*, August 1994, pp. 62–68.

Baker, Beth. "Harmful Algal Blooms." *BioScience*, January 1998, p. 12.

Barker, Rodney. 1998. *And the Waters Turned to Blood: The Ultimate Biological Threat*. New York: Touchstone Books.

Betina, Vladimir. 1989. *Mycotoxins: Chemical, Biological, and Environmental Aspects*. Bioactive Molecules, Vol 9. Oxford, UK: Elsevier Science Ltd.

Bhat, Ramesh V. "Moulds that Can Kill." *World Health*, March 1987, pp. 20–22.

Dinehart, S.M., et al., "Caripito Itch: Dermatitis from Contact with *Hylesia* Moths." *Journal of the American Academy of Dermatologists*, November 1985, pp. 743–747.

Falconer, Ian. "Harmful Effects of Blue-Green Algae on Human Health." *Australian Biologist*, Volume 1, 1997, pp. 107–110.

Franklin, Deborah. "The Poisoning at Pamlico Sound." *Health*, September 1995, p. 108 ff.

Fuller, John G. 1969. *The Day of St. Anthony's Fire*. London: Hutchinson.

Hagmann, Michael. "A Mold's Toxic Legacy Revisited." *Science*, April 14, 2000, pp. 243–244.

Halstead, Bruce W. 1984. *Paralytic Shellfish Poisoning*. Geneva: World Health Organization.

Herbert, H.J. "Polluting the Coast." Associated Press, April 5, 2000.

Iffy, L., et al. "Ergotism: A Possible Etiology for Puerperal Psychosis." *Obstetrics and Gynecology*, March 1989, pp. 475–477.

Kawamoto, F., and Kumada, N. "Biology and Venoms of Lepidoptera." In Tu, A.T. (Editor). 1995. *Handbook of Natural Toxins*, Volume 2. New York: Marcel Dekker.

Kendrick, B. 1992. *The Fifth Kingdom*, 2nd ed. Newburyport, MA: Focus.

Matossian, Mary Kilbourne. 1989. *Poisons of the Past: Molds, Epidemics, and History*. New Haven, CT: Yale University Press.

Meinesz, Alexandre. 1999. *Killer Algae*. English translation by Daniel Simberloff. Chicago: University of Chicago Press.

Mitchell, John. 1979. *Botanical Dermatology: Plants and Plant Products Injurious to the Skin*. Vancouver, BC: Greengrass.

"Sea Lion Deaths Linked to Toxic Algae Bloom." Associated Press, January 8, 2000.

"Widespread Red Tide Outbreak Hits Florida's Coasts." Reuters News Service, October 13, 1999.

POISONOUS ANIMALS, PLANTS, AND FUNGI

As we said earlier, a poisonous organism is one that causes poisoning if you ingest it. The previous section contains some borderline cases; biology is always like that. For example, if you eat a peanut butter sandwich derived from peanuts that once supported a population of *Aspergillus* fungi, you are being poisoned, but only by the metabolic garbage that the fungi left behind. But if you go out into a field, gather a basket of toadstools, and serve them for dinner, that is an example of what the word "poisoning" usually connotes. You are consuming the fungus itself as a source of food, not its products as an accidental contaminant.

Poisonous Mammals

The meat of many mammals (such as cats) is unpalatable to most humans, but not actually poisonous. In some mammals, however, the liver stores vitamin A in such high concentrations that it can harm the unwary hunter who tries to eat it. In 1857, the Arctic explorer Elisha Kane became ill after eating polar bear liver. Less exotic sources also will do the trick; chicken liver has caused vitamin A toxicity in toddlers who have eaten as little as four ounces per day for four months. Symptoms may include headache, vomiting, loss of appetite, and swelling.

Vitamin A and other fat-soluble vitamins tend to accumulate in the body and can reach high levels, a problem that is less likely with water-soluble beta-carotene (a vitamin A precursor). Birth defects have resulted from vitamin A overdoses in pregnant women. At high enough levels, even beta-carotene can be lethal. People have actually turned orange and died after drinking enormous quantities of carrot juice.

Poisonous Birds

In 1992, scientists reported that a New Guinea bird called the hooded pitohui (*Pitohui dichrous*) and four related species have a highly potent toxin called homobatrachotoxin in their feathers and skin. This alkaloid is closely related to the chemicals found in the skin of arrow-poison frogs, discussed later in this chapter. In the pitohui, however, the toxin apparently is present in low concentrations; people have eaten small amounts of the skin without serious effects. One researcher reported numbness and burning in his mouth when he licked his hands after handling pitohui feathers.

The muscle and internal organs of the bird also contain the toxin, but in even smaller amounts. Local people in New Guinea apparently have tasted the bird on occasion, and their name for it ("the rubbish bird") suggests that it is unpalatable rather than deadly.

Poisonous Reptiles

At least two species of sea turtles, the hawksbill (*Eretmochelys imbricata*) and the leatherback turtle (*Dermochelys coriacea*), are poisonous if eaten. Their flesh contains chelonitoxin, which causes nausea, a burning sensation in the mouth, profuse salivation, tightness in the chest, difficulty in swallowing, and a skin rash, sometimes followed by liver enlargement, coma, and death. The case fatality rate is variously reported as about 7 percent or "high," depending on the source; in either case, there is no known antidote. Unfortunately for these turtles, their eggs are edible, and the hawksbill's shell was formerly considered valuable for the manufacture of combs. As a result of overcollecting, both turtles have joined the world's list of endangered and threatened species.

Apparently, some individual hawksbill turtles are poisonous and others merely bad-tasting. It is not clear if the level of toxicity depends on the turtle's recent food or on other factors. Fishermen in the Caribbean formerly tested a turtle for edibility by offering its liver to crows; if the birds rejected it, the rest of the turtle was thrown away.

Venomous (versus poisonous) reptiles were described earlier in the chapter.

Poisonous Amphibians

The skin secretions of many amphibians are poisonous. In a survival situation, amphibians represent an exception to the usual rule that most animals (unlike plants) are safe to eat.

North American newts in the genus *Taricha* contain a highly potent toxin called tetrodotoxin. The chemical was originally called tarichatoxin, until scientists discovered that it was the same as the previously discovered puffer fish poison (next section). Later, it turned up in another unrelated animal, the blue-ringed octopus. In all these species, symbiotic bacteria manufacture the toxin.

There is enough tetrodotoxin in a newt weighing ten grams (about one-third of an ounce) to kill 1500 mice. Under most circumstances, newts and people have little contact; but there seems to be nothing that someone has not done at least once. In 1981, on a dare, a 20-year-old man died after swallowing an Oregon rough-skinned newt (*Taricha granulosa*) with a whiskey chaser. In 1971, a 26-year-old man did the same thing, except that he swallowed five newts and promptly vomited, a reflex that saved his life.

People who ingest tetrodotoxin apparently can remain conscious for several hours, even though they appear dead. We know this only because some people have recovered and described their experiences. Tetrodotoxin is the same chemical that voodoo priests allegedly use (in carefully controlled doses) to create zombies—people who seem to die, but then return from the dead as mindless slaves.

Tetrodotoxin is not the only lethal amphibian toxin. The skin of the colorful South American arrow-poison frogs (*Dendrobates* and *Phyllobates*) contains batrachotoxin and other highly toxic chemicals that native people once used on their hunting darts.

Batrachotoxin, even in very small doses, affects the nervous system and can stop the heart.

For a discussion of some other toad toxins, see the sections in this chapter on venomous animals (above) and psychoactive substances (below).

Poisonous Fishes

At least 700 known species of marine fishes are considered poisonous, at least in certain seasons. Most of these species are nonmigratory and live in tropical oceans.

As an example, puffer fish (*Tetraodon* and relatives) or fugu is a favorite food in Japan, despite the fact that the skin and certain organs contain a powerful neurotoxin called tetrodotoxin (the same as tarichatoxin in the previous section). Puffer fish raised in captivity may lack the toxin, which is made by symbiotic bacteria, but wild ones are risky to eat. Every year, about 50 people in Japan die from eating fugu, and 100–200 people in Tokyo alone show signs of fugu poisoning. Fugu chefs must qualify for a government license, and the final examination requires the chef to eat his own fugu. A Japanese folk song reportedly contains the lyrics: "I want to eat fugu, but I don't want to die."

As noted in the section on *Taricha* newts, tetrodotoxin is unusual in that the victim may appear dead while remaining fully conscious. As recently as 1983, competent physicians in Japan have declared fugu victims dead somewhat ahead of schedule. In one such case, a man revived just as attendants were preparing to cremate him.

Another poisonous fish that deserves mention here is the tropical band-tailed goatfish (*Upeneus arge* and related species), or nightmare weke. People who eat its flesh—particularly from the head end, and during the summer months—sometimes report vivid hallucinations and nightmares, accompanied by sweating, weakness, and tightness in the chest. The Hawaiians reportedly called this fish the "Chief of the Ghosts."

Poisonous Plants

There are so many poisonous plants in the world that we must limit this discussion to a few of them. In 1993, in the United States alone, over 94,000 reported cases of poisoning resulted from the ingestion of toxic plants.

Table 7.6 lists several of the most toxic species, and Table 7.7 lists the plants responsible for most calls to poison control centers. Note that the two lists are completely different. The first list contains mostly wild plants, many of them so bad-smelling or foul-tasting that only the most determined "head" would go near them. The second list contains a high proportion of house and garden plants that children tend to swallow. A few of these, such as poinsettia, are not highly toxic, although they can cause an upset stomach.

A typical weed-grown vacant lot in southern California may contain castor bean, datura, and tree tobacco—three of the most poisonous plants on Earth—plus the odd nightshade, oleander, and others. In an era when every minor hazard creates a public uproar, these plants somehow pass unnoticed. Fortunately, most people have the good sense to leave them alone.

Several common foods (or inedible parts of food plants) also can cause illness; examples appear in Table 7.8.

Castor Bean. The beans of this plant (*Ricinus communis*, Figure 7.5) contain ricin, one of the most toxic chemicals known to science. Toxicology studies with mice have

Table 7.6
Some Poisonous Wild Plants and Fungi in North America

Common Name	Scientific Name	Notes
Castor Bean	*Ricinus communis*	Ricin; highly toxic
Rosary Pea	*Abrus precatorius*	Abrin; highly toxic
Tree Tobacco	*Nicotiana glauca*	Nicotine; highly toxic
Jimson Weed	*Datura meteloides*	Atropine; highly toxic
Water Hemlock	*Cicuta* sp.	Convulsant toxins
Oleander	*Nerium oleander*	Digitalis-like compounds
Carolina Yellow Jessamine	*Gelsemium sempervirens*	Solanine; mitotic poison
Nightshade	*Solanum* sp.	Solanine; levels vary
Crocus	*Colchicum* sp.	Colchicine; highly toxic
Monkshood	*Aconitum* sp.	Aconitine; highly toxic
Death Cap Mushroom	*Amanita phalloides*	Lethal in small doses

Source: Amdur et al. (1991).

Table 7.7
Plant Ingestions Most Often Reported to Poison Control Centers

Common Name	Scientific Name	Reported Exposures, 1993
Philodendron	*Philodendron* sp.	4,726
Pepper	*Capsicum annuum*	3,912
Dumb Cane	*Dieffenbachia* sp.	2,837
Poinsettia	*Euphorbia pulcherrima*	2,798
Holly	*Ilex* sp.	2,651
Pokeweed or Inkberry	*Phytolacca americana*	2,231
Peace Lily	*Spathiphyllum* sp.	2,086
Jade Plant	*Crassula* sp.	1,658
Pothos or Devil's Ivy	*Epipremnum aureum*	1,401
Poison Ivy	*Toxicodendron radicans*	1,308
Umbrella Tree	*Schefflera actinophylia*	1,141
African Violet	*Saintpaulia* sp.	1,137
Azalea or Rhododendron	*Rhododendron* sp.	1,029
Yew	*Taxus* sp.	969
Eucalyptus	*Eucalyptus* sp.	945
Pyracantha	*Pyracantha* sp.	894
Spider Plant	*Chlorophytum comosum*	787
Christmas Cactus	*Schlumbergera bridgesii*	781
English Ivy	*Hedera helix*	765
Climbing Nightshade	*Solanum dulcamara*	754

Source: Morbidity and Mortality Weekly Report, January 27, 1995.

shown that ricin is 6000 times more lethal than cyanide, and there is no known treatment other than supportive care. In a widely reported 1978 incident, an unknown assassin killed Bulgarian BBC correspondent Georgi Markov by injecting him with ricin on the tip of an umbrella.

Contrary to the plots of several television programs and stories, modern analysis methods *can* detect ricin at autopsy. In other words, it is not a safe way to kill someone and get away with it. Nor is it a nice way; the victim may survive for ten to 12 days with nausea, vomiting, bloody diarrhea, and circulatory collapse. Terrorists might put ricin in water or food, deliver it on pro-

jectiles, or even disperse it as a small particle aerosol. Inhaled ricin would cause symptoms (mainly nausea and shortness of breath) within eight hours and death in 36 to 72 hours.

Despite the potential for mischief, castor bean is widely cultivated for its oil, and the bushes grow wild in tropical and subtropical regions. In some places, the seeds are made into necklaces and sold as souvenirs. One seed, if chewed, is enough to kill a child.

Datura. Several forms of this plant grow in North America and throughout the world. One of the most poisonous is jimson weed (*Datura stramonium*), a familiar sight

Table 7.8
Unexpected Effects of Various Foods

Food	Effects
Apple	Seeds may release cyanide when digested (risk is minimal)
Apricot	Seed pit, leaves, stem, and bark contain cyanogenic glycosides
Bitter Almonds	Contain prussic acid; toxic
Chocolate	Contains theobromine, which is poisonous to dogs
Carrots	In huge doses, beta-carotene turns you orange and kills you
Elderberry Juice	Toxins in roots and leaves may contaminate the juice
Grapefruit Juice	Fine by itself; dangerous if combined with some medicines
Horseradish	In large doses, may cause collapse and confusion
Lima Beans	Contain cyanide; toxic if eaten raw in large quantities
Mango	May cause dermatitis in people sensitive to poison ivy
Nutmeg	Psychoactive and toxic in large doses
Parsnip	Skin contact followed by sun exposure causes burning
Pokeweed	Highly toxic if prepared incorrectly; delicious otherwise
Potato	Green areas may contain solanine (remove by peeling)
Red Beans	If undercooked, can cause anemia in susceptible persons
Rhubarb	Leaves are poisonous (high levels of oxalic acid)
Soursop (tropical fruit)	Seeds, leaves, bark, and roots are toxic enough to use as pesticide
Spinach	Handling raw leaves may cause dermatitis
Yam	Contain steroids; toxic if eaten raw in large quantities

Sources: Botanical Dermatology Database; *Morbidity and Mortality Weekly Report*, various; Amdur et al. (1991).

in vacant lots and along roadsides. The plant takes its name from the early Jamestown Colony in Virginia, where British soldiers made themselves sick by eating it in 1676. Ironically, it was not native to the area; the colonists had imported it from England to use in medicinal salves.

In 1813, when advised to plant datura in his garden, Thomas Jefferson wrote:

I have so many grandchildren and others who might be endangered by the poison plant, that I think the risk overbalances the curiosity of trying it. The most elegant thing of that kind known is a preparation of the Jamestown weed, Datura Stramonium, invented by the French in the time of Robespierre. Every man of firmness carried it constantly in his pocket to anticipate the guillotine.[9]

More recently, in 1983, a Canadian couple became severely ill when they accidentally used dried datura seeds as hamburger seasoning. The section on psychoactive substances, later in this chapter, contains additional comments on datura. This plant and its relatives are the source of a drug called atropine, widely used as a remedy for organophosphate poisoning, including the effects of certain chemical warfare agents.

Another form of datura is an ornamental vine called angel's trumpet (*Datura metel*), whose lovely flowers are a familiar sight in

[9]H.A. Washington (Editor), *The Writings of Thomas Jefferson* (New York: J.C. Riker, 1855).

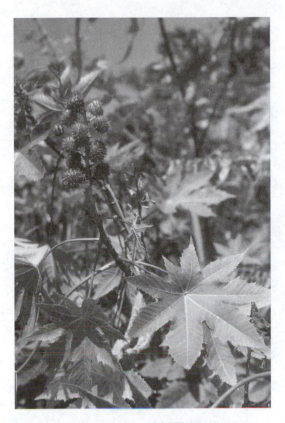

Figure 7.5. Castor Bean (*Ricinus communis*). (*Source*: Dr. Daniel L. Nickrent, Southern Illinois University, Carbondale.)

tropical gardens. It is extremely toxic. According to an often-repeated and possibly exaggerated story, a Hawaiian woman picked the flowers and then prepared a sandwich for her husband. Traces of plant juice from her fingers contaminated the food, and he died. Other poisonous garden plants also are called angel's trumpet, such as shrubs in the related genus *Brugmansia*, which has flowers that hang down (datura flowers generally stick up).

Dieffenbachia. This familiar house plant contains high levels of oxalic acid. It is not

deadly, but biting into a leaf causes immediate, severe burning pain and swelling of the mouth that may prevent speech. For this reason, the plant is often called the dumbcane. Small children are the usual victims, and ice cream is the traditional remedy.

Oleander. Like several other garden plants, this common ornamental shrub contains chemicals similar to the heart medication digitalis. Children who eat oleander leaves may experience nausea and a slow heartbeat with an irregular rhythm, in some cases leading to cardiac arrest. The dried leaves are just as toxic as the fresh ones.

Philodendron. For many years, this house plant has topped the list of plant ingestions most often reported to poison control centers in the United States. The leaves and stems, like those of its relative dieffenbachia, contain high levels of oxalic acid that cause a burning sensation in the mouth and throat. The effects of philodendron typically are more severe, however, and may also include nausea, vomiting, diarrhea, and swelling of the mouth or throat. In rare cases, the swelling may block the airway.

Poinsettia. Although poinsettia is not very poisonous, we must include it here because people fill their homes with these red-leaved plants every Christmas, and then frantically call poison control centers to report that their child or pet has eaten a leaf. In 1995, a survey of members of the Society of American Florists showed that two-thirds of them believed poinsettia to be lethal.

The poinsettia legend started in 1919, when an Army officer's two-year-old child died after allegedly eating a poinsettia leaf. The cause of death was never verified, and apparently no one else has ever died from eating this plant. The sap, if rubbed on the skin, can cause irritation and blisters; eating the leaves might also cause cramps and diarrhea. Reports indicate, however, that a 50-pound child would need to eat at least 500 poinsettia leaves in order to receive a lethal dose.

Pokeweed **(Phytolacca americana).** This controversial wild plant is both a cherished Southern vegetable and the source of an estimated 2000 human poisonings in the United States each year. The roots, mature leaves, and possibly the berries contain toxin saponins that can cause severe vomiting and diarrhea. At one time, Southerners used pokeweed roots to treat dogs with distemper; it is unlikely that the dogs ever had distemper again.

When properly prepared, however, poke leaves are delicious as a boiled green with bacon or salt pork. If you must eat the leaves, you need to preboil them, drain off the liquid, and then boil them a second time. Some cooks also chop the stalks and fry them like okra, and a few risk-takers use the young leaves raw in salads.

Poisonous Fungi

According to an unusual theory that circulates periodically on the Internet, fungi are not native to this planet. Their arsenal of powerful toxins, weird hallucinogens, and delicious flavors when sautéed with garlic are interpreted by some as evidence of extraterrestrial origin. Whatever the truth may be, people seek out fungi, and fungi respond.

Every year, poison control centers in the United States receive about 11,000 reports of toxic mushroom exposure. Most victims are among the following: (1) foreign visitors who eat wild mushrooms that resemble a familiar edible species; (2) small children who eat toadstools on their front lawns; (3) teenagers or adults who are trying to get a buzz; or (4) victims of attempted homicide or suicide.

Poisonous mushrooms contain four different types of toxins, depending on the species. Gastrointestinal toxins cause nausea, vomiting, cramps, and/or bloody diarrhea, sometimes leading to kidney failure. Disulfiram-like toxins are those that resemble a drug used to treat alcoholism; they can cause a severe drop in blood pressure and other symptoms, particularly if consumed with alcoholic beverages. Neurologic toxins may cause salivation, dizziness, behavioral changes, and hallucinations. Finally, protoplasmic toxins may cause vomiting, seizures, and death from kidney and liver failure.

Some mushrooms, such as the famous death cap (*Amanita phalloides*), contain a mixture of toxins representing more than one category. Other cases of apparent mushroom poisoning do not fall into any of these groups, and often have nothing to do with the mushrooms. Some of these may have been sprayed with pesticides, whereas other cases involve ordinary bacterial food poisoning resulting from improper cooking or storage.

Nearly all fatal mushroom poisonings in North America result from the death cap or its relatives. These mushrooms cause severe liver damage, and the victim may lapse into a coma and require a liver transplant. At least 100 mushroom species in North America are poisonous, however, and people who insist on gathering mushrooms should take a class (or several) and learn how to identify them. They should also consider the fact that some wildlife species depend on these fungi as a food source.

REFERENCES AND RECOMMENDED READING

Alber, J.I., and Alber, D.M. 1993. *Baby-Safe Houseplants and Cut Flowers*. Pownal, VT: Story Communications, Inc.

Betina, Vladimir. 1989. *Mycotoxins: Chemical, Biological, and Environmental Aspects*. Bioactive Molecules, Vol 9. Oxford, UK: Elsevier Science Ltd.

Bradley, S.G., and Klika, L.J. "A Fatal Poisoning from the Oregon Rough-Skinned Newt (*Taricha granulosa*). *Journal of the American Medical Association*, July 17, 1981, p. 247.

Champetier de Ribes, G., et al. "Intoxications par Animaux Marins Vénéneux à Madagascar (Ichyosarcotoxisme et Chélonitoxisme): Données Épidémiologiques Récentes. [Poisonings by Venomous Marine Animals in Madagascar (Ichthyosarcotoxism and Chelonitoxism): Recent Epidemiological Data]." Bulletin Société de Pathologie Exotique, Vol. 90, No. 4, 1997.

"Datura Poisoning from Hamburger, Canada." *Morbidity and Mortality Weekly Report*, Vol. 33, No. 20, 1984, p. 282.

Davis, Wade. "Zombification." *Science*, June 24, 1988, pp. 1715–1716.

Dumbacher, J. P., et al. "Homobatrachotoxin in the Genus *Pitohui*: Chemical Defense in Birds?" *Science*, Vol. 258, 1992, pp. 799–801.

Ellis, David J. "Devil in Angel's Petals." *American Horticulturist*, May 1995, p. 7.

Fox, Barry. "Stalking the Safe Mushroom." *New Scientist*, January 18, 1992, p. 38 ff.

Gomez, Julie. 1997. *A Guide to Identifying Deadly Herbs*. Surrey, BC: Hancock House.

Halstead, Bruce W. 1988. *Poisonous and Venomous Marine Animals of the World*. 2nd ed. Princeton, NJ: Darwin Press.

"Hazards of Stalking the Wild Mushroom." *State of Alaska Epidemiology Bulletin No. 17*, August 21, 1998.

Kingsbury, John M. 1964. *Poisonous Plants of the United States and Canada*. Englewood Cliffs, NJ: Prentice-Hall.

Kingsbury, John M. 1966. *Deadly Harvest: A Guide to Common Poisonous Plants*. New York: Holt, Rinehart & Winston.

Knight, B. "Ricin—A Potent Homicidal Poison." *British Medical Journal*, Vol. 278, 1979, pp. 350–351.

Levy, Charles K., and Primack, Richard B. 1984. *A Field Guide to Poisonous Plants and Mushrooms of North America*. Brattleboro, VT: Stephen Greene Press.

Matossian, Mary Kilbourne. 1989. *Poisons of the Past: Molds, Epidemics, and History*. New Haven, CT: Yale University Press.

Mayor, Adrienne. "Mad Honey: Bees and the Baneful Rhododendron." *Archaeology*, November–December 1995, p. 32 ff.

Meier, J., and White, J. (Editors). 1995. *Handbook of Clinical Toxicology of Animal Venoms and Poisons*. Boca Raton, FL: CRC Press.

Mulligan, Gerald A. 1990. *Plantes Toxiques du Canada*. Ottawa: Agriculture Canada.

National Consumers League. 1998. *Food & Drug Interactions* (Brochure). Washington, DC: NCL.

"The Poisonous Poinsettia Myth." Stillwater, MN: Rose Floral & Greenhouse, Inc., 1997.

Rodahl, K. "The Toxic Effect of Polar Bear Liver." *Skrifter* (Norwegian Polar Institute), No. 92, 1949, 90 pp.

Rubin, H.R. and Wu, A.W. "The Bitter Herbs of Seder: More on the Horseradish Horrors." *Journal of the American Medical Association*, Vol. 259, 1988, p. 1943.

Rumack, B.H., and Spoerke, D.G. 1994. *Handbook of Mushroom Poisoning, Diagnosis and Treatment*. 2nd ed. Boca Raton, FL: CRC Press.

Russell, F.E. "Vitamin A Content of Polar Bear Liver." *Toxicon*, July 1967, pp. 61–62.

Rwiza, H.T., "Jimson Weed Food Poisoning: An Epidemic at Usangi Rural Government Hospital" (*Tropical and Geographical Medicine*, January–April 1991, pp. 85–90).

Segal, Marian. "Stalking the Wild Mushroom." *FDA Consumer*, October 1994, p. 20 ff.

Steingarten, Jeffrey. "Salad: The Silent Killer." *House and Garden*, June 1988, p. 172 ff.

Swaroop, S., and Grab, B. "Snake Bite Mortality in the World." *Bulletin of the World Health Organisation*, Vol. 10, 1954, pp. 35–76.

Tu, Anthony T. (Editor). 1995. *Handbook of Natural Toxins*. New York: Marcel Dekker.

ALLERGENS

Allergy is big business in the twenty-first century. On the one hand, it is definitely real, and its prevalence is increasing. About 10 percent of Americans have at least one clinically significant allergy. Asthma has reached epidemic levels, particularly among inner-city children; the overall prevalence of reported asthma rose by 75 percent between 1980 and 1994. The reason for this trend is not clear, despite theories ranging from measles shots to working mothers. On the other hand, allergy is high on the list of convenient scapegoats for people who feel sick, and for their doctors who have no idea why. A recent review by the American Council on Science and Health concluded, in part:

Many people who believe they have MCS [multiple chemical sensitivity] suffer greatly. In extreme cases, afflicted individuals perceive almost everything around them as allergy-causing and potentially life-threatening. . . . The American Council on Science and Health believes that false claims related to "multiple chemical sensitivity" and its associated pseudoscientific practices constitute a serious problem in our society.[10]

An associated industry called clinical ecology has arisen to serve the needs of this patient population. At latest count, some 400 practitioners in the United States and Canada were working with attorneys to secure damages for people who, in some cases, claim no symptoms, but who are worried about future illness from exposure to "chemicals." One heartbreaking book or article after another describes how its authors struggled to understand why they had cancer, or why their children were disabled, or why people must die at all, until an answer presented itself: allergy. Some of these explanations may be valid, but others mislead the public and discourage more productive lines of inquiry.

Food Allergies

In the 1960s, a popular book advanced the theory that food allergy was responsible for nearly all illness. The test was simplicity itself: take your pulse, eat the suspected food (in any desired amount), and take your pulse again. If the rate goes up, you are allergic to the food. People claimed to feel much better after taking the test and avoiding such foods, and it is easy to see why. "Pigging out" on any favorite food usually speeds up the heart rate temporarily. By avoiding foods they liked best, the subjects simply ate less, and thus improved their health in general. But self-denial has never been popular, and another fad soon bit the dust.

Some studies indicate that about 20 percent of Americans think they have food allergies, but estimates of the true prevalence of food allergies in this country range from 1 to 8 percent. People often confuse food allergies with two other phenomena: food *intolerance*, in which an individual cannot

---

[10]Thomas Orme, *MCS: Multiple Chemical Sensitivity* (New York: American Council on Science and Health, 1994).

digest certain foods, as in lactose intolerance; and foodborne *illness*, caused by food that contains pathogens or toxins (see Chapter 3).

A real food allergy, however, is as serious as any allergy, and can even cause death from anaphylaxis. Over 90 percent of confirmed food allergies are from the following group of proteins: wheat, peanuts, soybeans, cow's milk, or egg whites. By one estimate, over 100 U.S. residents die each year from allergic reactions to peanuts alone. Many people are also allergic to cashews or other nuts, shellfish, and fish. Children are about ten times as likely as adults to have food allergies, but most outgrow their allergies to milk, wheat, and eggs by age six. Allergies to nuts and shellfish, by contrast, are more likely to last into adulthood. As of 2001, researchers at Johns Hopkins University were testing a peanut allergy vaccine.

Animal Allergies

Biologists who have worked with wild mammals safely for years are sometime perplexed the first time they handle a laboratory rat or rabbit and promptly break out in hives. Apparently, the difference has to do with hygiene. Wild mammals diligently groom themselves and one another, and they can control their surroundings.

A chipmunk's burrow, for example, has a sort of bathroom, a side chamber in which the occupant deposits its wastes. Even after a long winter underground, the animal is remarkably clean; when it needs a new nest, it makes one. A rat or rabbit in a small cage, by contrast, cannot go anywhere, and it continually walks back and forth through its own urine and feces. The strong allergic reactions in laboratory workers have been traced to particles of dried urine that flake off the animals' hair. Air-conditioning systems can even pick up these particles and circulate them through a building. (Laboratory workers who try to avoid the problem by wearing gloves often end up with a latex allergy, instead.)

Many other allergies result from dander shed by cats, dogs, and other house pets. In 1993, President Clinton was criticized for being allergic to the First Cat, and for banishing the animal to another part of the White House.

Insects and parts of insects are another frequent cause of allergies. Cockroach antigens appear to be the most common cause of asthma in inner-city children. There are more exotic examples; people who raise mushrooms may become allergic to mushroom flies, and museum curators often develop similar reactions to dermestid beetles. Arthropods other than insects, such as dust mites and their droppings, are widespread allergens. Bakers sometimes develop a skin rash from contact with mites in flour.

Many insects, such as cone-nosed bugs and ticks (see Chapter 5) and the venomous insects that appear earlier in this chapter, also can cause allergic reactions in sensitized individuals. Bee venom, for example, is not highly toxic in itself, but about 50 people die in the United States each year from anaphylaxis after a bee sting.

A recent study showed that the typical U.S. resident eats about a pound of insect parts every year, because many foods contain insects that were ground up during processing. Some authors have concluded that the food industry must therefore be responsible for the epidemic of allergies in this country. In fact, insects and their wastes are present in most plant and animal products, whether processed or not. In the 1960s, some vegetarians who moved to the United States from India soon developed a vitamin B_{12} deficiency, although they ate the same foods as before. The reason was that the locally purchased fruit no longer contained live grubs and other arthropods, a good source of the vitamin. (B_{12} does not normally occur in plant foods except in the form of inactive analogs.)

Plant, Pollen, and Fungus Allergies

As early as the twelfth century A.D., the Jewish philosopher Maimonides noted that people often had attacks of wheezing in damp weather. This was an accurate observation of the effects of fungal spores on sensitized individuals. Various plant products cause similar effects.

There are so many possible antigens in these categories that we can list only a few common examples (see Table 7.9). Some people sneeze and scratch year-round, others during a specific season, and still others not at all. The author can safely roll in a patch of poison oak, but cannot go near a tumbleweed.

***Poison Ivy, Poison Oak*, and *Poison Sumac*.** The first two plants are closely related and have similar effects, but occur in different parts of North America. Poison ivy (*Toxicodendron radicans*) occupies most of the continent, except for Nevada and parts of California. Poison oak (*Toxicodendron*

toxicarium) grows in the Pacific, eastern, and southern states; some botanists recognize additional species. Both poison ivy and poison oak have leaves in groups of three that tend to turn red in the fall. Poison sumac (*Toxicodendron vernix*) grows mainly in bogs and swamps east of the Mississippi River.

The famous Captain John Smith described poison ivy dermatitis in 1609: "The poisoned weed is much in shape like our English ivy, but being touched, causeth redness, itching, and lastly, blisters, and which, howsoever after a while pass away of themselves, without further harm."[11]

Robert Louis Stevenson described the western counterpart, poison oak, on his first trip to California in 1880:

[We were] continually switched across the face by sprays of leaf or blossom. The last is no great inconvenience at home; but here in California it is a matter of some moment. For in all woods and by every wayside there prospers an abominable shrub or weed, called poison-oak, whose very neighbourhood is venomous to some, and whose actual touch is avoided by the most impervious.[12]

In the United States, the various forms of *Toxicodendron* affect an estimated five to nine million people each year. It is the single greatest cause of Worker's Compensation claims, injuring many Forest Service employees and other outdoor workers. On the basis of lost work hours, poison oak is considered the most hazardous plant in California, although it is not toxic.

The leaves of poison oak, poison ivy, and poison sumac contain an otherwise harm-

[11]Quoted in A.M. Klingman, "Poison Ivy (*Rhus*) Dermatitis" (*AMA Archives of Dermatology*, Vol. 77 [1958], pp. 149–180).
[12]Robert Louis Stevenson, *The Silverado Squatters* (London: Chatto and Windus, 1883).

Table 7.9
Some Respiratory Allergenic Plants

Common Name	Scientific Name
Trees:	
Acacia	*Acacia* spp.
Palo Verde	*Cercidium* spp.
Arbor Vitae	*Thuja orientalis*
Bayberry	*Myrica gale*
Bottlebrush Tree	*Callistemon citrinus*
Bald Cypress	*Taxodium distichum*
Cedar	*Cedrus* spp.
Juniper (Chinese Juniper, Red Cedar)	*Juniperus* spp.
Elderberry	*Sambucus glauca*
American Elm	*Ulmus americana*
Eucalyptus (Blue Gum)	*Eucalyptus* spp.
Hackberry	*Celtis occidentalis*
Red Maple	*Acer rubrum*
Melaleuca	*Melaleuca quinquenervia*
Mulberry	*Morus* spp.
Oaks	*Quercus* spp.
Orange Tree	*Citrus sinensis*
Date Palm	*Phoenix dactylifera*
Canary Island Date Palm	*Phoenix canariensis*
Olive Tree	*Olea europaea*
Queen Palm	*Cocos plumosa*
Brazilian Pepper Tree	*Schinus terebinthifolius*
Australian Pine (Beefwood)	*Casuarina equisetifolia*
Pines	*Pinus* spp.
Common Privet	*Ligustrum vulgare*
Willow	*Salix* spp.
Grasses:	
Bahia Grass	*Paspalum notatum*
Bermuda Grass	*Cynodon dactylon*
Johnson Grass	*Sorghum halpense*
Orchard Grass	*Dactylis glomerata*
Redtop	*Agrostis gigantea*
Perennial Ryegrass	*Lolium perenne*
Salt Grass	*Distichlis spicata*
Timothy	*Phleum pratense*
Weeds and Garden Plants:	
Aster	*Aster* spp.
Baccharis (Mulefat, Broom)	*Baccharis* spp.
Careless Weed	*Amaranthus palmeri*

(*continued*)

Table 7.9   (Continued)

Common Name	Scientific Name
Castor Bean	*Ricinus communis*
Common Cattail	*Typha latifolia*
White Clover	*Trifolium repens*
Yellow Dock	*Rumex crispus*
Eastern Dog Fennel	*Eupatorium capillifolium*
Lamb's Quarters	*Chenopodium album*
Marsh Elder (Burweed)	*Iva xanthifolia*
Mexican Tea	*Chenopodium ambrosioides*
Common Yellow Mustard	*Brassica campestris*
Pickleweed	*Salicornia virginica*
Spiny Pigweed	*Amaranthus spinosus*
English Plantain	*Plantago lanceolata*
Ragweed	*Ambrosia* spp.
Russian Thistle	*Salsola kali*
Salt Bush (Wing Scale)	*Atriplex* spp.

Sources: Austin, D.F., *Respiratory Allergenic Plants*, <http://www.fau.edu/envsci/allergy.html>, 1998; University of Arizona Health Sciences Center.

less oil called urushiol, which causes an allergic skin rash in 75–85 percent of people. Burning the plants releases droplets of the oil on particles of dust and ash, and inhaling these droplets can cause a severe reaction in some individuals. In the eighteenth century, doctors used an extract of poison oak to treat herpes lesions. Native Americans reportedly used it to remove warts, and also poisoned arrows with it; some California tribes ate it. Today's herbalists somehow use the sap both as a stimulant and as a sedative. Homeopathic doctors use it as a treatment for muscle pain, sometimes causing severe allergic contact dermatitis in the process.

Latex Allergy. Natural latex rubber is a plant product, although it may not look like one. An estimated 6 percent of the general public, 20 percent of health-care workers, and 65 percent of children with spina bifida are allergic to latex. The most likely candidates for this allergy are people who have frequent contact with latex gloves, rubber tubing, contraceptive diaphragms, and other latex products, or those with other allergies such as hay fever.

Only about 1 percent of latex rubber consists of proteins, but at least 60 of its 240 proteins can cause allergic reactions. The practice of applying cornstarch to latex gloves makes the problem worse, because the latex proteins attach to cornstarch particles and may then become airborne. Contact dermatitis is the most frequent reaction, but hives and asthma may occur; latex condom allergies have even been mistaken for sexually transmitted infections (see Chapter 5). At least 15 deaths and many severe injuries have resulted from latex allergy.

People have gone into anaphylactic shock while receiving barium enemas with rubber-tipped catheters; at least one woman had a similar reaction to a latex catheter during labor, and her child was brain-damaged as a result of oxygen deprivation. Manufacturers are working to develop synthetic alternatives, with the goal of eliminating the routine use of latex products in hospitals.

Pollen Allergies. A 2000 study showed that ragweed—one of the most important pollens for allergy sufferers—now produces nearly twice as much pollen as it did a century ago. By the twenty-second century, its output may double again. The reason for this change, as for so many adverse changes recently reported in the press, appears to be global warming. Some plants grow better with higher temperatures and more carbon dioxide; others do not. It is unclear why weeds so often land in the first category and desirable plants in the second.

Fungus Allergies. A 1999 study by Mayo Clinic researchers showed that the vast majority of chronic sinus infections probably result from the immune system's overreaction to at least 40 different varieties of household fungi. At the time this book was published, doctors were optimistic that an effective treatment might be available within the next few years— excellent news for the estimated 37 million Americans with this condition.

The ubiquitous mold *Aspergillus flavus*, previously discussed as a pathogen (see Chapter 4) and as a source of toxins, is also a potent allergen for many people.

Other Allergens

Many obscure and unexpected materials can act as triggers for asthma attacks. In one case reported in 1986, a woman was allergic to a pancreatic enzyme powder that she mixed with her dog's food every evening near the return vent of her air-conditioning system.

Recently, some tabloids and equivalent media have claimed that the thinning of Earth's protective ozone layer will make allergies worse. That statement is true only for one type of allergy called photoallergic dermatitis—a skin rash that appears after exposure to sunlight, in a person who is already allergic to a chemical that reacts with light. For example, if someone who is allergic to sulfanilamide takes the drug and then goes out in the sunlight, a skin rash will later appear; more ultraviolet light could make the rash worse. But the ozone layer has no known connection to hay fever, asthma, or other types of allergies. (In theory, a major reduction of the ozone layer could suppress everyone's immune system, thus curing hay fever the hard way.)

REFERENCES AND RECOMMENDED READING

Barrett, Stephen. 1993. *Unproven "Allergies": An Epidemic of Nonsense*. New York: American Council on Science and Health.

Brasher, Philip. "The Ragweed Ratio." Associated Press, August 16, 2000.

Brown, A.F., and Hamilton, D.L. "Tick Bite Anaphylaxis in Australia." *Journal of Accident and Emergency Medicine*, March 1998, pp. 111–113.

Clark, William R. 1997. *At War Within: The Double-Edged Sword of Immunity*. New York: Oxford University Press.

Davis, Calvin L. 1979. *Insects, Allergy and Disease: Allergic and Toxic Responses to Arthropods*. Oshawa, Ontario: C.L. Davis.

Duerksen, Susan. "A Menace Uncovered: Debilitating, Sometimes Deadly Latex Reactions Pose Medical Peril." *San Diego Union-Tribune*, April 15, 1996.

Dumke, N., and Crook, W. 1992. *Allergy Cooking With Ease*. Lancaster, PA: Starburst Publishers.

Frazier, C. 1980. *Insects and Allergy and What to Do about Them*. Norman, OK: University of Oklahoma Press.

Garner, Lisa A. "Poison Ivy, Oak, and Sumac Dermatitis." *The Physician and Sportsmedicine*, Vol. 27, No. 5, May 1999.

Howarth, Peter, and Reid, Anita. 2000. *Allergy-Free Living*. London: Mitchell Beazley.

Millar, Myrna. 1995. *The Toxic Labyrinth: A Family's Succesul Battle against Environmental Illness*. Vancouver, BC: Nico Professional Services Ltd.

Nesse, Randolph M., and Williams, George. "Nothing to Sneeze At." *The Sciences*, November–December 1994, pp. 34–38.

Ponikau, J. U., et al. "The Diagnosis and Incidence of Allergic Fungal Sinusitis." *Mayo Clinic Proceedings*, September 1999, pp. 877–884.

Radetsky, Peter, and Phillips, Bill (Editors). 1997. *Allergic to the Twentieth Century: The Explosion in Environmental Allergies, from Sick Buildings to Multiple Chemical Sensitivity*. Boston: Little, Brown.

Sasseville, D., and Nguyen, K. H. "Allergic Contact Dermatitis from *Rhus toxicodendron* in a Phytotherapeutic Preparation." *Contact Dermatitis*, Vol. 32, 1995, pp. 182–183.

van der Valk, Pieter, and Maibach, Howard I. (Editors). 1996. *The Irritant Contact Dermatitis Syndrome*. Boca Raton, FL: CRC Press.

Walling, Anne D. "Latex Allergy: A Serious Risk to Patient and Health Worker." *American Family Physician*, August 1999.

Warren, C.P.W., and Dolovich, J. "Human Asthma Due to a Dog's Drugs." *American Journal of Medicine*, Vol. 81, 1986, pp. 939–941.

PSYCHOACTIVE AND ADDICTIVE SUBSTANCES OF BIOLOGICAL ORIGIN

Poisons are poisons, whether a person swallows them accidentally or pays for the privilege. This section will focus on the toxicology and history of the chemicals most often involved in what is commonly called substance abuse, but will largely skip the sociological issues. (Drugs of nonbiological origin, such as the amphetamines, are not included either.)

Which is worse, alcohol or tobacco? That depends on your definition of "worse." Tobacco advocates note that, although their product may kill its users (and a few innocent bystanders), at least it does not make them drive on the wrong side of the road or pick fights in bars. It is comforting to know that a person heavily intoxicated with nicotine can still perform the most exacting work, such as that of a surgeon or air traffic controller. Defenders of alcohol respond by citing controversial evidence of long-term health benefits resulting from moderate alcohol consumption.

Some sources claim that nearly all society's ills, from domestic abuse and other crimes to homelessness and mental illness, result from drug and alcohol addiction. It is a temptingly simple explanation. But people have always used drugs and alcohol, and have always committed crimes, and have always gotten sick. Thus, it is difficult to test the hypothesis by separating one phenomenon from the other.

Alcohol. In about 2500 B.C., a wave of technologically advanced immigrants whom we now call the Beaker People, of mixed Spanish and African ancestry, brought the first alcoholic beverage to the British Isles. It was a fermented honey product called mead, and the locals no doubt welcomed their new friends with open arms. The Beaker People also introduced metalworking and sheep raising to a backward society, but no matter; we remember them for their drinking vessels.

Alcohol, like gun control and food, is an emotional topic that discourages rational debate. One camp hates alcohol and blames it for everything. Another firmly believes (despite equivocal research findings) that moderate drinkers are healthier than non-drinkers—"moderate" being defined as no more than two cans of beer, glasses of wine, or mixed drinks per day for a person under age 65.

The principal claim in favor of alcohol is that it tends to prevent heart disease among people in their forties or older. Such studies, however, often fail to consider that some abstainers might avoid alcohol due to a pre-existing health condition, or that light social drinking may reflect a cheerful, relaxed personality that also is conducive to good health. In other words, like most topics in this book, it isn't quite that simple. But now that drinking is "in," some authors have embraced it with evangelical fervor: "Although moderate drinking has potential health benefits for some people, no one should ever feel pressured to drink alcoholic beverages for health reasons. Those who choose to abstain can attempt to reduce their risk of coronary heart disease in other ways."[13]

The American Heart Association has recently tried to put the matter in perspective: "Without a large-scale, randomized, clinical end-point trial of wine intake, there is little current justification to recommend alcohol (or wine specifically) as a cardioprotective strategy."[14]

Fans and critics of alcohol alike agree that heavy drinking severely damages the liver and other organs, causing diseases such as cirrhosis and liver cancer. It is also a major factor in traffic fatalities and domestic abuse.

Caffeine. Long ago, on an Ethiopian hillside, there lived a plant that would one day change the world. Today, caffeine is the world's most readily available addictive and psychoactive drug, and 90 percent of Americans consume it in one form or another. Coffee is not the only source; caffeine is an ingredient in most soft drinks, and it also occurs naturally in tea and chocolate.

Studies of caffeine, like those of alcohol and tobacco, often are poorly designed, strongly biased, and inconclusive. Reading them, we would sometimes like to shake the investigators. We will not add to the confusion by trying to distill into two paragraphs the body of research that has alternately indicted caffeine and then cleared it again. Once suspected of causing heart trouble, pancreatic cancer, impotence, birth defects, and menstrual cramps, caffeine enjoys a good reputation for the moment.

There is a consensus that caffeine is addictive; that it evolved, like nicotine, as a bug repellent; and that it seems to have no measurable, long-term adverse effects on the human body. But the notion of being addicted or dependent on any chemical is troubling, and it would be a great service to humanity if someone would figure out what (if anything) caffeine is *really* doing to us.

Cocaine. Although the only known source of this drug today is a New World

---

[13]K. Meister, *Moderate Alcohol Consumption and Health* (New York: American Council on Science and Health, 1999).
[14]Ira J. Goldberg, et al., "Wine and Your Heart" (*Circulation*, January 23, 2001, pp. 472–475).

plant (*Erythroxylon coca*), recent studies have detected traces of cocaine in ancient Egyptian mummies. No one knows if this finding reflects an early transatlantic drug trade, an extinct plant source, or some improbable contamination. For all we know, perhaps a museum worker spilled a bottle of Coca-Cola on a mummy in the early 1900s, when the beverage actually contained this drug.

There are many different names for cocaine and many ways to ingest or absorb it. Native Americans once chewed the coca leaves, but this practice evidently is passé. Modern users have access to a highly concentrated extract of the plant, which they may smoke in rock form (cocaine powder plus baking soda and ammonia); or inject into the bloodstream in liquid form, sometimes mixed with heroin; or drink, mixed with alcohol; or snort into the nose as a powder; or apply to the mucous membranes of the mouth, vagina, or rectum. A recently developed anticocaine vaccine appears to have backfired. It reduces the effects of cocaine, but not the craving for it, thus prompting vaccinated users to take several times the usual dose.

Cocaine users report a "rush" followed by extreme mood swings. In high doses, cocaine can produce the sensation of insects crawling under the skin, sometimes followed by seizures, vomiting, psychosis, cerebral hemorrhage, cardiac arrest, and death (Table 7.10). It may be superfluous to add that the drug can destroy the septum of the nose and also land the user in prison with many new friends.

Heroin. American adolescents often are the target of criticism for academic or other shortcomings, but they are doing at least one thing right: as of 2000, less than 2 percent of young people ages 12–17 had ever tried heroin. At about age 17, however, things apparently go wrong. The average age of a first-time heroin user in the United States is now 17.6, down from 27 just a decade ago. Authorities attribute this trend to the greater availability and lower price of the drug. The romanticized death of heroin addict Kurt Cobain in 1994 did not help matters, nor did a recent book that explains how to extract opium—used in the manufacture of heroin—from ordinary garden poppies.

Table 7.10
Drug-Related Emergency Room Visits, U.S.

Year	Marijuana/Hashish	Heroin/Morphine	Cocaine
1990	15,706	33,884	80,355
1991	16,251	35,898	101,189
1992	23,997	48,003	119,843
1993	28,873	63,232	123,423
1994	40,183	64,013	142,878
1995	45,271	70,838	135,801
1996	53,789	73,846	152,433
1997	64,744	72,010	161,087

Source: U.S. Department of Health and Human Services.

The traditional way to use heroin is to inject it intravenously, but some users have begun to smoke or snort it like cocaine. Heroin overdose deaths in the United States appear to be increasing; over 20,000 such deaths were reported between 1994 and 1998.

In 2000, an epidemic of deaths among heroin addicts in the British Isles was traced to a batch of heroin contaminated with the bacterium *Clostridium novyi*. Related bacteria cause botulism and other forms of food poisoning (see Chapter 3), but this species rarely causes human illness. Earlier reports linked the same epidemic to anthrax. Poor quality control often is a problem in illegal drug preparation.

Marijuana and *Hashish*. Marijuana is unique among illegal drugs in that many doctors and celebrities defend it and propose its immediate legalization. A synthesis of available data, however, suggests that both the dangers and the benefits of marijuana have been exaggerated.

Marijuana is dangerous in at least two important ways. First, smoking anything can damage the lungs, and we are only issued two at birth. Second, marijuana users sometimes go to jail, or at least end up with a criminal record that makes it hard to get a security clearance or to work in certain professions. Decriminalizing the drug would solve only the second problem. Certain other risks also may be associated with marijuana. At least one study has linked sudden death syndrome (SIDS) in infants to marijuana smoking by parents, but the connection is not clear. Other studies have shown that college students who smoke marijuana are at increased risk for meningitis.

But suppose a person lives in the Netherlands, where marijuana is perfectly legal and is sold freely in coffee shops; and suppose they eat the drug, in some palatable form, rather than smoking it. Is it still dangerous? Now we are in a gray area. Detractors believe that marijuana dulls the brain, and some U.S. journalists have claimed that Dutch teenagers are mindless drones. Records show, however, that Dutch high-school students score (excuse the word) much higher than American teenagers on standard tests of mathematics and science achievement—and surveys show that only about 30 percent of Dutch teenagers have tried marijuana anyway, despite its legality. Nearly the same percentage of American students in grades nine through 12 have smoked marijuana at least once. Thus, it would be premature to conclude that the drug itself either helps or hinders school achievement.

Surveys in the Netherlands also have shown that most people who try marijuana do not continue using it, nor do they "graduate" to harder drugs. The rate of cocaine use by American teenagers is six times higher than among their Dutch counterparts. The limited data available suggest that marijuana is not highly addictive, nor does it promote the use of other drugs, nor do most people even find it appealing. It has been described as a bad-smelling, harsh-tasting smoke.

A report in *New Scientist* claims that, in 1997, the World Health Organization suppressed a report by WHO staff that concluded that marijuana is less harmful than either alcohol or tobacco. But any mind-altering drug is bound to have some adverse effects, for the simple reason that our brains usually work fairly well if left alone. Any particulates or gases, other than those normally found in Earth's atmosphere on a clear day, are likely to cause some damage if dragged repeatedly through the human respiratory tract.

The medicinal use of marijuana is a separate issue. Many chemicals not sold in coffee shops are available by prescription, and many doctors feel that more objective research on marijuana should focus on identifying any real benefits and separating them from the hype.

Tobacco. Visitors to California often admire a common roadside tree or shrub with attractive heart-shaped leaves, cylindrical yellow flowers, and a fragrance reminiscent of Raleigh, North Carolina. The foliage looks neat and attractive because the leaves contain a deadly poison that has evolved as a built-in insecticide; Native Americans reportedly used it to kill head lice. The plant is commonly known as tree tobacco (*Nicotiana glauca*), and its poison is, of course, nicotine. Farmers recognized more familiar domestic varieties of tobacco as a valuable cash crop so early in our nation's history that the whole idea now seems almost normal.

The first written reference to the practice of smoking tobacco appears in the journal of Columbus, dated November 6, 1492: "The two Christians met on the way many people who were going to their towns, women and men, with a firebrand in the hand, [and] herbs to drink the smoke thereof, as they are accustomed.[15]

Nicotine rarely kills people directly, except under unusual circumstances; for example, it was once a fairly common practice to force children to eat cigarettes as a punishment for unauthorized smoking.[16] The main hazard associated with nicotine is the fact that it is highly addictive. The cigarette, in the words of the tobacco industry, is a nicotine delivery system (see Chapter 10). Studies have shown that even "light" cigarettes contain eight times as much nicotine as indicated on the product label.

Many people report that nicotine has a soothing or stimulating effect that helps them concentrate or relieves depression. Not unexpectedly, a 2000 study showed that psychiatric patients consume nearly half of all cigarettes smoked in the United States. Sigmund Freud was his own worst patient, smoking more than 20 cigars per day and eventually suffering from mouth cancer and angina. Although nicotine itself raises blood pressure and contributes to heart disease, other ingredients in tobacco smoke are worse, such as the nitrosamines and hydrocarbons that cause cancer. The frequent combination of alcohol and tobacco further increases the risk of certain cancers, as the alcohol appears to serve as a cocarcinogen. Aside from causing cancer and lung disease, tobacco has some unexpected effects; children exposed to secondhand cigarette smoke, for example, have over three times the average rate of bacterial meningitis.

Tobacco, in fact, kills an estimated one-half of all its consumers (see Table 7.11). In a delightfully candid 2001 report, cigarette

[15]Christopher Columbus, *The Journal of Christopher Columbus*, English translation by Cecil Jane (New York: Crown Books, 1989).
[16]P. Clark, et al., "Anti-tobacco Socialization in Homes of African-American and White Parents, and Smoking and Nonsmoking Parents" (*Journal of Adolescent Health*, May 1999, pp. 329–339).

Table 7.11
Tobacco-Related Deaths Worldwide, 1998

WHO Region:	Both Sexes	Males	Females
All Member States	4,023,000	3,241,000	782,000
Africa	125,000	112,000	13,000
The Americas	772,000	472,000	300,000
Eastern Mediterranean	182,000	160,000	22,000
Europe	1,273,000	1,066,000	207,000
Southeast Asia	580,000	505,000	75,000
Western Pacific	1,093,000	927,000	166,000

Source: World Health Organization (estimates to nearest thousand).

manufacturer Philip Morris concluded that smokers' premature deaths had saved the Czech Republic over $30 million per year in health care and pension costs. Now consider the impact on a larger nation such as China, where two-thirds of men become smokers before age 25. If present trends continue, about 100 million of China's 300 million young men will die prematurely from tobacco-related causes. Tobacco will be the world's leading cause of death by the year 2030, with an annual toll estimated at 10 million.

Over 80 percent of smokers say they want to quit smoking, but only about half of them stop even briefly, and 75 percent of those resume smoking within a year. A small percentage quits permanently, but no one seems to know how, although genetic factors may be involved. For the majority, one possible solution is a nicotine vaccine that is presently being tested in rats. As noted in the discussion of cocaine, however, there is a risk that a vaccine will simply increase the amount of drug that users need to obtain the desired result. To paraphrase a very old

television commercial, they would smoke more but enjoy it less.

Observers have noted that the aboriginal tribes of the Americas used tobacco for both ceremonial and recreational purposes, without suffering from an excess of lung disease. But life in a hunter-gatherer society was difficult and usually short, and it is possible that people died of something else before tobacco had time to kill them. Or perhaps the pre-Columbian people of North America, unlike their European counterparts and uprooted descendants, had the self-discipline to use addictive drugs sparingly. Yet another theory holds that the tobacco plant changed in the hands of foreigners, thus fulfilling a great chief's curse on the people who destroyed his land and culture. Whatever the truth may be, tobacco has killed more human beings than all the imported diseases and genocide campaigns in the history of North America.

Perhaps we should thank that same curse for the junk foods that make us fat and clog our arteries, such as chocolate, corn chips, potato chips, and french fries. All three New

223

World crops—cacao, maize, and potatoes—were healthful in their original versions, before Europeans started meddling with them. The bounty of the Americas overwhelmed its invaders' defenses as surely as any disease or drug.

Datura. This name refers to a group of wild and cultivated plants that contain atropine and other toxic and medicinal alkaloids. Although highly poisonous, these plants often are involved in substance abuse because of their hallucinogenic properties. The "sacred visions" of datura commonly involve picking at imaginary insects, possibly an overrated experience. Reports also indicate that users of datura, unlike people who take LSD and other drugs, frequently are not aware that their hallucinations are drug-induced. That property of datura, combined with its high toxicity, makes datura extremely dangerous.

Jimson weed (*Datura stramonium*), a common wild plant, is the most often abused form of datura in North America. In a typical case in 1994, four male teenagers in El Paso, Texas drank tea made from Jimson weed, then fell asleep in the desert. Two of them woke up, one with hallucinations and the other unaffected. Family and police found the other two dead.

Other Drugs. This section will describe two "minor" drugs with interesting origins. Both are illegal in the United States.

Peyote, a hallucinogenic drug made from the mescal cactus (*Lophophora williamsii*), was used for centuries in Aztec religious rites. Starting in the late nineteenth century, the practice spread northward into the United States. The Comanche chief Quanah Parker persuaded his tribe to adopt the peyote ritual as an alternative to war or alcohol, thus starting the Native American Church, whose 250,000 members today enjoy the legal right to use peyote. In Quanah's words: "The white man goes into his church house and talks about Jesus, but the Indian goes into his tipi and talks to Jesus."[17] The use of peyote remains controversial, however, as some people of European descent have falsely claimed Native ancestry in order to gain access to the drug.

Bufotenine and related toxins are present in the skin secretions of many frogs and toads. Some of the larger species, such as the Colorado River toad of Arizona (*Bufo alvarius*) and the nearly cosmopolitan cane toad (*Bufo marinus*), contain enough of these chemicals to cause drooling and convulsions in dogs that mouth them. In 1986, a five-year-old Arizona boy placed a Colorado River toad in his mouth and spent a week in the hospital with seizures. Dogs and children have enough sense to spit out an object that clearly is bad for them; some adults, however, have figured out a way to scrape the venom from the toad's back, dry it, and then either smoke it or inhale it like snuff. Bufotenine is a controlled substance, and in the late 1990s several people in California and Florida were arrested for having it in their possession. One user described the effect of this toxin as "an insect-cicada sound that ran across my mind and seemed to link my body to the earth."

[17]W.E. Washburn, *The Indian in America* (New York: Harper & Row, 1975).

REFERENCES AND RECOMMENDED READING

"Batch of Heroin Contaminated with *Clostridium* Bacteria." Associated Press, June 15, 2000.

Beeching, Jack. 1975. *The Chinese Opium Wars*. New York: Harcourt Brace Jovanovich.

Brownlee, S., and Roberts, S. V. "Should Cigarettes be Outlawed?" *U.S. News and World Report*, April 18, 1994.

Campbell, Julia. "Heroin Blight." ABCNews.com, July 10, 2000.

Chaloupka, Frank. 1998. *The Demand for Cocaine and Marijuana by Youth*. Cambridge, MA: National Bureau of Economic Research.

Douglas, Clifford E. 1994. *The Tobacco Industry's Use of Nicotine as a Drug*. New York: American Council on Science and Health.

Fisher, Mary. 1996. *My Name Is Nancy*. New York: Scribner.

Freedman, A. M. "Philip Morris Memo Likens Nicotine to Such Drugs as Cocaine, Morphine." *Wall Street Journal*, December 8, 1995.

Hitt, M., and Ettinger, D.D. "Toad Toxicity." *New England Journal of Medicine*, Vol. 314, 1986, p. 1517.

"Indians Want State to Give Them Confiscated Hallucinogen." Associated Press, July 23, 2000.

Iversen, Leslie L. 2000. *The Science of Marijuana*. New York: Oxford University Press.

Jarvis, M.J., et al. "Nicotine Yield from Machine-Smoked Cigarettes and Nicotine Intakes in Smokers: Evidence from a Representative Population Survey." *Journal of the National Cancer Institute*, January 17, 2001, pp. 134–138.

"Jimson Weed Poisoning." *Morbidity and Mortality Weekly Report*, January 27, 1995.

Karch, Steven B. 1998. *A Brief History of Cocaine*. Boca Raton, FL: CRC Press.

Klonoff-Cohen, H., and Lam-Kruglick, P. "Maternal and Paternal Recreational Drug Use and Sudden Infant Death Syndrome." *Archives of Pediatric and Adolescent Medicine*, July 2001, pp. 765–770.

Koppel, Naomi. "Philip Morris Report Attacked." Associated Press, July 17, 2001.

Kriz, P., et al. "Parental Smoking, Socioeconomic Factors, and Risk of Invasive Meningococcal Disease in Children: A Population Based Case-Control Study." *Archives of Disease in Childhood*, August 2000, pp. 117–121.

Lasser, Karen, et al. "Smoking and Mental Illness: A Population-Based Prevalence Study." *Journal of the American Medical Association*, November 22/29, 2000, pp. 2606–2610.

Lerman, C., et al. "Evidence Suggesting the Role of Specific Genetic Factors in Cigarette Smoking." *Journal of Health Psychology*, January 1999, pp. 14–20.

Mackenzie, Deborah. "Vraag een Politieagent . . . Go Ahead, Ask a Cop for Dope, the Dutch Don't Mind." *New Scientist*, February 21, 1998.

National Institute on Drug Abuse. 1999. *Cocaine Abuse and Addiction*. Washington, DC: National Institutes of Health.

Norris, M., et al. 1998. *Shattered Lives: Portraits from America's Drug War*. El Cerrito, CA: Creative Xpressions.

Olson, Cheryl K., and Kutner, Lawrence. 2000. *A Comparison of the Health Effects of Alcohol Consumption and Tobacco Use in America*. New York: American Council on Science and Health.

Pendergrast, Mark. 1999. *Uncommon Grounds*. New York: Basic Books.

Ross, Emma. "In China, Smoking Takes Terrible Toll." Associated Press, November 20, 1998.

Sharfstein, J. "Blowing Smoke: How Cigarette Manufacturers Argued that Nicotine is Not Addictive." *Tobacco Control*, Vol. 8, 1999, pp. 210–213.

"A Shot in the Arm: A Tobacco Vaccine Lowers Blood Levels of Nicotine." ABCNews.com, August 7, 2000.

Spillane, Joseph. 2000. *Cocaine: From Medical Marvel to Modern Menace in the United States, 1884–1920*. Baltimore, MD: Johns Hopkins University Press.

Watson, Ronald R. 1995. *Alcohol, Cocaine, and Accidents*. Totowa, NJ: Humana Press.

Wright, Karen. "Vaccine Counters Cocaine but Can't Stop the Craving." *Discover*, August 18, 1999.

Zimmer, Lynn, and Morgan, John P. 1997. *Marijuana Myths, Marijuana Facts*. New York: The Lindesmith Center.

OUTLOOK FOR THE TWENTY-FIRST CENTURY

In the developed world, venomous and poisonous organisms are minor biohazards at best, and that situation is unlikely to change in the foreseeable future. Certain annoying species, such as the Africanized killer bee and red fire ant, will most likely continue to expand their geographic ranges in North America. Meanwhile, more available and affordable antivenoms could save many lives in Third World countries.

Substance abuse has reached epidemic proportions worldwide. The United Nations has made a good start with a plan to reduce worldwide cultivation of three plants: the coca bush, the cannabis (marijuana) plant, and the opium poppy. But some observers have noted that the demand for these plants, at least in the United States, may be only a symptom of a more fundamental problem—namely, a societal mindset that converts a desire for almost anything, be it drugs, alcohol, tobacco, food, sex, love, or even achievement, into a crisis requiring intervention. Twenty years ago, an American woman risked criticism if she ate cookies in public; today, food is in and dieting is out, and overweight high-school counselors impose penalties on female students for being too thin. There is even an Internet Web site devoted to Chap-Stick® addiction. ("It was such a relief to discover that I'm not alone!")

Psychologists have recently found that some school antidrug programs backfire by focusing too much attention on drugs. Evidence suggests that the children (and adults) who resist substance abuse most effectively are the ones who simply have better things to do.

The Good Old Days

Poisons have ranked among our allies since ancient times. But many poisons, when first discovered, were used quite carelessly, with unintended consequences. Cocaine was an ingredient in soft drinks until the early 1900s, and a blister beetle extract called cantharides, more popularly known as "Spanish fly," was a renowned aphrodisiac as recently as the 1950s. In the following account, it is not entirely clear whether the young man ingested the substance accidentally or not:

There is an instance mentioned of a robust youth of twenty who by a mistake took a half ounce of cantharides. He was almost immediately seized with violent heat in the throat and stomach, pain in the head, and intense burning on urination. These symptoms progressively increased, were followed by intense sickness and almost continual vomiting. In the evening he passed great quantities of blood from the urethra with excessive pain in the urinary tract. On the third day all the symptoms were less violent and the vomiting had ceased. Recovery was complete on the fifteenth day.[18]

Although medical books of that era vary in accuracy, the same book contains a remarkably shrewd assessment of the lethality of North American snakes:

The common snakes of the deadly variety in the United States are the rattlesnake, the "copperhead," and the moccasin; and it is from the bites of one of these varieties that the great majority

---

[18]G.M. Gould and W.L. Pyle, *Anomalies and Curiosities of Medicine* (New York: Bell Publishing Co., 1896).

of reported deaths are caused. But in looking over medical literature one is struck with the scarcity of reports of fatal snake-bites. This is most likely attributable to the fact that, except a few army-surgeons, physicians rarely see the cases. The natural abode of the serpents is in the wild and uninhabited regions.[19]

Doctors did not understand the cause of allergies in those days, but they knew certain foods and other substances could produce alarming reactions in susceptible persons. Here is an 1896 description of a wheat allergy:

If [a patient] ate flour in any form or however combined, in the smallest quantity, in two minutes or less he would have painful itching over the whole body, accompanied by severe colic and tormina in the bowels, great sickness in the stomach, and continued vomiting, which he declared was ten times as distressing as the symptoms caused by the ingestion of tartar emetic. In about ten minutes after eating the flour the itching would be greatly intensified, especially about the head, face, and eyes, but tormenting all parts of the body, and not to be appeased. These symptoms continued for two days with intolerable violence, and only declined on the third day and ceased on the tenth. In the convalescence, the lungs were affected, he coughed, and in expectoration raised great quantities of phlegm, and really resembled a phthisical patient.[20]

FROM THE AUTHOR'S FILE CABINET

Biologists, like professionals in any other field, sometimes become careless. If their work involves handling venomous or toxic organisms, the results can be poor.

In 1957, the world lost one of its greatest herpetologists, Karl P. Schmidt, to an unnecessary bite from an African boomslang snake. In a log of these events and the sequelae, Dr. Schmidt admitted his carelessness in handling the snake; but even after multiple hemorrhages, vomiting, and inability to urinate might have suggested that something was wrong, he did not seek medical help. His chronicler, another herpetologist, explained:

That Dr. Schmidt's optimism was extremely unfortunate is proved by his death, but it must be admitted that there was some justification: The boomslang was very young [26 inches] and only one fang penetrated deeply. However, almost two decades ago careful experimentation . . . showed that boomslang venom has an extraordinarily high toxicity, even higher than those of such notorious snakes as cobras, kraits, and mambas.[21]

In 2001, a professional snake handler in Florida was bitten by a taipan (see Table 7.5), but survived with the help of antivenom flown in from the San Diego Zoo. And in 1999, a comparable incident nearly claimed the life of herpetologist Howard Reinert. Colleagues found him unconscious after a bite from a caged timber rattlesnake (*Crotalus horridus*); he survived with treatment, but was unconscious for five days. After his recovery, however, the press quoted him as saying that the bite was dangerous only because he was allergic to the venom. Herpetologists often downplay the risk associated with venomous snakes; in many areas, the timber rattler is an endangered species

---

[19]Ibid.
[20]Ibid.
[21]C.H. Pope, "Fatal Bite of Captive African Rear-Fanged Snake (*Dispholidus*)" (*Copeia*, December 22, 1958, pp. 280–282).

that needs all the public relations support it can get. The public needs to know, however, that rattlesnakes can cause severe injury and must be treated with respect.[22]

Researchers must sometimes risk their lives in order to contribute to our knowledge of venomous reptiles, but amateur collectors are another story. Many of them regard deadly snakes as status symbols, and somehow obtain permits to own these animals without the justification of research. Now and then, one of these snakes bites its owner under grotesque circumstances. Most victims—the owners, we mean—are saved, thanks to improved medical care. In 1999, a California man narrowly escaped severe disfigurement when friends at a party dared him to kiss a pet rattlesnake. In 2000, a Florida teenager stuck his tongue out at a coral snake, which he had mistaken for a harmless kingsnake, and was bitten on the tongue.

But professionals, as we said, can be equally careless. Over 25 years ago, one of the finest young men in herpetology died as he had lived—without a seat belt. No biological hazard caused his death, with the possible exception of alcohol. Months before the accident, however, he told the author that he often allowed his infant son to play with a live Gila monster. His theory was that the child, if exposed to such animals early enough, would learn not to fear them. Suffice it to say that the child survived (possibly with a mild case of salmonellosis). Parents can expose their children to wildlife in positive ways through field trips, books, and nature documentaries.

REFERENCES AND RECOMMENDED READING

Brogan, Joe. "Coral Snake Bites Boy on Tongue." *Palm Beach Post*, April 5, 2000.

"College of New Jersey Professor Bitten by Rattlesnake." Associated Press, September 22, 1999.

"Rattler's Kiss Nearly Fatal for Carlsbad Man on Dare." *San Diego Union-Tribune*, July 30, 1999.

[22]In two reported cases, people who were bitten by wild timber rattlers killed the snakes and took them to the hospital for identification, only to be fined for harming an endangered species.

CHAPTER 8

Predators and Other Biological Hazards

It has been related that dogs drink at the river Nile running along,
that they may not be seized by the crocodiles.
—Phaedrus, *Fables, Book 25* (A.D. First Century)

This chapter describes three categories of headline-grabbing biological hazards that actually claim relatively few lives: animals that kill people for the purpose of eating them; animals that show aggressive behavior toward humans for some other reason; and mechanical biohazards, defined as any biological entity that causes physical or economic harm to humans simply by being in the wrong place. Since some of the examples overlap slightly with the contents of other chapters, Table 8.1 provides a cross-reference.

PREDATION ON HUMAN BEINGS

The idea of being eaten, or perhaps the idea of someone else being eaten, has always intrigued movie audiences. The formula "a big _____ invaded _____ and started eating people" really packs them in, as witness the partial list of motion pictures in Chapter 12.

In reality, only a few animal species are frequent predators on human beings. Thanks to Hollywood, the example that immediately comes to mind is the great white shark, but statistics show that shark attacks are rare and seldom lethal.

Sharks

A shark that attacks a human swimmer frequently lets go again, although the person may be injured or dismembered in the process. In a typical year, there are 50–60 reports of shark attacks worldwide and about 12 deaths. The record to date was 2000, with 85 attacks but only ten deaths. About two-thirds of reported incidents occur in the coastal waters of North America, and at least one-third of those are in Florida (see Tables 8.2, 8.3).

In June 2000, an unidentified shark attacked and seriously injured two men in shallow water off the coast of Alabama; one

Table 8.1
Cross Reference: Related Topics in Other Chapters

Topic	Chapter	Notes
Infections	5	Animal bites and scratches transmit several diseases.
Livestock predation	6	Predators kill some livestock.
Venoms	7	Many animal species cause injury by envenomation.
Wildlife management	9	Control measures can prevent some injuries.

man lost an arm. Officials described the incident as the state's first unprovoked shark attack in 25 years, and only the second recorded since 1900. In 1997, a tiger shark (*Galeocerdo cuvier*) bit off the foot of a teenage surfer in Hawaii. Off the coast of South Africa, most shark attacks on human beings are attributed to the smaller Zambezi or bull shark (*Carcharhinus leucas*), which lives in all tropical and subtropical coastal areas and sometimes swims up rivers; in North America, it has occurred as far as 1750 miles up the Mississippi River.

One of the most highly publicized recent shark attacks occurred in July 2001, when a bull shark severed the arm of an eight-year-old Florida boy. When more than a dozen other shark attacks occurred along the same stretch of beach, the media promptly declared the "Summer of the Shark." In reality, despite the individual tragedies and their concentration in Florida, the total numbers of reported shark attacks and fatalities during 2001 were no higher than usual. The University of Florida's International Shark Attack File reported only 76 unprovoked

Table 8.2
Deaths and Injuries Resulting from Animal Incidents, United States

Type of Incident	Deaths Per Year (Average)	Injuries Per Year (Average)
Horse-related Injury	219	70,000
Vehicle Collision with Deer	100	7,000
Dog Bite	20	800,000
Shark Bite	3	50
Alligator Attack	1	20
Cougar Attack	1	14
Bear Attack	1	8
Bison Attack	1	6
Wolf Attack	0	0

Sources: University of Pittsburgh study, reported by Associated Press, 1998; U.S. Centers for Disease Control and Prevention.

Table 8.3
Partial List of Shark Attacks (Worldwide), 1554–1997

Common Name	Scientific Name	Number of Attacks
Great White Shark	*Carcharodon carcharias*	311
Tiger Shark	*Galeocerdo cuvier*	104
Bull (Zambezi) Shark	*Carcharhinus leucas*	69
Grey Nurse Shark	*Carcharias taurus*	53
Requiem Shark	*Carcharhinus sp.*	42
Shortfin Mako	*Isurus oxyrinchus*	38
Great Hammerhead	*Sphyrna mokarran*	31
Blue Shark	*Prionace glauca*	30
Nurse Shark	*Ginglymostoma cirratum*	23
Wobbegong	*Orectolobus barbatus*	23
Blacktip Shark	*Carcharhinus limbatus*	22
Lemon Shark	*Negaprion brevirostris*	21
Caribbean Reef Shark	*Carcharhinus perezi*	16
Blacktip Reef Shark	*Carcharhinus melanopterus*	14
Bronze Whaler Shark	*Carcharhinus brachyurus*	11
Grey Reef Shark	*Carcharhinus amblyrhynchos*	10
Sandbar Shark	*Carcharhinus plumbeus*	7
Spinner Shark	*Carcharhinus brevipinna*	6
Oceanic Whitetip Shark	*Carcharhinus longimanus*	5
Dusky Shark	*Carcharhinus obscurus*	5
Thresher Shark	*Alopias sp.*	5
Leopard Shark	*Triakis semifasciata*	4
Silky Shark	*Carcharhinus falciformis*	4
Sevengill Shark	*Notorhynchus cepedianus*	4
Porbeagle Shark	*Lamna nasus*	3
Scalloped Hammerhead	*Sphyrna lewini*	2
Whitetip Reef Shark	*Triaenodon obesus*	2
Smalltooth Sandtiger	*Carcharias ferox*	2
Basking Shark	*Cetorhinus maximus*	2
Galapagos Shark	*Carcharhinus galapagensis*	1
Ganges Shark	*Carcharhinus gangeticus*	1
Tope Shark	*Galeorhinus galeus*	1
Cookiecutter Shark	*Isistius brasiliensis*	1
Mako Shark	*Isurus sp.*	1
Piked Dogfish	*Squalus acanthias*	1
Silvertip Shark	*Carcharhinus albimarginatus*	1
Bignose Shark	*Carcharhinus altimus*	1
Horn Shark	*Heterodontus francisci*	1
Sixgill Shark	*Hexanchus griseus*	1
Whale Shark	*Rhincodon typus*	1
Greenland Shark	*Somniosus microcephalus*	1
Smooth Hammerhead	*Sphyrna zygaena*	1

Source: University of Florida Museum of Natural History, International Shark Attack File

shark attacks worldwide in 2001, as compared with 85 in 2000.

Other famous shark attacks have involved the great white shark (*Carcharodon carcharias*), which often occurs in cooler waters. Between 1952 and 2000, great whites attacked 79 people off California's coast and killed eight of them. The recent range expansion of the great white shark is one of many phenomena that some environmental scientists have attributed to global climate change. In 1998, the media reported that a 20-foot great white had attacked a cabin cruiser in the Adriatic Sea, apparently attracted by the blood of a small sand shark that was tied to the side of the boat.

A popular theory holds that sharks sometimes mistake people for seals, schools of fish, or other "normal" prey, and then let go when they recognize their mistake. On the surface, this might sound like the usual human chauvinism, but in biological terms it actually makes some sense. When any predator goes after its prey, it expends a great deal of energy and also risks injury if the prey fights back. The best prey, then, is a Shmoo-like creature with no natural weapons and huge stores of energy in the form of fat. Humans have no natural weapons, but we do have technological ones; a shark that ventures near a crowded beach is likely to suffer at the hands of people who want to kill, photograph, study, or hug it. Worse, even the plumpest human does not contain nearly as much fat as a seal. From a nutritional standpoint, we are junk food. Individual sharks that frequently attack humans may be in poor health, reflected in a sort of beer-and-pizza mentality.

Other Fishes

A horror movie entitled *Grouper* would most likely be a box-office flop, because the name does not conjure up the proper image. Underwater nature documentaries often show human divers interacting with these large, colorful, placid-looking fish. The problem with groupers is that they sometimes grow *very* large, and on occasion they have swallowed divers. There are reports of groupers so large that they could easily swallow not only a man, but (at least in theory) a man in a Volkswagen. Not even the grouper's manner of predation would lend itself to drama. The fish simply opens its huge mouth and sucks in some water, and the prey vanishes.

In August 2000, workers at a fish market in Brisbane, Australia, cut open a 97-pound flowery cod—a marketing name in Australia that refers to several fish species, including some of the large groupers—and were surprised to find a human head inside. Judging by the size of this fish, however, it most likely found the gentleman already dead.

Although the most obvious species to include in this section might seem to be the piranha (*Serrasalmus* sp.), there is little evidence that these small fish make a practice of eating people. The stories apparently started when Theodore Roosevelt visited Brazil in 1913 and heard about a 12-year-old boy who had recently been devoured alive by piranha. Roosevelt repeated the tale in an account of his travels, along with a remarkable description of a small pond filled with caimans (small crocodiles) and piranha that survived by eating one another. Suffice it to say that the former President was not a biologist, and that Hollywood, like any good omnivore, saw an opportunity and exploited it.

The piranha exists, and it eats meat—usually dead, but sometimes alive. A solitary piranha may often take a nip out of a wading person's leg, and large schools of piranhas have occasionally skeletonized injured cows or, presumably, humans. But scientists who have worked for decades in the Amazon swear that they have never seen a piranha attack.

Crocodiles and Alligators

Nile Crocodile (**Crocodylus niloticus**). This is one of the world's largest carnivores, reaching lengths of 18 feet and weighing nearly a ton. As its prey often include animals as large as wildebeest and Cape buffaloes, it should surprise no one that crocodiles can easily kill and eat human beings. The available data suggest, in fact, that the Nile crocodile and its Asian relatives are among the very few predators that eat humans on a regular basis. (We should forgive crocodiles for their dining habits, as recent studies suggest that the crocodile's highly efficient immune system may hold clues to help solve the problem of antibiotic-resistant bacteria.)

Reports indicate that many of the Nile crocodiles that attack humans are immature animals under eight feet long and weighing less than 200 pounds. Like sharks, these animals often release people after biting off a convenient body part. Estimates vary, but it appears likely that Nile crocodiles kill between 100 and 300 people each year in Africa.

Saltwater or *Indopacific Crocodile* (**Crocodylus porosus**, *Figure 8.1*). Even

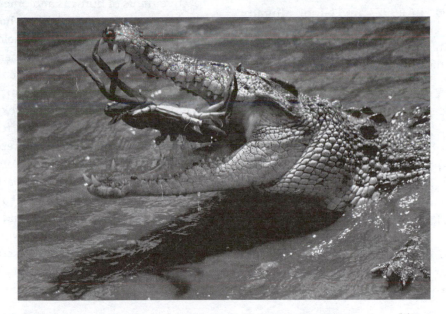

Figure 8.1. Saltwater crocodile (*Crocodylus porosus*). (*Source*: Adam Britton, crocodilian.com.)

larger than the Nile crocodile (up to 23 feet and 2200 pounds), the saltwater crocodile of northern Australia, Indonesia, and Malaysia is protected by law as an endangered species. It eats people, too; for a famous example, see the Ramree Island story later in this chapter. Some books indicate that the saltwater crocodile kills as many as 1000 people every year, but this estimate may refer to old records, and its accuracy is unknown. Queensland residents have recently complained that protection of the saltwater crocodile has endangered their livestock and children, but the real magnitude of the problem is unclear.

American Alligator (**Alligator mississippiensis**). The official state reptile of Florida is smaller than the Old World crocodiles, but still large enough to watch. In Florida alone, it bites an average of 18 people each year, and at least eight deaths resulted from such attacks between 1940 and 2000. In 1997, an 11-foot alligator grabbed and shook a man who was snorkeling in Florida; it seems reasonably certain that this was a predation attempt, although the man survived. His later comment to the press might have been either a joke or a statement of a common belief about predators: "When he tasted me, I think that's why he let me go."[1] In 2000, a nine-foot alligator seized a 14-year-old Florida boy and pulled him under water, but he managed to escape.

Most victims who die in alligator attacks appear to be small children or the elderly. In a 1997 case, a large alligator seized a three-year-old Florida child who was wading at the edge of a lake. The alligator was later shot and killed with the dead child in its mouth. A game warden investigating this tragedy made the interesting comment that the alligator probably thought the child was "just another animal" rather than a person.

The U.S. Fish and Wildlife Service listed the American alligator as endangered in 1967, but downgraded its status to threatened (less endangered) in 1975 and finally delisted it in 1987. The species still retains "special status" because of its resemblance to the American crocodile (*Crocodylus acutus*), which joined the endangered species list in 1975. In other words, there was concern that people might accidentally kill a rare American crocodile when their intention was to hunt alligators.

Whenever a large, potentially dangerous animal receives legal protection, the result is likely to be a heated debate over the respective rights of humans and other species. The outcomes of such debates have been mixed, but courts often have upheld human rights. In 1990, for example, a man named Kermit George had his arm bitten off by a large alligator while swimming in a Florida lake. The U.S. Forest Service had known of the alligator's presence, but had refused to post warning signs, despite the recommendations of its own staff, on the grounds that the signs might cause unnecessary public concern or put the alligator at risk. Mr. George sued the government, and the federal district court ruled in his favor: "If this Court were to hold that the discretionary function exception barred this suit, it would, in effect, be elevating the well-being of an

---

[1]"Victim Tells About Alligator Attack," Associated Press, October 5, 1997.

alligator to a level deserving more protection than that of a human."[2]

The 1961 book *Black Like Me* presents a similar dilemma from the viewpoint of a low-income African-American man struggling to feed his family in rural Alabama:

"Why don't you kill some of them? The tails make good meat. I could show you how. We learned in jungle training when I was in the Army."

"Oh, we can't do that," he said. "They stick a hundred-dollar fine on you for killing a gator. I'm telling you," he laughed sourly, "they got all the loopholes plugged. There ain't a way you can win in this state."

"But what about the children?" I asked. "Aren't you afraid the gators might eat one of them?"

"No. . ." he said forlornly, "The gators like turtle better than they do us."[3]

Other Crocodilians. There are about 23 species of crocodiles, alligators, and their relatives in the world. Several species occur in Latin America and the Caribbean, and occasionally they make headlines by attacking people. In 1999, a ten-foot-long American crocodile (*Crocodylus acutus*) in Jamaica killed a 70-year-old woman in an apparent predation attempt. This species also occurs in southern Florida, but it is rare, as noted above.

Other Large Reptiles

Komodo Dragon **(Varanus komodoensis).** This endangered lizard occurs on only one small group of islands in the world, and it does not eat people very often. A Swiss tourist named Baron Rudolf von Reding Biberegg

is said to have been eaten by Komodo dragons in 1974, but the circumstances are unclear. Some individual dragons apparently are friendly to humans, whereas others display odd behavior such as stealing clothing from tents. People have trained these lizards to jump through hoops and do other tricks. In 2001, a caged Komodo dragon at the Los Angeles Zoo bit a newspaper executive's toe; the incident became headline news for weeks, because the gentleman was the husband of actress Sharon Stone.

The Komodo dragon weighs up to 300 pounds and can easily kill prey by the usual process of biting and swallowing, but it has a backup method available. Its teeth are so heavily contaminated with bacteria and fragments of rotting meat that its saliva is actually poisonous. This is not a venom in the strict sense, but any animal that it bites will most likely die of the infection. After the prey begins to decompose, the Komodo dragon can smell it from several miles away. One source indicates that people have survived Komodo dragon bites with antibiotic treatment, only to die of related bacterial infections a few years later.

Large Snakes **(various species).** On rare occasions, large snakes such as pythons have tried to swallow young children. Usually the snake is a pet and the victim is an unguarded infant. Domestic animals also are susceptible; in 2001, a 200-pound pet python in California reportedly ate the household's 30-pound pit bull. Attacks by wild pythons are harder to verify. In 1999, the news media reported that a ten-foot python (species unknown) attacked a seven-year-old boy who was

---

[2]*George v. United States*, 735 F. Supp. 1524 (M.D. Ala. 1990).
[3]John Howard Griffin, *Black Like Me* (New York: Houghton Mifflin, 1961).

camping in Australia with his father. A snake of that size could not possibly swallow a child, and it is not clear what happened. A hospital treated the boy for puncture wounds and released him in good condition.

Despite early travelers' tales of 130-foot snakes gulping entire elephants—together with the faithful manservant who was riding the elephant at the time, and his howdah—there are no reliable reports of snakes swallowing humans larger than infants, and even those incidents are rare and hard to verify. Pet snakes become habituated to human presence and may be more aggressive than wild ones. Men who engage in feats of daring for nature documentaries, wading around half-naked in rivers full of anacondas, sometimes also report an uncomfortable choking sensation.

Mammals

The following paragraphs refer to attacks on humans by wild mammals under more or less natural conditions. Similar incidents involving zoo specimens are discussed later in the chapter.

African Lion (**Panthera leo**). Every year in Africa, wild lions kill an estimated 30–40 humans. Aside from these sporadic cases, unusual outbreaks of lion predation also occur at times. Some lions that become "maneaters" may be unable to capture their usual prey because of damaged teeth or other physical problems.

In 1898, for example, two lions killed and ate 135 railway workers in Kenya, an incident portrayed in the 1996 motion picture *The Ghost and the Darkness*. Biologists have recently examined the skulls of those two lions and concluded that both suffered from broken teeth and abscesses that might have prevented them from hunting more difficult prey. A similar case occurred in Tanzania between 1932 and 1945, when three or four specific prides killed an average of 100 people per year. More recently, a 1999 press release from Tanzania stated that a severe drought had forced older lions and leopards to hunt for food closer to human settlements.

Once this behavior becomes established, as in the 1930s, lion attacks on humans tend to increase as cubs learn from their elders' example. In 1945, a game warden and his scouts ended an outbreak by shooting 18 of the offending lions. The Tanzanian government now has a policy of eliminating any lions that kill humans.

Gray Wolf (**Canis lupus**). The unpopularity of the wolf in North America stems largely from its predation on livestock. There are few, if any, reliable reports of wolves killing adult humans in the United States. Children are within the size range of prey for this animal, however, and a few incidents have occurred. In 2000, a wolf attacked a six-year-old boy in Alaska and bit him repeatedly. The boy escaped, and it was not clear whether this was a predation attempt or the wolf had rabies. It may be significant (or not) that the wolf was wearing a radio collar, described as "tight."

Elsewhere in the world, the relationship between humans and wolves is less cozy. In a widely publicized incident in 1996, a wolf pack in India killed at least 46 children and injured dozens more. Such behavior by wolves was unprecedented in recent memory, and the first wildlife biologists on the scene confidently reported that wolves could not be responsible. Villagers, even eyewitnesses, blamed the deaths on were-wolves or Pakistani terrorists; in the confusion, some 20 people were lynched. Eventually, more reliable witness accounts and forensic evidence left no room for doubt, and the wolves were hunted and killed. A century earlier, wolf attacks on humans were commonplace in India. In the state of Uttar Pradesh in 1878 alone, British officials reported that wolves had killed 624 people.

Grizzly Bear or *Brown Bear* **(Ursus horribilis).** The scientific name of this species means just about what it looks like: "horrible bear." The bear is not horrible, in the colloquial sense, but it can be a frightening and worthy adversary if crossed. Grizzlies are more likely than other bears to make a meal of a human being, although this is still a rare event. One source indicates that Alaskan brown bears (the same species as the grizzly) killed only 24 people in Alaska between 1900 and 1993. In 2000, a brown bear killed and partly ate a man who was camping in Alaska near the Canadian border.

Several authors, however, note that grizzly bear attacks have increased in recent years. It is not clear whether this trend reflects the growing human population, enhanced media coverage, or a real change in behavior. Probably the most convincing explanation—which also applies to the smaller black bear—is that humans encourage these animals to approach populated areas by making garbage available as a food resource. Bears that have lost their fear of humans are more likely to attack than wild bears. Another theory, advanced in the 1980s, was that tranquilizers used for tagging and relocating bears turned some of

them violent, like a person having a bad drug reaction.

Hyena **(Hyaena hyaena,** *the striped hyena,* **and Crocuta crocuta,** *the spotted hyena).* These animals have a bad reputation in many cultures, perhaps reinforced by their hunched posture and scruffy appearance. The authors of medieval bestiaries claimed that hyenas arose from the unnatural mating of cats and dogs, and that they lured people out of their houses by imitating human voices.

Whatever their secret, these predators are fairly successful. Between October 1998 and January 1999, hyenas killed a total of 50 people in southern Ethiopia, including 35 children. Three other fatal attacks were reported in October 1999. Sporadic attacks apparently occur throughout the hyenas' range in Africa, southern Asia, and India. In 1995, an American woman camping with friends in Kenya was attacked in her tent and badly injured by a hyena.

Jaguar **(Panthera onca).** Jaguars and humans have coexisted in the Americas for thousands of years. As jaguars are considerably larger than mountain lions and can easily kill a full-grown cow, they must have eaten people on occasion, and yet documented examples are hard to find. Jaguars, unlike most cats, are good at catching fish and can even kill crocodiles; perhaps they simply do not need us. But like so many animals that threaten humans or their livestock, the jaguar is now an endangered species.

A popular book about a man's alleged travels in the Amazon reports several incidents of jaguars—and caimans, and giant snakes, and ocelots—eating people, but the book is largely a work of fiction. In another value-added story, a South American missionary tells how a jaguar mauled and bit two Indians, who then fired 16 shots into the animal at point-blank range before it died. Conservation groups report that hunters exaggerate the jaguar's ferocity as an excuse to kill it and get the valuable pelt. Arturo Caso, a jaguar researcher in Mexico, writes that he has never documented a human attack by this species, other than incidents involving recently trapped or sedated jaguars. Sr. Caso also notes, however, that he has heard many stories of jaguars attacking people in Mexico and Brazil in former times.

An ambiguous clue comes from the Tsáchila people of Ecuador, who refer to the jaguar as their "Brother of the Big Hand" and tell stories of jaguars coming out of the forest to play with children. These traditions might mean that the people fear jaguars, or that they do not.

Leopard **(Panthera pardus)** and *Snow Leopard* **(Panthera uncia).** In India, leopards kill an estimated 60 people each year. In an unusual incident in South Africa in 1998, a leopard reportedly mauled six people in broad daylight before the driver of a passing truck killed the animal with a screwdriver. The news media have also reported isolated leopard attacks in Nepal in 1989, in Tanzania in 1999, and—strangest of all—in Wales in 2000.

In the latter case, the victim was an 11-year-old boy who told British tabloids that he was attacked by a large black cat with blood on its face. This might be a description of a black leopard (or panther) that the boy had inadvertently surprised in the middle of its dinner; since the victim was a child, however, and an "expert" identified

the animal solely from scratches on the boy's face, it is possible that a large black house cat was responsible. (The expert was not a scientist or physician, but an advocate of the big cat theory.)

For decades, people in England and Wales have claimed to see large cats roaming the countryside, but most scientists and officials have dismissed these reports as something akin to Bigfoot sightings in the United States. There are some good photographs, but their authenticity is unknown. Some of the eyewitness accounts have been confused; in one case, three witnesses who saw an animal in Kent identified it as a large black cat, an ostrich, and a gorilla, respectively. The 2000 incident, if verified, would be the first physical evidence of the legendary cat's existence. If there really are feral big cats in the British Isles, they are not a native population, but most likely the descendants of escaped zoo animals or pets.

Mountain Lion or *Cougar* **(Felis concolor).** During most of the recorded history of North America, there were few reports of mountain lion attacks on human beings. In California, for example, there were two fatal attacks in 1890 and 1909, but no further attacks for the next 77 years. (In the 1909 incident, the lion had rabies, and the victims died of the disease rather than the injuries.)

Recent fatal attacks have, however, occurred in California, Colorado, Montana, and other states. Nationwide, there were on average three mountain lion attacks per year (most of them non-fatal) until 1970, when the rate increased to the present average of 14 per year. The increase has been attributed to habitat destruction, hunting restrictions, and more frequent encounters between mountain lions and people in sub-urban areas.

As of 2000, available records list a total of 13 fatal mountain lion attacks in the United States and several more in Canada, most of them since 1990. Contrary to the popular belief that mountain lions only hunt children, about half the victims have been adults. In 1994, for example, a mountain lion killed and ate a tall, well-conditioned female athlete who was training alone on a trail in northern California.

Two such deaths and nine injuries have occurred since 1986 in California, where mountain lion (and human) populations have increased since a ban on lion hunting took effect in 1972. Before that ban, hunters and wildlife managers together killed an average of 55 mountain lions each year in California; state wildlife officials alone now kill about 120 per year in response to "problem" reports. Some of these problem lions become privately owned rugs or trophies, while others end up in museum collections. Thus, the 1972 law has actually increased the level of mountain lion hunting in California, while eliminating its recreational value.

A six-year-old Montana boy who survived a mountain lion attack in 1998 showed more wisdom than most adult victims or observers of animal attacks. When asked why the cat had mauled him, he replied: "I was the last person in line. He was hungry."[4]

Tiger **(Panthera tigris).** Although the Asian tiger is now an endangered species, until recently it was one of the world's leading predators of human beings. A book published in 1896 states that tigers and leopards together killed 2893 people in India in 1894. Between 1978 and 1984, tigers killed and ate 138 people in India's Kheri District of Uttar Pradesh, but nationwide statistics apparently are not available. As recently as 1998, a Sumatran tiger killed four people in Jakarta, Indonesia, before it could be trapped and placed in a zoo. Tigers in eastern Russia also have caused some recent deaths.

REFERENCES AND RECOMMENDED READING

Aho, Karen. "Wolf Attacks 6-Year-Old near Yakutat." *Anchorage Daily News*, April 27, 2000.

"Alligator Chomps Snorkeler." Associated Press, October 6, 1997.

Ambrose, Greg. 1996. *Shark Bites: True Tales of Survival*. Honolulu: Bess Press.

Baldridge, Henry David. 1974. *Shark Attack*. New York: Berkley Medallion Books.

"Bear Kills, Eats Man in Alaska." Associated Press, July 17, 2000.

Benchley, Peter. "Great White Sharks." *National Geographic*, April 2000, pp. 2–29.

Blair, Lawrence. 1988. *Ring of Fire*. London: Bantam Press.

"Boy Attacked by 'Panther' in South Wales." Reuters News Service, August 26, 2000.

Brandt, John H. 1989. *The Hunters of Man: True Stories of Man-Eaters, Man-Killers and Rogues from Southeast Asia*. Alamosa, CO: Jungle Tracks Pub.

"Burmese Python Devours 30-pound Pit Bull." AP Wire Service, October 6, 2001.

Burns, John F. "India Fighting Plague of Man-Eating Wolves." *New York Times*, September 1, 1996.

Capstick, Peter H. 1978. *Death in the Long Grass*. New York: St. Martin's Press.

Capstick, Peter H. 1993. *Maneaters*. Huntington Beach, CA: Safari Press.

[4]"Boy Attacked by Lion," Associated Press, August 3, 1998.

Predators and Other Biological Hazards

Caso Aguilar, Arturo. "Problem Jaguars: Myth or Reality?" *Revista de Ducks Unlimited de México*, Summer 1997.

Ciofi, Claudio. "The Komodo Dragon." *Scientific American*, March 1999, pp. 84–91.

Conrad, L. "The Maul of the Wild." *Emergency Medical Services*, March 1994, p. 71 ff.

Corbett, Jim. 1946. *Man-Eaters of Kumaon*. New York: Oxford University Press.

Corbett, Jim. 1948. *The Man-eating Leopard of Rudraprayag*. New York: Oxford University Press.

Corbett, Jim. 1955. *The Temple Tiger, and More Man-Eaters of Kumaon*. New York: Oxford University Press.

"Cougar Attacks Increasing in West." Associated Press, August 8, 1998.

Danielson, Jack, et al. "Dinner Bell Bears." *Outdoor Life*, January 1988, p. 56 ff.

Danz, Harold P. 1999. *Cougar!* Athens, OH: Swallow Press.

"Deaths as a Result of Tiger Attacks." *Cat News*, September 6, 1999.

East, Ben (Editor). 1970. *Danger! Explosive True Adventures of the Great Outdoors*. New York: E.P. Dutton.

"Editor Attacked by Komodo Dragon." Associated Press, June 10, 2001.

Edwards, Hugh. 1989. *Crocodile Attack*. New York: Harper & Row.

Ellis, Richard. 1994. *Monsters of the Sea*. New York: Knopf.

Ewing, Susan, and Grossman, Elizabeth (Editors). 1999. *Shadow Cat*. Seattle: Sasquatch Books.

Floyd, T. "Bear-Inflicted Human Injury and Fatality." *Wilderness and Environmental Medicine*, Summer 1999, pp. 75–87.

Garnett, S., and Ross, Charles A. (Editors). 1989. *Crocodiles and Alligators*. New York: Checkmark Books.

Lutz, Richard. 1996. *Komodo, the Living Dragon*. Salem, OR: Dimi Press.

MacCormick, Alex. 1998. *Shark Attacks*. New York: St. Martin's.

"Man a Possible Victim of a Grizzly Bear Attack." Associated Press, May 21, 1998.

"Man-Eating Lions Needed Dentists." Associated Press, June 21, 2000.

Masterman, Sue. "Antibiotic Dundee." ABCNews.com, May 26, 2000.

McMillion, Scott. 1998. *Mark of the Grizzly*. Guilford, CT: Falcon Publishing Co.

McRae, Bill. "Are We Creating Crazed Bears?" *Outdoor Life*, January 1986, p. 56 ff.

Mitchell, Garry. "Shark Attack." Associated Press, June 10, 2000.

Ngowi, Rodirique. "Big Cats Kill 21 in Tanzania." Associated Press, November 5, 1999.

Olsen, Jack. 1969. *Night of the Grizzlies*. New York: Putnam.

Ross, Ian. "Encounters with a Silent Predator." *Natural History*, December 1994, p. 57 ff.

"Russian Hunters Kill Man-Eating Tiger." Associated Press, December 23, 1997.

"The Russians Are Coming." *Discover*, March 1990, p. 16.

"Seafood Surprise: Human Head Found Inside Giant Cod in Australia." Reuters News Service, August 29, 2000.

St. John, Allen. "Bearanoia." *Audubon*, January–February 1993, p. 20 ff.

Taylor, V., and Taylor, R. 1990. *Sharks: Silent Hunters of the Deep*. New York: Reader's Digest.

"Teen Survives Gator Attack." United Press International, July 12, 2000.

"Teenager Loses Right Foot to Shark in Attack." Associated Press, October 29, 1997.

"Three Ethiopians Eaten by Hyenas." AFP (Agence France-Presse), October 29, 1999.

Torres, Steve. 1997. *Mountain Lion Alert*. Guilford, CT: Falcon Publishing Co.

"Villagers Trap Tiger Suspected of Killing Four People in Indonesia." Associated Press, January 3, 1998.

Wikramanayake, Eric. "Journey to the Land of the Dragon." *Smithsonian*, April 1997.

Willwerth, James. "Get Off My Turf." *Time*, August 24, 1998.

"Woman, 70, Killed by Crocodile in Jamaica." Reuters News Service, September 11, 1999.

Worth, Nick. "When Cats Go Bad." *Outdoor Life*, January 1991, p. 56 ff.

Zahl, Paul. "Seeking the Truth about the Piranha." *National Geographic*, November 1970.

NONPREDATORY ATTACKS ON HUMAN BEINGS

Animals frequently injure humans for reasons other than predation. Dogs bite hundreds of thousands of people each year in the United States, but rarely consume them. Horses and other livestock also cause many injuries. According to the U.S. General Accounting Office (GAO), rodents injure about 27,000 Americans each year. Most attacks by wildlife are probably related to the animal's perception of the human as a threat.

In the absence of comprehensive environmental planning, more U.S. residents can expect to find moose, bighorn sheep, bobcats, and other visitors in their yards as suburbs encroach on former wilderness. The results of such encounters depend largely on individual attitudes. Some people will burble in delight and rush out to hug the visitor (which might see the situation differently), while others grab their varmint guns and start shooting up the neighborhood. In either case, the results often are unsatisfactory.

Nonpredatory Attacks by Fishes

Moray Eel (**Muraenidae, about 80 species**). All divers and snorkelers are aware of the risk posed by moray eels, but attacks are relatively infrequent, despite the eels' sharp teeth, powerful jaws, and large size (up to 11 feet). One of the most often-cited cases occurred in 1948, when a marine biologist speared a moray eel and the animal responded by biting his elbow. It took three months for the man to recover the use of his arm, but it is not clear whether the damage resulted mainly from the eel's bite or from the tourniquet that was applied as a first-aid measure during transport to the hospital.

Barracuda (**Sphyraena barracuda**). This fish can be up to six feet long and has caused severe injuries to some divers, but it is probably too small to perceive humans as prey. More often, barracudas approach spearfishers and try to appropriate their catch. Barracuda also are attracted to splashing and to bright colors, and have occasionally bitten or even killed humans who were swimming. Barracuda are prized as sport fish, but they are among the warm-water fish that sometimes cause ciguatera poisoning (see Chapter 7).

Nonpredatory Attacks by Amphibians

The only amphibians large enough to inflict serious mechanical injury on a human being are the giant salamanders of China and Japan (*Andrias davidianus* and *A. japonicus*, respectively). There are few, if any, verifiable records of such attacks. Their smaller North American cousin the congereel also has a painful bite, but the only reported bites have occurred when someone was handling a captive salamander.

Nonpredatory Attacks by Reptiles

Alligator Snapping Turtle (**Macroclemys temmincki**). This North American turtle is one of the world's largest freshwater turtles, sometimes weighing over 200 pounds. Its normal habit is to lie on the bottom of a river or lake with its mouth open, wiggling a worm-like appendage in its mouth to attract fish. Of course, it must surface from time to time like any other reptile. When annoyed, this turtle can make a real mess of an unwary fisherman or diver. Reports indicate that its jaws can easily sever a broom handle or a person's arm.

Its smaller relative the snapping turtle (*Chelydra serpentina*) weighs up to 50 pounds, and also has very strong jaws that have bitten off people's fingers. In 1999, a snapping turtle severed the big toe of a nine-year-old Ohio boy; the neighbors pitched in and organized a turtle soup cook-off to help pay the medical bills. These turtles are particularly inclined to bite when on land, and will sometimes strike repeatedly with their long necks, almost like snakes. The best way to avoid this problem is to leave all wild turtles strictly alone. Most turtles are harmless, but people find them so attractive (as pets or as soup) that many species have become endangered. A few species, like this one, can be dangerous, and all are a good source of salmonella.

Crocodiles **and** *Relatives*. Most crocodilians, other than a few large species discussed earlier in this chapter, are either too small or otherwise uninclined to hunt human beings. Although American alligators have killed or injured a number of people, more often they eat dogs or simply become a nuisance. Each year in the southeastern United States, state agencies issue trapping permits to individuals for the removal of 12,000–15,000 "nuisance alligators."

In 1999, floods in Villahermosa, Mexico brought an invasion of rather small crocodiles that blocked traffic and created a minor hazard; a few were as long as eight feet, but no attacks on humans were reported. In 2000, a fairly small 50-pound alligator in Mississippi struck a police officer with its tail and made national news. The officer,

who was not injured, was simply trying to relocate the animal and possibly forgot about the Miranda Act.

Whether the next two stories are true or not, the press reported them in 1998, and they are too good not to share:

- A 77-year-old sleepwalker in Florida awoke to find himself standing in a pond surrounded by several fairly small alligators. He fought them off with his cane until his shouts for help attracted a neighbor.

- An Ohio man left his 12-foot-long pet python, Gidget, soaking in the bathtub while he went to visit a neighbor. Whether by accident or design, Gidget nudged the faucet handle, and the tub overflowed and damaged the downstairs apartment. Police then arrested the snake's owner for harboring a dangerous animal.

Nonpredatory Attacks by Birds

In Massachusetts in 2000, the media reported that roving flocks of wild turkeys were attacking people, tearing up gardens, and depositing large quantities of feces in suburban Boston. These birds became extinct in Massachusetts in about 1850, but state wildlife officials began reintroducing them in the 1970s. Since most of the birds' original habitat had been converted to farmland, they moved into the suburbs, where people started feeding them. No serious injuries have occurred, but the birds have become a nuisance and a possible disease threat. Individual "problem turkeys" have been captured and relocated.

In 1997, an ostrich on a farm in South Africa attacked an elderly couple, seriously injuring the man and kicking the woman to death.

Nonpredatory Attacks by Domestic and Caged Mammals

Dogs. At latest count, the United States alone has at least 60 million dogs, including unowned packs of semi-wild dogs as well as licensed pets.

In 1998, researchers at the University of Pittsburgh determined that dogs bite nearly 4.5 million U.S. residents every year. Of these, an estimated 800,000 are injured seriously enough to need medical care. Some 334,000 seek emergency room treatment, and 15–20 deaths result in a typical year—more than all the people killed by shark attacks worldwide. About one-third of all homeowner's insurance claims involve dog bites. Children are bitten more often than adults, and males more often than females. Baseball and softball injuries are the only category of injuries that result in more hospital visits than dog bites. Some occupational groups also are at high risk; for example, dogs bite about 2700 letter carriers every year.

As of 2000, dog bites ranked as the second most expensive health problem in the United States (after sexually transmitted diseases). Curiously, both problems may be indirectly related to the phases of the moon. At least one recent study has shown a statistically significant excess of dog bites on full-moon days.

Most of these numbers reflect the behavior of ordinary pet dogs, but the worst and most highly publicized incidents involve American pit bull terriers, rottweilers (Figure 8.2), or trained attack dogs of various breeds. The fear of crime has led many people to purchase such dogs for protection. Unfortunately, the dog cannot necessarily

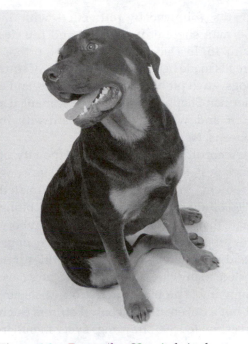

Figure 8.2. Rottweiler. Hospitals in the United States treat several hundred thousand people each year for dog bites. Although rottweilers and pit bulls top the list, most individual dogs of both breeds make good pets. (*Source*: PhotoDisc, Inc.)

tell when its owner is really in danger. The pit bull and some other breeds were selectively bred for generations to produce an aggressive fighting dog, and it is not surprising that some individuals retain this quality, even though many others are excellent, well-behaved pets.

In 2000, the American Veterinary Medical Association announced that the rottweiler had replaced the pit bull as the most dangerous dog breed in the United States, having caused 33 known human fatalities between 1991 and 1998, as compared with 21 for pit bulls. During the interval 1979–1998, pit bulls led the pack with 66 mauling deaths, followed by rottweilers with 37, German shepherds with 17, and huskies with 15. In December 2001, the top three breeds made headlines when a pack of stray dogs—two pit bulls, two rottweilers, and a German Shepherd mix—severely mauled a man and woman on the boardwalk in Queens, New York.

According to press reports, the city of Bucharest, Romania has the worst stray dog problem in the world. An estimated 100,000–200,000 dogs roam the city, biting more than 50 people per day. When authorities proposed killing some of the stray dogs, residents and even foreign celebrities protested. Many cities in the United States have comparable problems; in Detroit, Michigan, about a dozen animal control officers catch an estimated 500 stray dogs every month in an effort to reduce the damage caused by packs of unowned dogs. New laws in several states also impose stiff penalties on irresponsible dog owners.

In one of the most bizarre incidents recorded in this book, authorities in Guatemala arrested and jailed a dog named Baloo in 1998 and proposed to put it on trial for allegedly participating in the murder of a bishop. The United Nations, the European Union, and the Roman Catholic Church all issued statements of support, demanding the dog's release.

Other Pets. In 2000, a 400-pound pet tiger owned by a Texas family bit off the right arm of a three-year-old boy, and: "No charges were expected, as authorities believed the attack was an accident."[5] It is not clear whether this statement refers to the family, who certainly did not own the tiger

by accident, or the pet, for simply acting like a tiger.

Horses. Although the raw numbers (Table 8.2) show that horses kill more people each year than any other animals in the United States, it is difficult to interpret these numbers. The horse, unlike a bear or wolverine, in most cases has a person riding voluntarily on its back. A horse might throw its rider for many reasons beyond the horse's immediate control; if the horse stumbles on a steep trail, for example, or is startled by a vehicle, or if the rider simply falls off, the horse is not exactly the "cause" of the injury. Of the 200 or more people who die in horse-related accidents each year, an estimated two-thirds could be saved by wearing helmets.

Other Livestock. Almost any animal can be dangerous under some circumstances. In 2000, an Oklahoma man was gored to death while feeding his penned herd of European red deer (*Cervus elaphus*), and a cow went on a car-wrecking spree in England. The police inspector assigned to the latter incident remarked: "Who's to say what goes through a cow's mind?"

Zoo Animals. Large cats frequently injure zoo personnel and visitors who insist on sticking their arms into the animals' cages. In 2000, a volunteer at a wildlife refuge in Colorado had her arm bitten off by a caged Siberian tiger. In 1998, a jaguar escaped from a zoo in western France and killed a three-year-old boy.

Similar incidents have involved captive animals other than carnivores. In 1998, a caged tapir in Oklahoma bit off the arm of a zoo worker in an apparent effort to pro-

[5]"Pet Tiger Attacks Boy," Associated Press, March 16, 2000.

tect her calf. The arm was badly damaged and could not be reattached; the worker also suffered facial injuries and a punctured lung. In 1999, a hippopotamus killed the director of the Pessac Zoo in Brittany. Zoo and circus elephants also have caused a number of deaths.

Nonpredatory Attacks by Wild Mammals

African Elephant **(Loxodonta africana).** When anything as large as an elephant becomes upset, the results are memorable. Most stories of such attacks involve retaliatory strikes on big game hunters in a bygone era, but several modern photographers and wildlife biologists have had close calls with enraged elephants charging their jeeps. In 2000, the Namibian government reported that elephants had killed an American tourist who was taking photographs. There are also stories of elephants covering people with leaves or debris for no known reason.

Badger **(Taxidea taxus).** Some of the most frightening animal attacks in the literature have involved an animal less than two feet long. Such attacks are rare, and in every known case the badger was minding its own business. In one incident, a field biologist had his head near the entrance to a burrow when a badger suddenly jumped out and inflicted severe facial injuries. Farmers are well aware that badgers can kill animals as large as horses. Loyal fans of *Wind in the Willows* and the "Frances" books should consider the fact that people have recruited badgers (like bears) for centuries for the so-called sport of baiting, in which a pack of dogs attacks a captive wild animal. This practice, while indefensible, proves that badgers are capable of fighting back. Give these animals a wide berth and do not corner them.

Bison **(Bison bison).** Between 1984 and 1999, bison or buffalo killed at least two people in the United States and injured 56 others. This phenomenon is nothing new; bison have been killing and injuring people for at least 15,000 years, as discussed later in this chapter. In the recent incidents, however, the people were not hunting the bison, but more likely trying to persuade them to pose for photographs in a national park.

Black Bear **(Ursus americanus).** This species represents one of the borderline cases between predation and opportunistic snacking. Black bears sometimes attack people in campgrounds and wilderness areas, and in some cases partially eat their victims; but it is not clear whether these incidents start as predation attempts, or the bear kills the person for some other reason and then sees an available food source. In 1997, a black bear in British Columbia killed a woman and mauled her two children. The same bear also killed an experienced bear hunter who tried to rescue the family, and injured a second man who arrived on the scene and was finally able to shoot the bear. Although such incidents are rare, they are not reassuring. The survivors were not aware of anything they had done to provoke the incident, other than to walk through the woods.

At least one recent study concluded that most black bear attacks are predacious. By contrast, some wildlife biologists who study black bears insist that these animals never attack humans without severe provocation. The problem appears to lie in defining "provocation" from the viewpoint of a bear.

In several documented cases, victims (sometimes asleep inside tents) had their scalps severely mauled for no apparent reason. It is possible that some hair-care products have a smell that bears find threatening. Another theory holds that bear attacks are just the latest in a series of problems attributed to menstruating women. Someone drew this conclusion when bears in a park attacked two women who happened to have their periods at the time; a more objective study (Kelly 1994) has debunked the theory, but it has survived as an urban legend nonetheless, and many park rangers believe it.

Other factors that contribute to bear attacks may be naive wildlife management practices and the widespread public perception of bears as cuddle toys. These influences, in effect, train some individual bears to perceive humans as easily removed obstacles standing between themselves and garbage can access.

Bobcat **(Felis rufus) and** *Lynx* **(Felis lynx).** Although bobcats and lynxes are predators that occasionally attack people, they are too small to perceive humans as likely prey. In one such attack in 2000, a wild bobcat attacked a Minnesota woman as she walked across her front lawn. Authorities speculated that the woman might have interrupted the animal's efforts to kill her pet cat, or that it might possibly have had rabies. Again, as in earlier examples, spectators' comments are helpful in understanding common beliefs about animals and their alleged motives. One biologist told the reporter: "If that bobcat had attacked with malicious intent, it could have seriously maimed her."[6]

Cape Buffalo **(Syncerus caffer).** Most books on Africa—older ones, anyway—claim that the Cape buffalo is the most dangerous of all big game animals, but nearly all verifiable incidents seem to involve wounded buffalo that have turned on their hunters. In some parts of Africa, rinderpest epidemics (see Chapter 6), ironically, have saved this species from extinction by discouraging human occupancy. Buffalo can contract the disease, but it is less dangerous than human hunters and cattle ranchers.

Coyote **(Canis latrans).** Coyotes have occasionally attacked small children, but it is not clear whether these were predation attempts or the animals had rabies. One recent case involved a four-year-old boy on Cape Cod, Massachusetts, whose mother hit the animal on the head and dragged it away from the child.

Hippopotamus **(Hippopotamus amphibius).** In Egypt's First Dynasty (3100–2890 B.C.), a ruler named Narmer unified Upper and Lower Egypt, reigned for 62 years, and was killed by a hippopotamus. During the next 5000 years, over one million people probably died the same way. Even today, by some estimates the hippopotamus kills several hundred Africans every year, often by biting them in half or overturning their boats, or occasionally both.

Hippos do not eat meat, but they seem to dislike having boats bump them, and they have a strong sense of territory. A female hippo with young might mistake a boat for a threatening crocodile and treat it accordingly. Some of those killed are hunters, who often cannot resist the opportunity to collect a half-ton of meat with one shot. Hunters

---

[6]C. Niskanen, "Bobcat Attack of Human May Be First in Minnesota" (*St. Paul [MN] Pioneer Press*, July 21, 2000).

who miss soon discover how fast a large animal can move.

Despite this uneasy relationship, people do not seem to hate and fear the hippo as so many do the crocodile, probably because hippos look round and cute. Like bears, they are favorite zoo attractions, cartoon characters, and stuffed toys.

Monkeys (**various species**). According to a 1998 report from India, the city of Srinigar was invaded by hordes of monkeys that attacked people, raided restaurants, and ransacked houses. In a similar 1998 incident, monkeys invaded a soccer match in Somalia and attacked the players and spectators. Monkeys appear to be an ongoing problem in New Delhi, where an estimated 7000 rhesus macaques roam the city and routinely break into houses and public buildings. In one entertaining incident, the monkeys allegedly stole a stack of classified documents from a government office and scattered them on the front lawn.

Polar Bear (**Thalarctos maritimus**). Although polar bears are widely believed to be highly dangerous and aggressive as bears go, there are only a few confirmed reports of this species attacking humans. In 1998, a very thin polar bear approached a tourist camp in Norway and was shot almost immediately. Although it had not threatened anyone, the occupants were legitimately concerned, as polar bears had killed at least three Norwegians in 1994 and 1995.

Wolverine (**Gulo luscus**). These large weasel-like mammals are serious livestock predators in some countries, but attacks on humans are rare and usually involve a dis-

pute regarding the ownership of a meat cache. Despite the wolverine's documented ability to kill prey as large as a 300-pound caribou, these animals live mainly on carrion and on smaller animals such as porcupines.

Really Big Invertebrates

In the days of wooden ships, sailors occasionally reported attacks by enormous squid up to 50 feet long, usually depicted dragging down the masts and eating the luckless crew (see Figure 8.3). Here is a typical nineteenth-century account of a pearl diver's close call:

These loathsome monsters—call them squids, or devil-fish, or what you will—would sometimes come and throw their horrible tentacles over the side of the frail craft from which the divers were working. . . . The terrible creature was after him, however, and to the horror of the onlookers it extended its great flexible tentacles, enveloped the entire boat, man and all, and then dragged the whole down into the clear depths.[7]

Such animals exist, and in the past few years many have washed ashore on beaches or turned up in commercial fishing nets in the oceans near New Zealand. These giant squids belong to the species *Architeuthis dux*, which is believed to live in deep water. It is not clear, however, why a squid would attack a ship. It is possible that the sailors in question had seen a dead giant squid and were merely speculating as to what a live one might do. In any case, the giant squid has the dubious honor of being the only real animal

[7]Louis de Rougemont, *The Adventures of Louis de Rougemont, as Told by Himself* (Philadelphia: J.B. Lippincott, 1900).

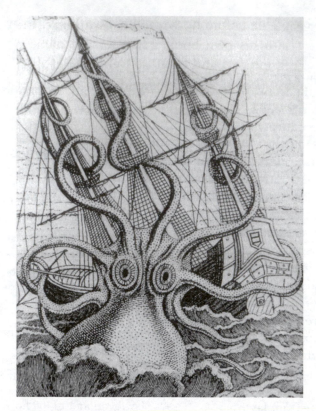

Figure 8.3. Nineteenth-century artist's conception of the giant squid. (*Source*: Pierre Denys de Montfort. 1802. *Histoire Naturelle, Générale et Particulière, des Mollusques, Animaux Sans Vertèbres et a Sang Blanc*. [Natural History, General and Particular, of Mollusks, White-Blooded Animals Without Bones.] Paris: L'Imprimerie de F. Dufart.)

that regularly appears on television programs of the "stranger than science" variety.

There are more recent reports of 13-foot-long Humboldt squids (*Dosidicus gigas*) pulling sailors out of their boats in Mexico's Sea of Cortez, but the most lurid example we could verify involved three squid that mugged a diver who was working on the 1998 PBS documentary series "Secrets of the Ocean Realm." The animals dragged him under, stole his collecting bags and bottles, his computer, and a gold chain from his neck—flashing complex patterns of color all the while—and left him decorated with sucker

marks before releasing him unharmed. Worse things have happened on land.

REFERENCES AND RECOMMENDED READING

"Alligator in Big Black River Whacks Officer with Its Tail." Associated Press, June 29, 2000.

"Alligators Wake Up Sleepwalker." *London Telegraph*, November 26, 1998.

Avis, S.P. "Dog Pack Attack: Hunting Humans." *American Journal of Forensic Medicine and Pathology*, September 1999, pp. 243–246.

"Bear Kills Two, Injures Two in British Columbia." *Boston Globe*, August 17, 1997.

Bixby-Hammett, D.M., and Brooks, W.H. "Common Injuries in Horseback Riding." *Sports Medicine*, January 1990, pp. 36–47.

"Boy Killed by Jaguar at Zoo." Associated Press, December 6, 1998.

Collins, Amy. "Murder by Pit Bull?" ABCNews.com, July 19, 2000.

"Dog Bite Injuries Become an Epidemic, CDC Reports." Associated Press, October 11, 1998.

Ellis, Richard. 1998. *The Search for the Giant Squid*. New York: Lyons Press.

"Floridians Warned to Watch Out for Alligators." Reuters News Service, April 27, 1999.

Floyd, T. "Bear-inflicted Human Injury and Fatality." *Wilderness and Environmental Medicine*, Summer 1999, pp. 75–87.

Frame, George W., and Frame, L.H. "The Dangerous Hippo." *Science Digest*, November 1974, pp. 80–86.

"Giant Squid Surface in Large Numbers Off New Zealand." Reuters News Service, October 18, 1999.

Gilbert, D. "Wolverines—What to Do If a Demon of the North Comes a' Calling?" *Smithsonian*, 1993, Vol. 23, pp. 136–140, 142–146, 148.

"Her Final Moments: Bear Dragged Athlete During Fatal Attack." Associated Press, July 6, 2000.

Herrero, Steven. 1988. *Bear Attacks: Their Causes and Avoidance*. New York: Lyons Press.

Hughes, Jay. "Tapir Bites Off Zoo Worker's Arm." Associated Press, November 21, 1998.

Kaniut, Larry. 1984. *Alaska Bear Tales*. Seattle: Alaska Northwest Books.

Kaniut, Larry. 1990. *More Alaska Bear Tales*. Seattle: Alaska Northwest Books.

Kaniut, Larry. 1997. *Some Bears Kill!* Huntington Beach, CA: Safari Press.

Kelly, Diane. "Menstruation and Bears." Posted on <http://www.urbanlegends.com>, April 11, 1994.

Kneafsey, B., and Condon, K.C. "Severe Dog-Bite Injuries, Introducing the Concept of Pack Attack: A Literature Review and Seven Case Reports." *Injury*, January 1996, pp. 37–41.

LaGuardia, Anton. "Leopard Killed with Screwdriver." *Electronic Telegraph*, London, October 2, 1998.

Lamb, Christina. "UN Backs Dog Jailed for Killing Bishop." *Electronic Telegraph*, London, December 6, 1998.

Langley, R.L., and Hunter, J.L. "Occupational Fatalities Due to Animal-Related Events." *Wilderness and Environmental Medicine*, Fall 2001, pp. 168–174.

Long, John (Editor). 1997. *Attacked! By Beasts of Prey and Other Deadly Creatures: True Stories of Survival*. New York: McGraw-Hill.

Lopez, Luis. "Crocodiles Creep into Mexican City." Associated Press, October 15, 1999.

McClam, Ed. "Bad Dog." Associated Press, September 15, 2000.

Nettleton, Philip. "Rampaging Cow Killed by Police." Associated Newspapers Ltd., October 23, 2000.

"Ostrich Kicks 63-Year-Old Woman to Death in South Africa." Associated Press, December 29, 1997.

"Pessac: The Zoo Director Killed by a Hippopotamus." *Le Télégramme*, November 2, 1999.

"Polar Bear Attacks Tourists." Telegraph Group Ltd., August 10, 1998.

"Python Leaves the Tap On." Associated Press, January 28, 1998.

Randall, J.E. "How Dangerous Is the Moray Eel?" *Australian Natural History*, June 1969, pp. 177–182.

Sparano, V.T. "Bears and People Who Won't Listen." *Outdoor Life*, November 1993, p. 10.

"Street Life in Bucharest: Watch Out for That Dog!" Associated Press, November 26, 1997.

Woodward, Calvin. "A View of Wildlife in which People are the Victims." Associated Press, January 11, 2002.

Zaidle, Don. 1997. *American Man-Killers: True Stories of a Dangerous Wilderness*. Huntington Beach, CA: Safari Press.

Zaidle, Don. "Killer Cougars." *Outdoor Life*, February 2001, pp. 44–49.

MECHANICAL BIOHAZARDS

Readers may be surprised to learn that one of the most expensive biological hazards in the world is the problem of collisions between animals and various human transportation devices. A few other hazards also qualify as mechanical in nature, as discussed in the following paragraphs.

This book will skip plants that cause injury by mechanical means alone. Of course, humans can impale themselves on a shin-dagger agave, stick themselves on rose thorns, or slip on a banana peel. Some of these cases are borderline; thorns, for example, may teach avoidance by inoculating a wound with bacteria or fungi, which act as a pseudo-toxin like the gunk on a Komodo dragon's teeth.

Aircraft Collisions with Birds

According to the U.S. Department of Agriculture's National Wildlife Research Center, in the period 1990–1998 there were about 2500 reported collisions each year between civil aircraft and birds or other wildlife. These reports are voluntary, and investigators believe the actual number may be five times higher. In 2001, the GAO studied this problem and estimated that 6000 collisions between birds and aircraft occurred in 2000 alone.

Although most of these collisions occur in the air, some happen on the runway during takeoff. About 60 percent of bird strikes have no effect on flight, but many others cause substantial damage (see Figure 8.4), and 19 planes have been destroyed. The total price tag for such collisions now exceeds $300 million per year.

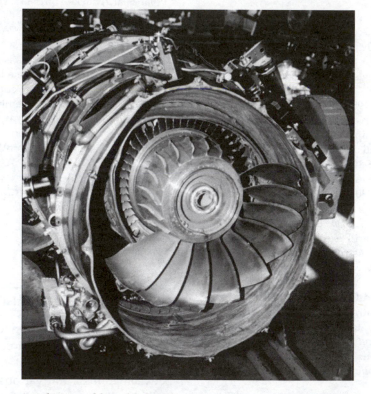

Figure 8.4. Jet engine destroyed by a bird strike. (*Source*: Transport Canada.)

The first known bird-strike accident was in 1912, when a small plane hit a gull and fell into the ocean, killing the pilot. In 1960, 62 people died when a plane at Boston's Logan Airport collided with a flock of starlings and other birds during takeoff. Altogether, more than 100 civilians in the United States have died in such accidents since the early 1900s. Worldwide, the estimated total is 350.

Another 600–800 collisions per year involve military planes, and several fatalities have occurred (see Tables 8.4 and 8.5). On September 23, 1995, an AWACS Air Force Surveillane plane took off from Elmendorf Air Force Base in Alaska and struck a flock of Canada geese. The fuel ignited and the plane crashed near the end of the runway, killing all 24 crewmen aboard.

One innovative plan is to equip planes with low-frequency radar that can "warn" birds of their approach. Another, already in use at some airports, is to use trained border collies and other dogs to chase away birds. Some airports use trained falcons, instead, but this is an expensive solution. JFK airport alone, for example, pays $1 million for three years of falcon protection, including the trainers' salaries.

Deer on Roads

If it sounds as if we are really reaching for a hazard here, consider the numbers. According to the National Highway Transportation Safety Administration, there are at least 350,000 collisions between vehicles and deer each year in the United States alone, with an average repair bill of $2000. Thus, the cost of automobile repairs alone exceeds $700 million per year. Add to that the value of the lives of the 100 people who typically die each year in such accidents every year—insurance companies somehow assign a value of $700,000 to each life—plus the unknown costs of treating survivors' injuries, plus the cost of paying contractors to scrape thousands of dead deer off the nation's highways, and total annual costs easily exceed $1 billion. (In 2001, a study by the GAO confirmed this estimate.)

Many Americans like to hunt deer and are willing to accept the tradeoffs associated with predator control, hunting restrictions, and the resulting high deer populations. Many nonhunters support the same practices because they simply like deer. But vehicle collisions are not the only cost. As noted in Chapter 5, the emergence of Lyme disease and other tickborne infections in the United States may also be related to the abundance of deer.

Table 8.4
U.S. Air Force Wildlife Strikes by Year
(1985–1999)

Year	Count	Cost
1985	2717	$5,452,151.00
1986	2850	18,081,085.00
1987	2728	241,008,061.00
1988	2642	3,353,576.00
1989	3064	24,408,483.00
1990	2955	6,471,984.00
1991	2772	17,656,528.00
1992	2284	26,050,141.00
1993	2445	13,150,533.00
1994	2364	15,811,416.00
1995	2649	84,864,258.19
1996	3102	8,773,172.15
1997	2733	9,811,982.59
1998	3504	30,306,458.62
1999 (to August)	1045	3,665,264.47
Total:	39854	$508,865,094.02

Source: U.S. Air Force, BASH Program.

Table 8.5
U.S. Air Force Wildlife Strikes by Species (1985–Aug 1999)

Common Name	Count	Cost
Horned Lark	877	$2,764,273.31
Mourning Dove	408	705,381.84
Turkey Vulture	369	33,761,132.31
Barn Swallow	332	407,233.00
Red-Tailed Hawk	300	12,388,000.00
American Robin	231	1,585,650.00
Meadowlark	211	56,666.74
Killdeer	208	152,722.00
Rock Dove	205	1,056,278.00
Chimney Swift	163	134,139.00
Common Nighthawk	149	68,608.00
Western Meadowlark	145	210,609.00
American Kestrel	141	120,480.31
European Starling	137	10,453,391.00
Sparrow	134	62,073.00
Mallard	117	2,790,477.00
Black Vulture	112	7,748,436.00
Swift	110	97,256.00
Eastern Meadowlark	96	335,982.00
Blackbird	89	97,350.00
Bat	78	43,012.00
Yellow-Rumped Warbler	75	6,532.00
Herring Gull	73	3,548,116.59
Skylark	69	19,745.20
Swainson's Thrush	63	16,772.00
Red-Winged Blackbird	62	235,058.00
Cattle Egret	61	104,777.00
American Crow	60	112,325.00
Cliff Swallow	57	2,257,180.00
Snow Bunting	57	255,558.00
Starling	57	68,188.00
Canada Goose	54	81,311,165.00
Swallow	52	3,010.00
Tree Swallow	45	$3,508.00
Purple Martin	44	1,402.00
Ring-Billed Gull	36	203,188.00
Scissor-Tailed Flycatcher	36	1,854.00
Laughing Gull	35	268,135.00
Hawk	32	132,992.50
Song Sparrow	30	6,257.96
Northern Pintail	29	120,088.00
Sharp-Shinned Hawk	28	2,116,815.00
American Coot	28	123,571.00

Table 8.5   (Continued)

Common Name	Count	Cost
Snow Goose	27	4,981,722.00
Black-Headed Gull	27	659,494.00
White-Throated Swift	26	60,646.35
Swainson's Hawk	26	1,284,849.00
Sandpiper	25	0.00
Vesper Sparrow	24	16.00
Lesser Golden Plover	24	4,492.00
House Sparrow	24	2,069.00
Lapwing	24	91,760.00

Source: U.S. Air Force, BASH Program.

Other Animals on Roads

Anything can cross a road, but most animals are not large enough to present a significant hazard to the driver. Deer are the main problem, as noted above, but cars also collide with hundreds of black bears, moose, livestock, and other large mammals every year. In New Hampshire in 1997 alone, 246 moose died in vehicle accidents.

In one spectacular case in Canada in 1998, a moose landed on the hood of a car and crashed through the windshield, splitting its body cavity open in the process and spewing the contents. Although the moose was the only casualty, the hospital staff must have been confused when the family arrived covered with moose intestines and blood. A fire chief investigating the incident noted that there was a moose lung on the front seat of the car.

Bears Vandalizing Houses and Cars

In 1998, wildlife officials in Colorado killed a black bear and her three cubs after they had broken into 15 houses in three weeks, apparently searching for food.

In Yosemite National Park, in 1998 alone, foraging black bears broke into more than 1000 vehicles and caused over $600,000 in damage. Remarkably, the bears showed a strong preference for small Honda and Toyota sedans. Mother bears were observed teaching their cubs how to insert their claws just above the rear side door and pull the door frame down to knee level, thus creating a ramp for easy access. The next step was to claw through the back seat and into the trunk.

When one couple threw a chair at a bear that was breaking into their vehicle, it simply ignored them, circled the car, and broke another window. One bear learned how to break into cars while the owners were registering at the campground; another managed to fold down a back seat and press a button to open a cooler. Park officials considered euthanizing these bears—this author might have recommended teaching the bears a trade, instead—but by 1999, nonlethal measures such as bear-chasing dogs, bearproof food lockers, and public education campaigns had reduced the number of such incidents by half.

At about the same time, the advertising industry created its classic image of a bear that breaks into an Airstream trailer after confusing its shape with that of a Hostess Twinkie, and asks the universe: "Where's the cream filling?"

Other Mechanical Biohazards

In 2000, a young woman was wading in chest-deep water near the Florida Keys when a houndfish (*Tylosurus crocodilus*) leaped out of the water and severely lacerated her neck with its serrated bill. This might sound like an attack, but it was not, any more than the geese in earlier examples were trying to eat the aircraft. These fish simply tend to jump when startled, and their random collisions can cause serious injuries. In a similar incident that same year, an arrowfish (species unknown) leapt from the ocean and killed a Chinese fisherman by piercing his lung with its sharp beak. In 2001, a Florida man died while operating a high-speed watercraft on a lake, when a flying duck collided with his head.

Some non-native animal and plant species that lack natural biological controls in their new homes may multiply until their sheer numbers create a hazard, as when the imported zebra mussel (*Dreissena polymorpha*) clogs pipes in the Great Lakes area, directly harming no one, but causing an estimated $3 billion worth of damage per year.

In December 1999, a major electrical blackout struck most of the city of Luzon in the Philippines after large jellyfish were sucked into a power plant cooling system. The timing of the event unfortunately inspired rumors of a Y2K systems failure (a bit ahead of schedule) or possibly the end of the world. The Philippine government reported that over 50 truckloads of jellyfish were removed from the cooling system.

REFERENCES AND RECOMMENDED READING

"Bears Learn to Avoid Tourists." Associated Press, November 15, 1999.

"Be Nice—Or Else!" ABCNews.com, July 19, 2000.

Blokpoel, H. 1976. *Bird Hazards to Aircraft: Problems and Prevention of Bird/Aircraft Collisions.* Ottawa: Clarke, Irwin & Co.

"Broward Personal Watercraft Driver Dies After Duck Strikes Head." AP Wire Service, November 19, 2001.

"Contractors Make a Killing Picking Up Deer Carcasses from Highways." Associated Press, July 23, 2000.

Dye, Lee. "Birds and Planes Don't Mix." ABCNews.com, October 20, 1999.

Fialka, John J. "Yosemite's Black Bears Are Choosing Specific Auto Models for Break-Ins." *Wall Street Journal*, January 13, 1999.

Michael, R.A. 1986. "Keep Your Eye on the Birdie: Aircraft Engine Bird Ingestion." *Journal of Air Law and Commerce* 51(4):1007–1010.

National Technical Information Service. 1988. *Bird Strikes and Aviation Safety, January 1970–July 1988* (Bibliography). Springfield, VA: NTIS, 143 pp.

Onion, Amanda. "Falcon Fleet." ABCNews.com, June 22, 2000.

"Power Company Blames Blackout on Jellyfish." Associated Press, December 11, 1999.

Rennie, David. "Arrowfish Skewers Angler." Telegraph Group Ltd., June 27, 2000.

Revkin, Andrew C. "When Birds of Man and Nature Meet." *New York Times*, September 15, 1997.

Thorpe, J. 1977. *Bird Strikes to Transport Aircraft Jet Engines.* London: Civil Aviation Authority.

Thorpe, J. 1984. *Analysis of Bird Strikes Reported by European Airlines, 1976–1980 Civil Aircraft over 5700 Kilograms Maximum Weight.* London: Civil Aviation Authority.

TranSafety, Inc. 1997. "Deer-Vehicle Collisions Are Numerous and Costly: Do Countermeasures Work?" *Road Management and Engineering Journal*, May 12, 1997.

Woodward, Calvin. "A View of Wildlife in which People are the Victims." Associated Press, January 11, 2002.

MAJOR OUTBREAKS

Earlier chapters presented examples of disease outbreaks in tabular form, but an "outbreak" of crocodile attacks, for example, requires a bit of explanation.

Although the hazards in this chapter are not diseases, the principles of epidemiology still apply. Various agencies (see Chapter 10) track the numbers and locations of incidents such as dog bites, wildlife attacks, and vehicle collisions with birds, just as the CDC tracks disease outbreaks. If an unusual cluster of such incidents appears, or if an upward trend is evident, these agencies often look for causes and preventive measures.

For some observed trends, the reason is apparent. The increasing (but still low) numbers of shark and bear attacks may reflect increasing opportunities for contact. In other cases, a few individual predators have learned to hunt humans for convenience. Yet no known art or literature survives from a time when humans stood below the top link on the food chain. Today, we are a routine host for many pathogens, but no longer a routine food in the diet of any predator. Thus, to recapture an earlier era, we must look for unusual circumstances that level the playing field, redefining our species once again as meat.

At least twice during World War II, predators killed large numbers of displaced military personnel. In the first incident, in 1945, British troops pursued about 1000 Japanese soldiers into a mangrove swamp on Ramree Island, off the coast of Burma. While the British waited for the Japanese to emerge from the swamp in full surrender, the crocodiles moved in:

The din of the barrage had caused all crocodiles within miles to slide into the water and lie with only their eyes above, watchfully alert. When it subsided the ebbing tide brought to them more strongly and in greater volume than they had ever known before it the scent and taste that aroused them as nothing else could—the smell of blood. Silently each snout turned into the current, and the great tails began to weave from side to side.[8]

And so forth. By morning, the swamp contained about 20 thoroughly demoralized Japanese soldiers and a lot of fat crocodiles. This is stirring stuff, told by an alleged eyewitness, but it is not clear how many of these soldiers died from bullet wounds or simply escaped before either the crocodiles or the Brits arrived. Something happened that night; but war is a nasty business, and by 1945, some Western readers unfortunately might have relished the thought of the enemy becoming sushi.

The Allies were not immune to predation either, for a comparable tragedy claimed several hundred American sailors when their ship, the USS *Indianapolis*, was torpedoed in the Pacific in 1945 after transporting the first atomic bomb to the island of Tinian. Readers may remember the story as

[8]Bruce Wright, *Wildlife Sketches Near and Far* (Fredericton, Canada: Brunswick Press, 1962).

Quint's monologue in the 1975 motion picture *Jaws*:

They didn't even list us overdue for a week. Very first light, chief, the sharks come cruisin'. So we formed ourselves into tight groups. . . . I don't know how many sharks, maybe a thousand! I don't know how many men, they averaged six an hour. . . . So, eleven hundred men went in the water, three hundred and sixteen men come out, the sharks took the rest, June the 29, 1945. Anyway, we delivered the bomb.[9]

REFERENCES AND RECOMMENDED READING

Kurzman, Dan. 1990. *Fatal Voyage: The Sinking of the USS* Indianapolis. New York: Atheneum.

OUTLOOK FOR THE TWENTY-FIRST CENTURY

Now that several major predators have legal protection from hunters, their numbers are likely to increase, but there is no reason to assume that more human deaths will result. Predators such as mountain lions eat humans only as a last resort anyway, and the same resource agencies that protect and manage these animals are supposed to design recovery plans that ensure protected habitat with an adequate food supply. In Australia, the recovery of the saltwater crocodile has not produced an epidemic of human disappearances.

Public debate is likely to continue regarding the wisdom of restocking locally extinct predators, such as the gray wolf and grizzly bear, in areas where they may harm livestock or hikers. A few years ago, when the government released Mexican wolves in Arizona over the protests of cattle ranchers, someone simply shot the wolves. In the opinion of many observers, the U.S. Endangered Species Act now serves largely as a vehicle for limiting urban sprawl and restricting human use of wilderness areas, rather than as a coherent framework for reducing biodiversity loss. Many scientists believe that a long-term solution will require laws that recognize the nature of biological species as well as the inevitability of human impacts.

The animals that cause the most human injuries are not bears or wolves in any case, but domestic dogs. If the threat (or perceived threat) of violent crime and terrorism continues to increase, particularly in large cities, more people are likely to purchase guard dogs, and more states will pass laws holding those owners accountable for the result.

THE GOOD OLD DAYS

An ancient painting in a cave at Lascaux, France, dated at approximately 14,000 years B.C., shows a man who has just been fatally gored by a wisent or European bison (*Bison bonasus*). We infer that the injury was fatal because the painting contains an image that scholars have interpreted as the man's soul ascending in the form of a bird. We may also infer that the man (and his chroniclers) had been hunting the bison before it attacked, as he appears to have dropped his spear and spear thrower, and the bison's guts are dragging (Figure 8.5). In other words, in today's parlance, the bison attack was provoked.

---

[9]P. Benchley and C. Gottlieb, Screenplay for *Jaws* (Universal City: Universal Pictures, 1975).

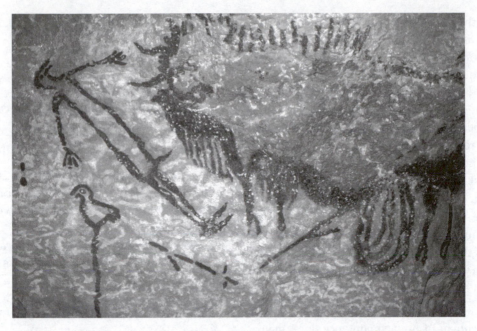

Figure 8.5. Cave painting of a bison attack, Lascaux, France. (*Source*: Charles and Josette Lenars/ Corbis.)

Most remarkably, archaeologists have found versions of this same painting at several locations in France and Spain, separated in time by thousands of years: the man, the bison, the spear, and the bird. Clearly, the story was a Paleolithic best-seller. But how shall we explain the audience appeal? *Jaws* was a hit in 1975 because it shocked complacent modern audiences who had always assumed nothing could eat them. At the time of the bison story, however, animal attacks and hunting accidents must have been commonplace. Why would crowds gather to hear about this one? Perhaps the man was famous, or perhaps it was more a catechism than a novel, holding the promise of immortality for every hunter who gave his life to feed his people.

By the twelfth century A.D., Europe had witnessed many changes, but the sport of kings had survived. The remaining herds of bison and other wild game animals had dwindled, but they were still worthy adversaries, and their ability to fight back was a major reward of the hunt:

I devoted much energy to hunting as long as I reigned in Chernigov. . . . Two bison tossed me and my horse on their horns, a stag once gored me, a boar tore my sword from my thigh, a bear on one occasion bit my kneecap, and another wild beast jumped on my flank and threw my horse with me. But God preserved me unharmed.[10]

[10]"The Testament of Vladimir Monomach" (circa 1125), in B. Dmytryshyn, *Medieval Russia: A Source Book*, 2nd ed. (Hinsdale, IL: Dryden Press, 1973).

257

Predators and Other Biological Hazards

By the 1600s, however, the European bison was nearly extinct and was the focus of a major conservation effort that lasted well into the twentieth century. In 1919, a man named Nikolaj Szpakowicz briefly distinguished himself by killing the last wild European bison. But a captive breeding program rescued the species, and several thousand now survive, at least in the status of tourist attractions in Poland's Bialowieza Forest.

The wisent's North American cousins continued to gore unlucky hunters on the eve of their near-extinction in the nineteenth century, as President Theodore Roosevelt observed:

A ranchman of my acquaintance once, many years ago, went out buffalo hunting on horseback, together with a friend who was unused to the sport, and who was mounted on a large, untrained, nervous horse. While chasing a bull, the friend's horse became unmanageable, and when the bull turned, proved too clumsy to get out of the way, and was caught on the horns, one of which entered its flank, while the other inflicted a huge, bruised gash across the man's thigh, tearing the muscles all out. Both horse and rider were flung to the ground with tremendous violence. The horse had to be killed, and the man died in a few hours from the shock, loss of blood, and internal injuries.[11]

Incredibly, visitors to Yellowstone National Park in the twenty-first century still try to pet or feed the few remaining bison, despite warning signs and some 16,000 years of experience. That herd alone injures several people every year, mortally in some cases.

REFERENCES AND RECOMMENDED READING

Ford, Peter. "Inside the Bialowieza Forest." *Christian Science Monitor*, August 3, 1998.
Leroi-Gourhan, André. 1967. *Treasures of Prehistoric Art*. New York: Harry N. Abrams, Inc.

FROM THE AUTHOR'S FILE CABINET

Death comes in many forms, and it need not stalk on four legs. It may sail on four wings, or hop on its haunches, or even fall through the air.

One spring evening in 1971, the author was driving near a freeway overpass in the East Bay area of northern California when she saw what appeared to be a four-winged bird with no feet, on a high-speed collision course with the driver's side window. Startled, she swerved onto the embankment and nearly rolled the car, while nearby drivers got out of the way as best they could. The bird or thing hit the car door with a surprisingly loud *thud*. By the time the car stopped and the dust settled, the creature had somehow broken in half; one piece now lay on the pavement, while the other crawled up the bank through the ice plant and was lost to view. The author got out to investigate and found a dead bird called a white-throated swift (*Aeronautes saxatalis*). A pair had been copulating in flight, as swifts do. The female presumably had died happy, while the male, being on top, had survived. No people were hurt, but several might easily have been.

At least one other college student (probably many) also happened to be driving on

---

[11]Theodore Roosevelt, *Hunting Trips of a Ranchman* (New York: G.P Putnam's Sons, 1885), Chapter 8.

a northern California highway on a spring night in 1971. He first realized that something was wrong when several cars ahead of him began sliding out of control on the pavement. There had been a recent rain, and hundreds of frogs had chosen that moment to migrate across the road from an adjacent field. Their squashed remains made a slippery surface; fortunately, no one was hurt on that occasion (other than the frogs), but similar incidents have caused occasional traffic pileups both in the United States and in Australia.

The third story that seems to belong here involves a 71-year-old Oregon woman who was driving on a mountain road in 1997, when she noticed two black angus bulls fighting on a cliff some 20 feet above the road. One of the bulls then lost its footing and fell off the cliff onto the car, but the driver lived to tell her tale: "The last thing I remember is the bull coming in through the windshield, and then I don't know—I must have lost consciousness for a few minutes. It was a lot of bull and a lot of shattered glass."[12]

[12]"Bull Falls Off Embankment, Totals Car," Associated Press, July 18, 1997.

CHAPTER 9

Hazard and Controversy

Did He who made the lamb make thee?
—William Blake, "Tyger, Tyger" (1794)

A unique property of biological hazards, not shared with geological or other natural hazards, is their ability to generate suspicion and controversy. Not even the most dedicated conspiracy theorist has yet blamed government bureaucrats or evil scientists for a storm or volcanic eruption, yet such claims routinely follow in the wake of every "new" disease outbreak, health-care fiasco, mutilated cow, or crop plague.

We have selected four such topics for discussion in this chapter. They are environmental protection and its human health and safety tradeoffs; health-related controversies, such as immunization, alternative medicine, and the origins of HIV; surrogate hazards; and biological warfare. The purpose of this chapter is to encourage discussion in classrooms and neighborhoods, not to present "right" answers (which do not necessarily exist). For a discussion of a fifth relevant topic, agricultural biotechnology, see *Recent Issues and Advances in Environmental Science* (Oryx Press, 2000).

MAN AND NATURE

Chapter 1 described the role of biological hazards in a hypothetical Bronze Age culture. Childhood diseases, mysterious epidemics, crop plagues, and predators were everyday problems. Even without knowing the right words, people must have wished they could purify the drinking water, kill crop pests and predators, and prevent the children from becoming sick.

Today, residents of the United States and other developed nations take all these services for granted—but the services are far from perfect. Instead of being grateful for a vaccine that protects 90 percent of recipients, we sue pharmaceutical companies, doctors, and the National Vaccine Injury Compensation Program on behalf of the other 10 percent. A worm in an artichoke or a snake in the backyard is an occasion for outrage. And yet a large minority has moved in the opposite direction, claiming that the original hazards are preferable to the safeguards. This movement has demanded that governments stop vaccinating children, chlorinating water, killing predators, and spraying crops. In some cases, the reasons are compelling. But which biological hazards do we really need to keep, and which ones are dispensable?

Every chapter in this book contains examples of the tradeoffs involved in controlling or eliminating biological hazards. Peru learned a hard lesson when its decision to stop chlorinating water contributed to the 1991 cholera epidemic. More than one nation has discovered that draining wetlands to control malaria and yellow fever can reduce biodiversity, and that restoring the lost wetlands may restore the original disease hazard (Figure 9.1); that diverting rivers to relieve drought can bring waterborne and vectorborne parasites; that antibiotics have steered the evolution of drug-resistant bacteria; and that pesticides make higher crop yields possible, but are highly toxic to exposed human populations. In the United States, we have seen that killing mountain lions and wolves can save cattle, but also allows deer and their ticks to proliferate. Compromise measures, such as training wild wolves to avoid livestock by making them wear electric-shock collars, appear to defeat both objectives; the wolves are no longer wild and free, nor is the anti-wolf contingent much happier.

Nathan Augustus Cobb, the great agricultural scientist, once speculated that if everything else in the world were somehow to vanish, leaving all the nematode worms hanging in space precisely where they had

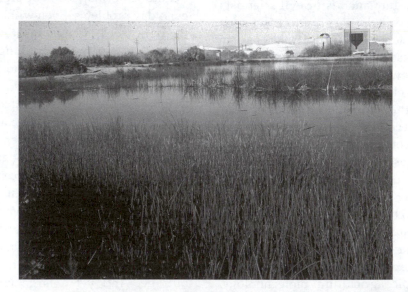

Figure 9.1. A restored wetland in Arizona. Mosquito control measures incorporated into the site design include (1) deep, open water to limit emergent vegetation, (2) mosquito fish and bacterial agents to control larvae, and (3) surveillance of mosquito and arbovirus activity. (*Source*: Dr. William E. Walton, University of California, Riverside.)

been, their bodies would reveal a clear tracing of the Earth and all its creatures.[1] In other words, these worms are so numerous and so greatly interwoven with the world that they are inseparable from it. But if we could perform the reverse miracle, by dipping the globe in a great vat of nematicide to kill these creatures, its very structure would collapse. Biological hazards, in fact, are very much like worms. Even if we think we hate them, they are inseparable from our lives.

Who owns the Earth? Several generations ago, the prevailing view was that people owned it and could do whatever they wanted with it. One generation ago, a more politically correct answer was that the Earth owns us, and that we must leave it alone. Today, there is a weak consensus that no one can ever own the Earth in quite the way that Bronze Age man might have dreamed. Take away the hazards, and the world is gone. Readers must decide for themselves how much wilderness is enough, and what sacrifices they will make in order to keep it.

In that spirit, Table 9.1 summarizes the "worst" biological hazards in each category covered in earlier chapters, and thus sets the stage for Table 9.2—a nonserious list of the "best" and "worst" places in the world to live, based on the sole criterion of biological risk. The intended point is that poor choices may result from too much emphasis on avoiding negative conditions rather than seeking out positive ones. Otherwise, squeaky-clean New Zealand would today be severely overpopulated, while the African cradle of our species, with its rich heritage of biological hazards, would stand empty.

REFERENCES AND RECOMMENDED READING

Anderson, Christopher. "Cholera Epidemic Traced to Risk Miscalculation." *Nature*, November 28, 1991, p. 255.

Bjørneboe, Jens. "Hemingway and the Beasts," pp. 5–14 in *Samlede Essays*. Oslo, Norway: Pax, 1996. English Translation by Esther G. Mürer.

Bolgiano, Chris. 1995. *Mountain Lion: An Unnatural History of Pumas and People*. Mechanicsburg, PA: Stackpole Books.

"Grizzly Encounters Pose Challenge to Western Parks." *National Parks*, January–February 1988, p. 14.

Lopez, Barry Holstun. 1978. *Of Wolves and Men*. New York: Charles Scribner's Sons.

McCombie, Brian. "A Bear of a Problem." *Field and Stream*, September 1999, p. 120 ff.

Mowat, Farley. 1963. *Never Cry Wolf*. New York: Dell Publishing Co.

Parent, G., et al. "Grands Barrages, Santé et Nutrition en Afrique: Au-delà de la Polémique. [Dams, Health and Nutrition in Africa: Beyond the Polemic.]" *Sante*, November–December 1997, pp. 417–422.

Patz, Jonathan A., et al. "Global Climate Change and Emerging Infectious Diseases." *Journal of the American Medical Association*, January 17, 1996, p. 217 ff.

HEALTH-RELATED CONTROVERSIES

Like the environmental tradeoffs in the previous section, the following issues are neither simple nor easily resolvable. Again, we present a brief summary of relevant facts and opposing viewpoints.

The Immunization Crisis

Two or three generations ago, vaccination was a miracle. Today, smallpox is gone from the world (except in two freezers), and polio

---

[1]N. A. Cobb, "Nematodes and Their Relationship" (*USDA Yearbook*, 1914, pp. 457–490).

Table 9.1
Worst Biological Hazards by Category

Category	Entity	Rationale
Waterborne Disease	Diarrhea	All forms of diarrhea kill nearly as many people as AIDS
Foodborne Disease	Diarrhea	All forms of diarrhea kill nearly as many people as AIDS
Airborne Disease	Tuberculosis	Presently kills more people than any other single infectious disease
Vectorborne Disease	Malaria	Has killed more people than any other known disease (perhaps half of all humans who have ever lived)
Sexually Transmitted Disease	HIV/AIDS	Arguably the worst infectious disease epidemic in history
Other Contact Disease	Measles	875,000 reported deaths, 1999
Agricultural Pest	Potato Late Blight	Historic impact; resistant strains; annual cost
Venomous Animal	Cobra	May kill thousands each year in India
Poisonous Plant	Philodendron	Not the most toxic by far, but the most often eaten
Fungus	*Aspergillus flavus*	Carcinogen, allergen, and pathogen
Contact Allergen	*Toxicodendron* sp.	Millions are affected each year
Food Allergen	Peanut	Over 100 deaths each year in the U.S. alone
Addictive Biological Substance	Tobacco	Enough said
Predator on Humans	Crocodiles	Over 1000 deaths each year in Africa and Southeast Asia
Domestic Animal	Domestic Dog	About 334,000 humans hospitalized with dog bites each year, U.S.
Other Biological Hazard	Deer on highways	Total annual cost exceeds $1 billion

and diphtheria are gone from four continents; public health agencies and pharmaceutical companies rightly congratulate themselves on these victories. Most couples no longer have eight or ten children in the hope that two or three might survive to adulthood. Meanwhile, a growing worldwide movement insists that vaccination is harmful and unnecessary. As usual in such situations, both sides may be partly right. Childhood vaccinations protect groups, but sometimes at the expense of individuals.

The antivaccination movement, like any other, has an extreme fringe that invites derision by the medical establishment. These extreme views make good tabloid headlines ("Flu Shots Cause Cancer"), but are unlikely to represent the millions of conscientious men and women who find some modern medical practices troubling, and who seek only to sort out the facts and protect their children. To put the matter in historical perspective, consider the polio vaccination campaign of the 1950s. Many parents voiced

Table 9.2
"Best" and "Worst" Places to Live

This table is intended as a light summary of the book's contents,
not as an indictment of any region or fauna.

Hazard You Wish to Avoid	Best Places	Worst Places
Infectious Diseases (not STD)	North America	Africa, India
Sexually Transmitted Diseases	Sweden	United States, Africa
Venomous Snakes	New Zealand, Ireland	Sri Lanka, Australia
Venomous Spiders	Alaska, northern Canada	Australia
Venomous Scorpions	Canada, New Zealand	Mexico and North Africa
Sharks	Deserts	Coastal waters of Florida
Crocodiles	Europe	Australasia and Africa
Large Wild Mammals	New Zealand, Ireland	Africa
Vicious Dogs	France	United States and Romania
Alcohol	Vietnam	Luxembourg
Tobacco	Papua New Guinea	Cyprus
Poisonous Plants and Fungi	Frozen food section	Everywhere; eat nothing
Everything	New Zealand	Africa

appropriate fears and concerns about the shots, but had their children immunized anyway, for the good of the community—while others insisted that the Salk vaccine had actually *caused* the polio epidemic, and that the vaccine's manufacturer was in cahoots with the Coca-Cola Company, whose sugary drinks somehow caused polio.

Even some U.S. doctors supported this strange notion, possibly because they resented Dr. Salk's hero status. And yet the idea contained a microscopic germ of truth—not the part about sugar, that is, but the cloud of suspicion that tends to overhang the pharmaceutical industry and privately funded research in general. Altruism rarely is the sole motive of any manufacturer, and an early version of the inactivated polio vaccine was rushed into human trials in 1954 before it was entirely safe. Whether the doctors were in a hurry to save lives, or the manufacturer and sponsors wanted to recover their investment, the outcome was the same: some batches contained live poliovirus that infected several hundred children, and the courts later awarded damages to some of them.

The alleged conspiracy with the Coca-Cola Company may refer to the fact that Coca-Cola, like any other major corporation, has contributed to various philanthropic causes over the years, including polio research in the 1950s. As recently as 2000, Coca-Cola's India office announced a partnership with Rotary International to combat polio in that country, but the news is scarcely sinister. And although it would be hard to deny that Americans consume too much sugar, there is no evidence that sugar causes polio or makes it worse. (A doctor drew that conclusion after he noticed that polio and sugar consumption both peaked in summer.)

The polio vaccine took it on the chin again in 1999, when the press revived an earlier finding that both the Salk and Sabin vaccines given before 1962 were contaminated with a monkey tumor virus called SV-40. This virus, as a result, now infects some 100 million people in the United States and Europe, and may increase their cancer risk. Unlike most antivaccination rhetoric, this claim was based on legitimate research findings published in a peer-reviewed journal. Fragments of the SV-40 virus have turned up in many cancer patients, particularly those with mesothelioma, a deadly tumor normally associated with asbestos exposure. Doctors have recently found SV-40 in younger patients who never received the contaminated vaccine, a fact that suggests the virus may be sexually or placentally transmitted.

At first, it seemed possible that the virus was an incidental passenger and not the cause of these tumors. A 1997 international workshop on SV-40 reached that conclusion. More recent studies, however, have dashed any such hope. Investigators compared mesothelioma patients in Finland (where the contaminated polio vaccine was not used) with those in the United States. As expected, most of the Finnish mesothelioma patients had occupational exposure to asbestos, and none tested positive for SV-40. But in the American sample, SV-40 turned up in 60 percent of mesotheliomas, and about half the patients had no known contact with asbestos.

But if polio vaccine contained one unwanted virus, why not another? In 1999, a well-researched book entitled *The River* revived another theory—previously published in 1992 in the magazine *Rolling Stone*, and in 1994 in the journal *Medical Hypotheses*—that the worldwide AIDS epidemic resulted from a contaminated polio vaccine used in Africa between 1957 and 1961. The authors of those publications claimed that medical researchers used chimpanzee kidneys rather than monkey kidneys to make some batches of the vaccine, and that the virus made the jump from chimps to humans as a result. Recent tests show that existing samples of that vaccine contain no chimpanzee DNA, but the samples may not represent all batches.

Vaccinating a population really means giving that population a disease, but in a milder form than it would otherwise take. Whenever doctors inject millions of people with a mixture of complex, inadequately understood biological materials, there is a risk. By all available standards, that risk is small compared with the outcome of a full-blown disease epidemic. Balancing those facts, however, is the perception of blame. If, for example, one million parents have their children vaccinated, and one child dies as a result, one parent (or two) will be devastated. Not only has the child died, but the parent *did* it, and the example will frighten other parents. If, on the other hand, the same million parents refuse the vaccine, and several hundred children die of a preventable disease, the parents may convince themselves that they are blameless. They did nothing; it was divine will or bad luck. When promoting vaccinations, public health officials might consider this viewpoint, instead of dismissing vaccination fear as a simple case of risk compression—that is, the human tendency to overestimate rare risks and to underestimate common ones, as discussed in earlier chapters.

The polio vaccine was neither the first nor the last that has raised concerns about contamination. In the first half of the twentieth century, some yellow fever vaccines contained both avian leukosis virus, which probably does not harm humans, and hepatitis B virus, which obviously does. Some people have even speculated that the 1918 influenza pandemic, and the encephalitis lethargica pandemic that occurred at the same time, might somehow have resulted from a bad batch of smallpox vaccine given to U.S. troops in World War I. As another example, some parents still refuse to have their children immunized against measles, either for religious reasons or because of unsubstantiated claims that the vaccine causes diabetes or autism. In 1991, a measles outbreak occurred in two faith-healing churches in Philadelphia and claimed the lives of six children.

At least two Internet Web sites currently promote the theory that the World Health Organization (WHO) created the AIDS virus and intentionally gave it to Africans during a smallpox vaccination program. (This is unrelated to the theory that HIV was a contaminant in an early polio vaccine.) The smallpox claim is unusual for the genre in that it cites a specific 1972 WHO publication as proof. That publication, however, says nothing of the kind; it simply reviews the evidence that certain naturally occurring viruses can damage the immune system. It is an interesting and prophetic paper, but scarcely a blueprint for world conquest.

During the late 1990s, the U.S. Department of Defense encountered some resistance to its anthrax vaccination program. Doubts persisted even after the October 2001 outbreak; at latest word, less than 3 percent of people exposed to contaminated mail had accepted the government's offer of anthrax vaccine. The vaccine's effectiveness against inhalation anthrax is unknown; other issues range from a general concern about personal liberty to a rumor that some batches were contaminated with the agent of bovine spongiform encephalopathy (BSE). Similarly, many parents have joined in a campaign against the diphtheria-pertussis-tetanus (DPT) vaccine, or more specifically its pertussis component. They note—correctly, in the opinion of some doctors—that the pertussis vaccine carries a significant risk, and that the disease itself is rarely dangerous in developed nations. Sweden, for example, banned the pertussis vaccine in 1979 (but reinstated it in 1995).

Worldwide, about 17 percent of infants with pertussis develop pneumonia, and about 300,000 die of related complications in Africa and Asia each year. Most of those children, however, do not have access to proper medical care. The most objective studies show that the vaccine is only about 70 percent effective in preventing pertussis, and that one in every 1750 children will develop serious complications from the vaccine. Some parents now claim, moreover, that these statistics hide subtle brain damage that may cause learning disabilities in a large percentage of vaccinated children.

Most medical researchers interpret these same facts differently. Infants receive their DPT shots at an age when they are growing rapidly and subject to many environmental influences. When two events occur at the same time, the public often assumes that one has caused the other—just as some doctors once believed that sugar caused polio. A recent book described an Australian family in which four children all developed seizure disorders soon after receiving their DPT shots in the 1970s, or, put another way, all four children developed those disorders at a similar age. No one knows if this tragedy resulted from a familial disorder that would have struck in any case, or a familial tendency to react badly to the DPT vaccine, or an unlikely cluster of rare accidents. But DPT shots do not affect most children this way, and for those parents who may be concerned, diphtheria and tetanus vaccines are available without the pertussis component.

The following anonymous message from an Internet support group member may put the controversy in a different light:

[The baby] started having fits of screaming that lasted for hours when he was a few days old, before he ever had a DPT shot. Nobody could find a reason. He did not seem any worse after the shots. He was healthy growing up, but had some problems that his teachers asked about. Later on he started having seizures and we are not out of the woods yet, but God makes everyone different. The doctors tried to blame it on bad parenting, which was not fair. It would have been so easy for us to turn around and blame the doctors and their shots.

It is true that vaccines have harmed some individuals and populations, usually because of contaminants that scientists had not yet developed the technology to detect, or risks that were not apparent from the available data. They used the best tools available in the hope of saving lives, and were successful more often than not. In 1990, the editors of the journal *Nature* wrote the following statement, in response to growing public concern and controversy about the BSE epidemic in England. The same words apply to the vaccination controversy or to any other:

Never say there is no danger. Instead, say that there is always a danger, and that the problem is to calculate what it is. . . . Never say that the risk is negligible unless you are sure that your listeners share your own philosophy of life.[2]

Alternative Medicine and Health Foods

Alternative medicine is another hot topic that involves biological hazards. Sometimes it alleviates these hazards, and sometimes it creates them. From the viewpoint of many doctors, however, there is no such thing as alternative medicine. A drug or other treatment, "natural" or otherwise, either works or it does not.

The only real difference between mainstream and alternative medicine is that the latter often uses methods and substances that have not been put to the test of science. Granted, this might seem to make little difference, as several mainstream drugs and vaccines have proven harmful after receiving FDA approval. More than anything else, the current popularity of alternative medicine may reflect consumer distrust of the health-care system. Horror stories saturate the media: doctors who remove the wrong lung; pharmacists who kill patients by dis-

[2] Quoted in F.A. Murphy, "Emerging Zoonoses" (*Emerging Infectious Diseases*, July–September 1998).

pensing the wrong drugs; insurance companies who limit dying patients to the cheapest available treatments, even if those treatments are known to be ineffective.

U.S. residents now spend an estimated $14 billion per year on self-prescribed herbal and vitamin supplements alone, which are largely exempt from regulation in the United States under the Dietary Supplement Health and Education Act of 1994. According to a recent study, more than two-thirds of cancer patients take these supplements, and 60 percent do not tell their doctors. In some cases, the herbal products may interfere with the patients' chemotherapy or vice versa.

There is an unfair tendency for advocates and critics alike to combine all alternative medicine under one aegis. Some of these methods and substances really work, others are harmless but ineffective, and a few are potentially deadly. If a certain herbal tea, for example, makes a person feel better and causes no damage, few doctors would object to it. Several herbal medicines, such as St. John's wort and kava, have gained some acceptance in the medical literature; in 2001, however, St. John's wort failed in a small clinical trial, and the FDA was investigating reports of kava causing liver damage. Ginkgo biloba and ginseng may slightly improve mental performance—as does ordinary caffeine. But recent studies have identified the following herbs as potentially unsafe, depending on the consumer and dose: borage, calamus, coltsfoot, comfrey, life root, sassafras, chaparral, germander, licorice, and ephedra (ma huang). Some people find it hard to believe that "natural" plants can be dangerous, but the examples in Chapter 7 should suffice as proof.

On the extreme fringe of alternative medicine we find, for example, practitioners who convince the gullible that their bodies are stuffed with parasites and filth, and then charge outrageous fees to "cleanse" them. One Web site advises people to search their own stool for parasites every day. It even provides a checklist of what to look for, including several parasites that we evidently missed in researching this book, such as "fish-type parasites that swim out of the colon in schools" and "fuzz balls."

Here are several examples of recent abuses that have tended to antagonize mainstream doctors on the subject of alternative medicine:

- In 1990–1992, an herb in a weight-loss preparation caused kidney failure or serious damage in over 100 patients at a Belgian clinic.

- Cancer patients who traveled to the Bahamas for alleged therapy to boost their immune systems were injected with a mixture of unregulated blood products contaminated with HIV and hepatitis B.

- A doctor recently read the labels on dietary supplements in his local health-food store, and reported in the *New England Journal of Medicine* that several of these preparations contained animal products of undocumented origin, including bovine testicles. These ingredients present an unknown risk of BSE, anthrax, or other disease transmission.

- In 1999, the FDA and the state of Missouri stopped the distribution of an alternative health-care product called Triax Metabolic Accelerator, which actually contained a potent and dangerous thyroid hormone that caused severe illness in several people.

- A homeopathic practitioner in 1999 recommended a spider venom—diluted with water until only the water remains—as treatment for Ebola hemorrhagic fever. Freedom of speech is not at issue here, but there is always the risk that a desperate physician or dying patient might take such advice seriously.

- A 2000 study of health food stores showed that store employees gave questionable advice to investigators posing as family members of cancer patients. An example is the "give way" test, in which the shopper selects the appropriate treatment by lifting bottles of various compounds. The person's arm is supposed to become tired when holding the right bottle.

- Soy products, which first became popular in health-food stores and are now standard ingredients in many foods and infant formulas, have recently become the target of an FDA investigation. Soy contains estrogen-mimicking chemicals that are known to cause adverse effects in laboratory animals.

- Many dietary supplements are manufactured under poor controls, making it impossible for consumers to determine what dose they are taking. A study of ephedra supplements showed that the total alkaloid content varied from 0 to 18.5 milligrams per dosage unit. Lot-to-lot variations in the content of various active ingredients sometimes exceeded 1000 percent.

- In 1983, a hostess in New York served bagels that had been enriched with 60 times the proper amount of niacin (a B vitamin). Although the baker's intention was to promote good health, 14 of 25 people who ate the bagels became severely ill with flushing and itching.

In light of such problems, how can the government protect consumers without infringing on their right to choose? There is no simple answer, but many authorities have suggested that improving the quality of mainstream health care might be a step in the right direction. Most consumers in developed nations already have access to the information resources they need to evaluate risks, but many prefer instead to follow the advice of an individual they trust. Whether that individual is a doctor or a health-food store clerk may depend largely on the credibility and compassion of each.

More AIDS Controversies

Two other health controversies deserve mention here, and both are related to AIDS: Who is at high risk and thus ineligible to donate blood? And if HIV exposure is a criterion, how shall we reconcile that policy with the apparently growing popular belief that HIV does not cause AIDS?

The safety and availability of the blood supply is a major health issue for the United States as well as for the rest of the world. Although improved blood testing methods since the early 1990s have greatly reduced the chance of HIV or hepatitis transmission in developed nations, eligibility restrictions have contributed to an intermittently serious blood shortage (Figure 9.2). Now that a high percentage of the population is ineligible to donate, it is uncertain if blood banks can maintain adequate supplies. If the eligibility criteria are relaxed, however, there is concern that people will stop using blood banks and rely instead on private donations.

At the time this book was written, no one who acknowledged membership in any of the following risk groups could donate blood products to a U.S. blood bank: any man who had sex with another man even once after 1977; anyone who had sex in exchange for money or drugs after 1977; anyone who had ever used intravenous drugs; anyone who was HIV-positive; anyone with cancer, multiple sclerosis, hemophilia, or certain noninfectious conditions, such as

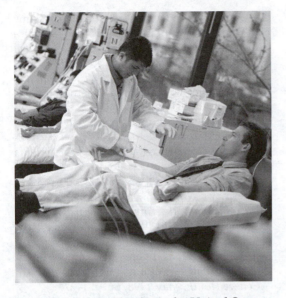

Figure 9.2. Blood banks in the United States face a shortage of donors. (*Source*: PhotoDisc, Inc.)

epilepsy; or anyone who had spent more than six months in England between 1980 and 1986 (during the BSE epidemic). As of 2001, the FDA reportedly was considering a ban on blood donations from deer hunters, based on the fact that three U.S. deer hunters died of Creutzfeldt-Jakob disease (CJD) after possible exposure to a prion disease. But a heterosexual person with an HIV-infected partner could donate blood after remaining HIV-negative for one year.

The issue here is not whether certain people have the right to give blood, but whether the risk factors are properly defined. A man who is honest enough to tell a blood bank that he is homosexual, but who has remained HIV-negative since 1977, is arguably a better risk than a woman with an HIV-positive husband. A man who ad-

mits that he injected heroin once 30 years ago, but now tests negative for HIV and hepatitis, might be a safer bet than another man who secretly visits prostitutes several times a week. The criteria, in other words, may be based partly on people's fears and dislikes rather than on scientific facts. The phrase "bad blood" has a dual meaning, in English as in other languages.

And yet many people now claim that HIV is not the cause of AIDS. If this is true, then why worry about contamination of the blood supply? As of 2001, even South African President Thabo Mbeki was leaning toward this viewpoint—a move that could compromise HIV treatment in his country and in others that might follow his lead. Some authors have claimed that scientists are afraid of alternative views, and are trying to suppress the truth about HIV; although most scientists love debate, AIDS research is a highly competitive arena. The problem here is that, while the debate continues, millions of people are dying. The cause of AIDS is as well understood as the cause of any other disease—imperfectly, in other words. Future studies may reveal that AIDS involves cofactors and environmental influences in addition to HIV. But most doctors feel that effective action is necessary here and now, not in some future Eden where all truths will come to light.

Sugar did not cause polio, nor did the malodorous miasmata of the night cause yellow fever. The advocates of those theories were not martyrs to the truth; they were simply wrong. Most had the good grace to yield in the face of evidence, while others went down fighting and took their patients with them.

REFERENCES AND RECOMMENDED READING

Allison, A.C., et al. "Virus-associated Immuno-pathology: Animal Models and Implications for Human Disease." *Bulletin of the World Health Organization*, Vol. 42, 1972, pp. 257–274.

Basser, Stephen. "Anti-immunisation Scare: The Inconvenient Facts." *Australian Skeptics*, March 1997. <http://www.skeptics.com.au/journal/anti-immune.htm>

Butel, J.S. "Simian Virus 40, Poliovirus Vaccines, and Human Cancer." *Bulletin of the World Health Organization*, Vol. 78, 2000, pp. 195–198.

Carbone, M., et al. "Simian Virus 40: The Link With Human Malignant Mesothelioma Is Well Established." *Anticancer Research*, March–April 2000, pp. 879–884.

Cohen, Cathy J. 1999. *The Boundaries of Blackness: AIDS and the Breakdown of Black Politics*. Chicago: University of Chicago Press.

Curt, G.A. "A Primer on the Perils of Unproved Treatments." *Journal of the American Medical Association*, January 24–31, 1986, pp. 505–507.

"Dozens Protest Anthrax Vaccine." Associated Press, January 29, 2000.

Elswood, B.F., and Stricker, R.B. "Polio Vaccines and the Origin of AIDS." *Medical Hypotheses*, Volume 42, 1994, pp. 347–354.

Foreman, Christopher H. 1994. *Plagues, Products, and Politics: Emergent Public Health Hazards and National Policymaking*. Washington, DC: Brookings Institution.

Fumento, Michael. 1990. *The Myth of Heterosexual AIDS*. Washington, DC: Regnery Publishing.

Gallo, Robert. 1993. *Virus Hunting: AIDS, Cancer, and the Human Retrovirus: A Story of Scientific Discovery*. New York: Basic Books.

Garrett, Laurie. 1994. *The Coming Plague: Newly Emerging Diseases in a World Out of Balance*. New York: Farrar, Straus & Giroux.

Goldberg, B., and Stricker, R. "Bridging the Gap: Human Diploid Cell Strains and the Origin of AIDS." *Journal of Theoretical Biology*, Vol. 204, 2000, pp. 497–503.

Green, S. "Immunoaugmentative Therapy: An Unproven Cancer Treatment." *Journal of the American Medical Association*, October 13, 1993, pp. 1719–1723.

Gurley, B.J., et al. "Content Versus Label Claims in Ephedra-Containing Dietary Supplements." *American Journal of Health-System Pharmacy*, May 15, 2000, pp. 963–969.

Hall, Robert, et al. 1998. *Immunisation: Myths and Realities*. 2nd ed. Canberra: Australian Government Publishing Service.

Haller, C.A., and Benowitz, N.L. "Adverse Cardiovascular and Central Nervous System Events Associated with Dietary Supplements Containing Ephedra Alkaloids." *New England Journal of Medicine*, December 21, 2000, p. 1833.

Hamerman, Warren J., et al. 1985. *Economic Breakdown and the Threat of Global Pandemics*. EIR Special Report. Washington, DC: Executive Intelligence Review.

Heiligenstein, E., and Guenther, G. "Over-the-Counter Psychotropics." *Journal of American College Health*, May 1998, pp. 271–276.

Hoey, John. "When the Physician Is the Vector." *Canadian Medical Association Journal*, July 14, 1998, pp. 45–46.

Hooper, Edward, and Hamilton, Bill. 1999. *The River: A Journey to the Source of HIV and AIDS*. Boston: Little, Brown & Co.

Klein, A. 1972. *Trial by Fury*. New York: Charles Scribner's Sons.

Klepser, T.B., and Klepser, M.E. "Unsafe and Potentially Safe Herbal Therapies." *American Journal of Health-System Pharmacy*, January 15, 1999, pp. 125–138.

Marcus, Adam. "Health Stores May Mislead Cancer Patients." *HealthScout*, August 14, 2000.

McClain, C. "St. John's Wort Fails in Study." *Arizona Daily Star*, April 18, 2001.

"Measles Hit Faith-Healing Churches." *Christianity Today*, April 8, 1991, p. 60.

Nortier, Joelle L., et al. "Urothelial Carcinoma Associated with the Use of a Chinese Herb." *New England Journal of Medicine*, June 8, 2000, pp. 1686–1692.

Norton, Scott A. "Raw Animal Tissues and Dietary Supplements." *New England Journal of Medicine*, July 27, 2000.

Papadopulos-Eleopulos, E., et al. "A Critical Analysis of the HIV-T4-Cell-AIDS Hypothesis." *Genetica*, March 1995, pp. 5–24.

Piot, Peter, et al. "The Global Impact of HIV/ AIDS." *Nature*, April 19, 2001, pp. 968–973.

Richardson, M.A., et al. "Complementary/Alternative Medicine Use in a Comprehensive Cancer Center and the Implications for Oncology." *Journal of Clinical Oncology*, July 2000, pp. 2505–2514.

Ross, Emma. "The Origins of AIDS." Associated Press, September 11, 2000.

Rubenstein, William B., et al. 1996. *The Rights of People Who Are HIV Positive.* Carbondale: Southern Illinois University Press.

Sandler, Benjamin P. 1951. *Diet Prevents Polio.* Milwaukee, WI: Lee Foundation.

Scannell, Kate. 1999. *Death of the Good Doctor: Lessons from the Heart of the AIDS Epidemic.* San Francisco: Cleis Press.

Tinsley, J.A. "The Hazards of Psychotropic Herbs." *Minnesota Medicine*, May 1999, pp. 29–31.

"Vaccine Worries Grow as Memory of Disease Dims." Associated Press, October 22, 1999.

Van der Vliet, Virginia. 1996. *The Politics of AIDS.* London: Bowerdean Pub. Co.

Vittecoq, D., et al. "Acute HIV Infection after Acupuncture Treatments." *New England Journal of Medicine*, January 26, 1989, pp. 250–251.

Yap, P.L. "Viral Transmission by Blood Products." *Irish Medical Journal*, April–May 1997.

SURROGATE HAZARDS

There appears to be a weak correlation between the things people say they fear, the things they logically should fear, and the things they really fear. Privately held fears that turn up in confidential surveys cover the whole spectrum from public speaking to cancer, but socially acceptable fears are another matter.

In 1999, tuberculosis killed nearly two million people worldwide, diarrhea killed another two million, and malaria one million. If there is a good way to die, it is not any of these. Tuberculosis victims essentially drown in blood; diarrhea is self-explanatory; and malaria brings miserable fits of headache, chills, fever, vomiting, and abdominal pain. And yet the news media rarely mention these diseases, instead warning readers of the most unlikely end-time plagues, such as Ebola fever or necrotizing fasciitis (see Chapter 5). Earthquakes, asteroids, comets, lake monsters, and unfriendly extraterrestrials are other front runners. Intestinal parasites also are favorites, perhaps because their faces are remarkably ugly. What all these popular hazards have in common is the low probability of their occurrence. No one really believes that a 25-foot tapeworm is curled up in their intestine (even if it is), or that bacteria will eat their arm.

For a few people, such fantasies are more than a harmless surrogate for real hazards. In a condition called delusional parasitosis, people believe that their bodies are crawling with invisible vermin. The following 2000 Internet posting may be representative, or not:

Hello! can you help my wife and I, please? We have a worm that attaches to our bones. mainly our lower sinel collum. goes in our ears, under the skin to our brain, mostly at night. and has come to our eyes and turned them blood shoot. apple sider vinigar makes them move. tolnaftate deaden them for a day. we can't stand more than a day of Mintezol but it drives the worms crazy. please help![3]

Some sufferers in this category may be mentally ill, but others appear to be misinterpreting common complaints such as allergic dermatitis, sciatica, "restless leg" syndrome,

---

[3]Downloaded September 18, 2001 from the Cutaneous Parasite Home Page.

and indigestion. It is also possible to have real parasites and delusions at the same time, as when a patient reports that his follicle mites are talking to him. Advertisements have begun to exploit these fears; excellent photographs of hookworms and tapeworms appear in a widely circulated brochure for herbal purgatives. Treatment of delusional parasitosis often is difficult, but experts advise the physician to start by carefully and respectfully ruling out any real infestation.

Pranksters often exploit these fears and semi-fears with biologically related hoaxes. Stories that once circulated by chain letter or word-of-mouth now reach millions via the Internet. In 2000, the CDC reported receiving several inquiries about a store clerk who allegedly contracted hantavirus and then somehow contaminated numerous soda cans and grocery packages. A similar mass e-mailing warned consumers that they might catch necrotizing fasciitis from Costa Rican bananas. Rumors of the nonexistent "Klingerman virus" made the rounds in 1999. Older stories, now full-blown urban legends, warned that deadly spiders might emerge by the trillion from "foreign" potted plants, or that human DNA (usually that of a recently terminated staff member) had turned up in the meat grinder of a certain hamburger chain.

These are verbal hoaxes, but there are also physical ones. In 2000, a microbiologist returning from a conference found that his handout materials included a note stating that he had been exposed to Q fever, with an attached packet of ominous-looking but apparently harmless powder. Between 1998 and 2000, many people and agencies re-

ceived similar notes and packets that warned of exposure to anthrax.

But not long after these hoaxes crossed some invisible threshold and ceased to be news, life imitated art, and letters filled with genuine anthrax turned up in several states. Suddenly, the long-awaited threat appeared to be real. And so we bought Cipro® and avoided junk mail—for a while—but continued eating at salad bars and swimming in the polluted blue waters of Santa Monica Bay.

REFERENCES AND RECOMMENDED READING

Blum, S.J., and Katz, H.L. "Itches, Illusions and Phobias." Chapter 27 in *Mallis Handbook of Pest Control*. Cleveland, OH: Franzak & Foster Co.

Borowitz, Andy. "Ridge: Northeast Battered by Five to Six Inches of Anthrax." *Newsweek*, January 9, 2002.

Bright, Chris. "Phytophobia." *American Horticulturist*, May 1994, p. 9.

Clark, Lee. 1999. *Mission Improbable: Using Fantasy Documents to Tame Disasters*. Chicago: University of Chicago Press.

Cowles, David L., and Cowles, Delys. 1997. *Miracle Victory over the Flesh-Eating Bacteria*. Salt Lake City: Gibbs Smith Publisher.

Glassner, Barry. 1999. *The Culture of Fear: Why Americans are Afraid of the Wrong Things*. New York: Basic Books.

Knutson, Roger M. 1996. *Furtive Fauna: A Field Guide to the Creatures Who Live on You*. Berkeley, CA: Ten Speed Press.

Knutson, Roger M. 1999. *Fearsome Fauna: A Field Guide to the Creatures that Live in You*. New York: W.H. Freeman.

Thornton, Bruce S. 1999. *Plagues of the Mind: The New Epidemic of False Knowledge*. Wilmington, DE: ISI Books.

Weintraub, Skye. 1998. *The Parasite Menace*. Pleasant Grove, UT: Woodland Publishing.

BIOLOGICAL WARFARE AND TERRORISM

Perhaps the most controversial biological hazard of our time is the use of pathogens, pests, or toxins as strategic weapons or instruments of terror (see Table 9.3). The United States and several other nations have developed such weapons, or have studied the agents for the purpose of developing defensive measures (Figure 9.3), which amounts to the same thing. There can be little doubt that this scenario presents a hazard; the issue is the level of risk.

Many wars throughout history have involved biological weapons that started disease epidemics (or were intended to start them). Many disease epidemics, conversely, have started rumors of biological weapons. Some of the weapons worked, and some of the rumors were true. But with every nation crying "Wolf!" at once, the truth in some cases may be hard to discern.

- In 1972, during the Cold War era, Cuba had an epidemic of swine fever and claimed that American agents had introduced the disease.

- In 1979, Zimbabwe had a major anthrax epi-

Table 9.3
Historical Examples of Biological Warfare and Terrorism

Date	Event
6th Century B.C.	Assyrians poisoned their enemies' wells with ergot of rye.
6th Century B.C.	Solon of Athens used hellebore (a purgative plant) to poison water.
74 B.C.	The Roman Lucullus defeated Mithridates by catapaulting hives of bees.
1346 A.D.	After some of its soldiers died of plague, the Tartar army threw the bodies over the walls of Kaffa, starting an epidemic and forcing a surrender.
1797 A.D.	Napoleon tried to infect the city of Mantua with swamp fever.
1862 A.D.	At the Battle of Antietam, the Southern Army fired on a row of beehives, releasing the bees and slowing the advance of Union troops.
1915 A.D.	A German-American physician in Washington, DC produced cultures of anthrax and glanders to infect Allied livestock and personnel.
1931 A.D.	The Japanese government tried unsuccessfully to infect a League of Nations commission with cholera.
1972 A.D.	Members of a right-wing organization in Chicago were arrested for possession of typhoid bacterial cultures.
1983 A.D.	The FBI arrested two men in the northeastern U.S. for manufacturing ricin.
1984 A.D.	The Rajneesh cult in Oregon contaminated salad bars with salmonella and sickened 750 people, in an effort to influence a local election.
1984 A.D.	French authorities found quantities of botulin toxin in a Paris laboratory operated by the Red Army Faction.
2001 A.D.	Some idiot mailed anthrax to media offices and public figures, killing five people and making 17 others sick, including a baby.

Sources: Electronic Dermatology Society; Canadian Security Intelligence Service; Oregon State University; Associated Press.

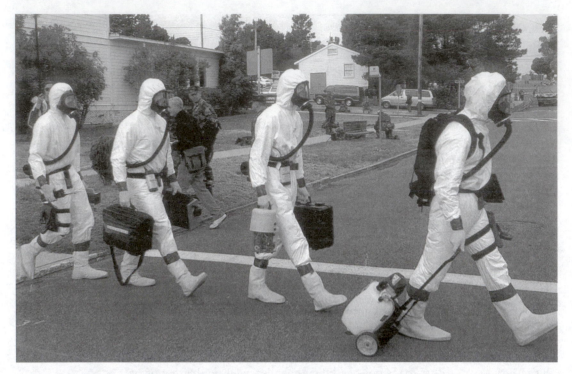

Figure 9.3 The Chemical-Biological Incident Response Force (CBIRF) responds to a mock emergency in California, 1999. (*Source*: AP/Wide World Photos/Ben Margot.)

demic during its civil war and blamed the white-dominated nationalist movement.

- In 1979, Cuba blamed the United States for a dengue epidemic.
- In 1980, during the Laotian civil war, Hmong refugees claimed that the Communist regime had deployed a chemical weapon called yellow rain.
- In 1993, when the first hantavirus outbreak occurred in the Southwest, many people thought a biological warfare agent must have escaped from an Army laboratory.
- In 1998, when doctors at a hospital in Libya accidentally infected 393 children with HIV, Libyan leader Moammar Gadhafi blamed the CIA and/or the Israeli government.
- In 1999, when West Nile encephalitis appeared in the United States, no less a periodi-

cal than the *New Yorker* interpreted the event as bioterrorism, possibly sponsored by Iraq.

Despite alternative explanations—the yellow rain, for example, apparently was bee urine—all these claims are at least slightly plausible; nations have done far worse things to one another and to their own citizens. But if even one such claim proves true, it will seem to lend credibility to the rest, when in fact these are independent events.

By contrast, some outbreaks that might be interpreted as suspicious pass almost unnoticed. Hawaii's first dengue fever epidemic in over 50 years, for example, occurred in the fall of 2001—near the time of the World Trade Center attack and the anthrax mailings—and dengue is a potential biological weapon. Like the West Nile outbreak, it was probably a natural event, but one raised eyebrows and the other did not.

By analogy, consider two prevalent beliefs in the United States in the 1970s: (1) that the tobacco industry had secretly adjusted nicotine levels in order to recruit addicts, thus causing an epidemic of lung disease; and (2) that the food industry was adding mind-control drugs to its products under the guise of preservatives, thus causing an epidemic of conformity. On the surface, neither claim seems more preposterous than the other. Could the enormously wealthy and respected tobacco industry really be plotting to turn its fellow Americans into junkies? Well—as it turned out—yes. But this conclusion has no bearing on the theory about food additives. Nicotine really is addictive, and cigarettes really are harmful; but there is still no evidence that soy lecithin or sodium benzoate can make us docile, mindless drones, whether anyone intended it that way or not.

Any epidemic, in wartime or not, seems so *wrong* that it is human nature to blame someone. An earlier section presented examples in which pharmaceutical manufacturers were the actual or suspected culprits. If the epidemic was plain bad luck, we are powerless to escape it next time, and if it was the will of God, the implications are huge. No, the bad guys must have done it. If no foreign power or corporation is available to blame, our own government or even a next-door neighbor will do. Here are examples of less plausible accusations:

- In 1350, Europeans blamed the Black Death on the Jews, and slaughtered many on the excuse of retaliation.

- In 1692, the people of Salem, Massachusetts hanged local witches (unpopular women) whom they blamed for several outbreaks of ergotism.

- In 1983, soon after the discovery of HIV/AIDS, some journalists blamed its existence on an Army experiment gone wrong.

- In 1997, an author who feared both biological warfare and the growing environmental movement speculated that environmentalists were plotting to unleash a biological weapon of mass destruction.

- In October 2001, there was widespread suspicion that Iraq or Iran must be responsible for the anthrax-filled letters mailed from New Jersey. (One target, the *National Enquirer*, claimed to have proof; as it turned out, the "proof" was a polite letter from a man in Iraq who had simply inquired about a subscription.)

- The author of a recent book and Web site claims that Iraqi women have smuggled vials of anthrax and plague into the United States for years, concealed in their vaginas.

Thus, for centuries, whichever nation or group happens to be unpopular at the moment becomes the target of a new wave of accusations of biological terrorism; and superimposed on each wave are the private nightmares of individuals.

Just how feasible is a large-scale biological attack? Despite many books that claim otherwise, no one really knows. There is a consensus that such weapons offer a cheap, easy way for a terrorist group to kill a limited number of people. In 1984, an Oregon cult spiked a salad bar with salmonella, giving 751 people diarrhea. Had they used botulin toxin instead, half of those 751 people might have died. But to produce the hundreds of thousands of casualties predicted in the tabloids, bioterrorists would need to clear some major technical hurdles.

The October 2001 anthrax mailings really changed nothing, other than to sell a few diehards on the germ theory of disease. The attack was effective, terrifying, and costly for the U.S. economy; yet only five people died, and the mailings soon stopped. The sender might just as easily have mailed hundreds of letters, but apparently did not—and the anthrax, quite disconcertingly, matched the variety produced by the U.S. Army. Perhaps this was not terrorism in the usual sense, but the act of some over-zealous American researcher who wanted to scare the government into upgrading its public health system. But a large-scale biological attack remains an unlikely scenario nonetheless. (Chemical weapons are another matter, but this book covers only the biological ones.)

For one thing, a biological attack beyond the salad-bar or envelope level would require considerable skill. To disperse bacteria over a city, for example, terrorists would need a nozzle capable of generating an aerosol cloud with particles in a specific size range. If the particles are too large, they fall out of suspension and drop to the ground, perhaps making a few cows sick; particles that are too small do not lodge in a person's lungs. The sprayers found on an ordinary crop-dusting airplane probably would not work for most biological agents. These agents also are vulnerable to heating, and most cannot survive delivery at supersonic speeds. A cruise missile might deliver biological agents effectively, but the United States and other nations have coastal radar and missile defenses to intercept such an attack.

Wind is another problem. In 1950, the U.S. Army released an aerosol of the bacterium *Serratia marcescens* over San Francisco to see how it would disperse. Mainly, it dispersed into a hospital's ventilation system and caused a dozen urinary tract infections and at least one death from endocarditis. (At the time, the Army was not aware that this bacterium is an opportunistic pathogen, but had chosen it for its bright red color.) The cloud might just as easily have blown out to sea. In an actual war, it might even have engulfed the attackers' own ground troops, and no vaccine is 100 percent effective.

If biological warfare is hard for the Army, how easy can it be for amateurs? The New Jersey saboteur of 2001 was clearly a professional and a rare exception. A recent study of all known domestic acts of biological terrorism between 1900 and 1998 showed that most were the work of inept clowns. In 1972, two college students decided to wipe out humanity with bacteria and then repopulate the earth with their own progeny. Their friends turned them in, and Armageddon was over. As another example, the Japanese cult that launched the 1995 Sarin attack on the Tokyo subway had tried similar attacks using anthrax and botulin toxin, but had failed every time. Bugs are easy to grow, but harder to deploy effectively.

Also, most nut cases and zealots alike prefer a weapon that makes a loud boom. The World Trade Center attack is a prime example. Biological weapons, by contrast, are silent and invisible; the perpetrator might need to wait days or weeks to tell if these weapons are even working. The cult that poisoned the salad bar in Oregon got caught only because one of its own members confessed, after health officials shrugged off the incident as a natural outbreak. Apparently, he could not stand being ignored. But individuals can afford to seek such gratification without fearing the long-term consequences—unlike a world leader, who might not retain the loyalty of his or her subjects, or the sympathy of the world community, after openly sponsoring a biological attack. The afterimages would simply be too ugly; a child dying of smallpox or hemorrhagic fever is still a child, regardless of nationality. Any government planning such an attack would more likely target an enemy's agricultural base, not its people.

Several nations have tried modifying bacteria to make them more lethal and to outwit vaccination programs. (A few days before the September 11 attacks, our own government announced that it was developing an enhanced strain of anthrax for defensive purposes.) Again, most world leaders realize that a genetically modified biological agent, once released into the environment, might have unanticipated long-term effects on their own people. Even the most carefully researched programs of biological control—the same thing as biological warfare, but against crop pests rather than humans—often have backfired due to the sheer complexity of living systems. In a recent experiment, scientists released an insect to kill a non-native weed, only to learn that the weed responded by releasing chemicals that, in turn, harmed native plants growing nearby. But the full potential for harm became clear in 2000, when Australian scientists accidentally created a lethal new virus while trying to develop a mouse contraceptive to control plagues.

In July 2001, the United States drew criticism when it unilaterally rejected the 1972 Biological and Toxin Weapons Convention (the full text appears in Chapter 10). By contrast, many scientists praised President Clinton's 1999 decision to preserve the world's last remaining samples of the smallpox virus—not because it is a species with the "right to live," as critics have sneered, but because of the possibility that nations other than the United States and Russia may have samples of their own. Studying the virus will increase scientific understanding of smallpox and other diseases, and will also make it possible to renew the vaccine supply in case of a future release. Some observers have proposed that vaccinating the entire U.S. population against smallpox would be less expensive than the years of debate that now appear inevitable; others note that the vaccine itself carries some risks, and that there is no real evidence that terrorists are likely to use smallpox as a weapon anyway. In December 2001, the U.S. Government announced that it would stockpile some 200 million doses of smallpox vaccine, but would make it available to the public only in the event of an outbreak. Research is also in progress to develop a safer smallpox vaccine.

REFERENCES AND RECOMMENDED READING

Alibek, K., and Handelman, S. 1999. *Biohazard*. New York: Random House.

"America the Vulnerable." *Time*, November 24, 1997.

Atiyah, Michael. "Science for Evil: The Scientist's Dilemma." *British Medical Journal*, August 14, 1999, p. 448 ff.

Atlas, Ronald M. "Combating the Threat of Biowarfare and Bioterrorism." *BioScience*, June 1999, pp. 465–477.

Benford, Gregory. "The Designer Plague (Ecoradicalism)." *Reason*, January 1994, pp. 36–41.

Burns, Robert. "Pentagon Plans to Proceed with Development of New Strain of Anthrax Bacterium." Associated Press, September 4, 2001.

Callaway, Ragan, et al. "Biological-Control Herbivores May Increase Competitive Ability of the Noxious Weed *Centaurea maculosa*." *Ecology*, June 1999, pp. 1196–1201.

"CDC Head: Bioterror Response Slowed by Neglected System." Associated Press, November 16, 2001.

Christopher, George W., et al. "Biological Warfare: A Historical Perspective." *Journal of the American Medical Association*, August 6, 1997.

Clarke, Robin. 1968. *The Silent Weapons*. New York: McKay.

Cohen, Philip. "A Terrifying Power." *New Scientist*, January 30, 1999, p. 10.

Cole, Leonard A. 1989. *Clouds of Secrecy: The Army's Germ-Warfare Tests over Populated Areas*. Lanham, MD: Rowman & Littlefield.

Cole, Leonard A. 1996. *The Eleventh Plague: The Politics of Biological and Chemical Warfare*. New York: W.H. Freeman.

"Cuba Case Tests Treaty: Bioweapons." *Bulletin of the Atomic Scientists*, November–December 1997, Vol. 53, No. 7.

"Dengue Fever Outbreak on Maui." Associated Press, September 22, 2001.

Duffy, David C. "Land of Milk and Poison." *Natural History*, July 1998, p. 4 ff.

Eitzen, Edward, et al. (Editors). 1999. *Medical Management of Biological Casualties Handbook*. Frederick, MD: U.S. Army Medical Research Institute of Infectious Diseases.

Falkenrath, Richard A., et al. 1998. *America's Achilles Heel: Nuclear, Biological, and Chemical Terrorism and Covert Attack*. Cambridge, MA: MIT Press.

"Foreigners Face Death Penalty in Case of 393 Children Injected with AIDS-Contaminated Blood." Associated Press, September 20, 2001.

Gould, Stephen Jay. "Above All, Do No Harm." *Natural History*, October 1998, pp. 16–24, 78–82.

Gunby, Phil. "Physicians Face Bioterrorism." *Journal of the American Medical Association*, April 7, 1999, p. 1162.

Harris, Sheldon. 1994. *Factories of Death*. London: Routledge.

Henderson, Donald A. "The Looming Threat of Bioterrorism." *Science*, February 26, 1999, p. 1279 ff.

Higgins, A. G. "U.S. Sole Nation to Reject Germ Warfare Treaty Draft." Associated Press, July 25, 2001.

Hinckle, Warren, and Turner, Will. 1981. *The Fish Is Red: The Story of the Secret War Against Castro*. New York: Harper & Row.

Horgan, John. "Were Four Corners Victims Biowarfare Casualties?" *Scientific American*, October 1993, p. 16.

"Iraq Sent Anthrax." *The National Enquirer*, November 6, 2001.

Jackson, R.J., et al. "Expression of Mouse Interleukin-4 by a Recombinant Ectromelia Virus Suppresses Cytolytic Lymphocyte Responses and Overcomes Genetic Resistance to Mousepox." *Journal of Virology*, February 1, 2001, pp. 1205–1210.

Joklik, W.K., et al. "Why the Smallpox Virus Stocks Should Not Be Destroyed." *Science*, November 19, 1993, pp. 1225–1226.

Kevan, Peter G., and Mardan, Makhdzir. "When Bees Get Too Hot, Yellow Rain Falls." *Natural History*, December 1990, p. 54.

Kilman, Scott. "Agro-Terrorism Still a Credible Threat." *Wall Street Journal*, December 26, 2001.

Lederberg, Joshua (Editor) and Cohen, William S. 1999. *Biological Weapons: Limiting the Threat*. BCSIA Studies in International Security. Cambridge, MA: MIT Press.

Lipton, Eric, and Johnson, Kirk. "Tracking Bioterror's Tangled Course." *New York Times*, December 26, 2001.

Lockwood, J.A. "Entomological Warfare." *Bulletin of the Entomological Society of America*, Vol. 33, 1987, No. 2, pp. 76–82.

Mangold, Tom, and Goldberg, Jeff. 2000. *Plague Wars: A True Story of Biological Warfare*. New York: St. Martin's Press.

McDermott, Jeanne. 1987. *The Killing Winds*. New York: Arbor House.

Miller, Judith, et al. 2001. *Germs: Biological Weapons and America's Secret War*. New York: Simon & Schuster.

Osterholm, M.T., and Schwartz, J. 2000. *Living Terrors: What America Needs to Know to Survive the Coming Bioterrorist Catastrophe*. New York: Delacorte Press.

Pile, James C., et al. "Anthrax as a Potential Biological Warfare Agent." *Archives of Internal Medicine*, March 9, 1998, pp. 429–434.

"Preparing for Chemical and Biological Terrorist Attacks." *Journal of Environmental Health*, Vol. 61, March 1999, p. 32 ff.

Pringle, Peter. "Bioterrorism Hits Home." *Nation*, May 3, 1999, p. 28.

Rogers, Paul, et al. "Biological Warfare against Crops." *Scientific American*, June 1999, p. 70 ff.

Rolicka, Mary. "Propaganda Value of Allegations of Biological Warfare in the Korean War." *Journal of the American Medical Association*, January 28, 1998, p. 274.

Rosenblatt, Joel. "Hazard a Guess: How Well Does the City Deal with an Actual Bio-terrorism Threat?" *New York*, March 15, 1999, p. 14.

San Nicolas, Claudine. "Case of Dengue Fever Discovered in Haiku." *Maui News*, October 1, 2001.

Shalala, Donna E. "Smallpox: Setting the Research Agenda." *Science*, August 13, 1999, p. 1011.

Stern, Jessica. 1999. *The Ultimate Terrorists*. Cambridge, MA: Harvard University Press.

Tucker, J.B. "National Health and Medical Services Response to Incidents of Chemical and Biological Terrorism." *Journal of the American Medical Association*, August 6, 1997, pp. 362–368.

Tucker, J.B., and Sands, Amy. "An Unlikely Threat." *Bulletin of the Atomic Scientists*, July/August 1999, pp. 46–52.

U.S. National Academy of Sciences, Institute of Medicine. 1999. *Assessment of Future Scientific Needs for Live Variola Virus*. Washington, DC: National Academy Press.

U.S. National Academy of Sciences, Institute of Medicine. 1999. *Chemical and Biological Terrorism: Research and Development to Improve Civilian Medical Response*. Washington, DC: National Academy Press.

Venter, A.J. "Plague War: Keeping the Lid on Germ Warfare." *Jane's Defense Weekly*, May 1, 1998.

Wiener, Stanley L. "Strategies for the Prevention of a Successful Biological Warfare Aerosol Attack." *Military Medicine*, May 1996, pp. 251–256.

Yu, V.L. "*Serratia marcescens*: Historical Perspective and Clinical Review." *New England Journal of Medicine*, April 19, 1979, pp. 887–893.

THE GOOD OLD DAYS

Although several examples in this chapter show that beliefs can cloud judgment, it does not follow that every visionary with a rejected theory must automatically be wrong. An old story that bears retelling is that of Ignaz Semmelweis, the Hungarian physician who discovered in 1847 that doctors and midwives could largely eliminate puerperal fever—a dangerous bacterial infection in a woman after childbirth—simply by washing their hands before delivery.

In Semmelweis' era, medical students attended most hospital births and also performed autopsies. Hand washing was not customary; a student might dissect a corpse, wipe the residue off his hands on a dirty apron, and then deliver a baby. About 10 percent of all new mothers died of the resulting infections. With or without the germ theory of disease, it might seem incredible that anyone would touch another person's body without first washing off the bad-smelling products of decay—but the training of medical students partly involved desensitizing the students to phenomena that they would otherwise find disgusting. Also, like people in any high-risk profession, these students and their role models might have indulged in a bit of denial. Thus, when Semmelweis proposed that hand washing could save lives, he became the target of ridicule that eventually led to his academic dismissal and confinement to a mental hospital.

Semmelweis had noticed that the death rate was far lower for women delivered by midwives, who washed their hands and, of course, did not perform autopsies. Granted, that observation alone did not prove a connection, but the hypothesis was easy enough to test. After Semmelweis ordered medical students to wash their hands, the postpartum death rate fell to less than 1.5 percent. But the prevailing view was that puerperal fever resulted from the unstable nature of pregnant women, and doctors were so committed to that view that hand washing was discontinued, and the death rate returned to its former level.

REFERENCES AND RECOMMENDED READING

Hoey, John. "When the Physician Is the Vector." *Canadian Medical Association Journal*, July 14, 1998, pp. 45–46.

Lillehei, C.W. "New Ideas and Their Acceptance." *Journal of Heart Valve Disease*, October 1995, Suppl. 2, pp. S106–S114.

Yates, E.L. "Semmelweis—Saddest Figure in Modern Medicine." *American Journal of Practical Nursing*, May 1966, pp. 114–117.

FROM THE AUTHOR'S FILE CABINET

A major controversy in the biohazard field is the proper relationship between wilderness and civilization, and the respective rights of the inhabitants of each.

Black bears (*Ursus americanus*) are not native to southern California, but in 1933 the California Department of Fish and Game (CDFG) stocked two mountain ranges in that area with "problem" bears removed from Yosemite National Park. The immigrants were fruitful and multiplied; they mauled only a few people, but quickly became a nuisance at campgrounds in the San Bernardino and San Gabriel Mountains. For the next 60 years, however, these bears did not colonize the adjacent San Jacinto Mountains, apparently because a low desert pass blocked their migration. Meanwhile, the state passed new laws that prohibited environmentally damaging actions (such as the introduction of non-native wildlife) without proper review and authorization.

In about 1997, rumors of bear sightings began to circulate in a small town in the San Jacinto Mountains. Long-time residents knew that the grizzly bear had been locally exterminated a century earlier, and that black bears had never lived in the area; most shrugged it off, reasoning that it was natural to see bears in the woods. A CDFG representative explained that the bears must have reached the mountains by crawling through a culvert under a freeway.

Every year thereafter, the local newspaper interviewed that same CDFG employee, who talked about bears and warned residents to take precautions. When reporters asked if the agency had released the bears, the CDFG man denied the possibility. Later, he began telling the newspaper that black bears had actually lived in the San Jacinto Mountains until the 1960s, and that their return was inevitable. Other CDFG staff disagreed, and expressed concern that the bears might damage the fragile mountain ecosystem or injure human residents.

A local biologist finally became suspicious, remembering that the pro-bear CDFG man had once remarked that he wanted to release bears in the San Jacinto Mountains but could not get permission. A records request to CDFG's legal office, and a call to the U.S. Forest Service, finally turned up the facts. Between 1997 and 1999, CDFG had, in fact, captured several black bears at various locations and transported them to the San Jacinto Mountains. The dates of these releases closely matched the bear sightings reported in the newspaper. Strangest of all, the CDFG employee who captured and released the bears was the same man whom the newspaper had interviewed.

A top CDFG official denied these events until shown his agency's own records, whereupon he responded that the bears had merely been "relocated," not "introduced." But these actions appeared to violate state and federal law as well as CDFG policy, and at latest word an investigation was in progress.

CHAPTER 10

Other Statistics and Primary Sources

> Thou shalt not be afraid for the terror by night; nor for the arrow
>   that flieth by day.
> Nor for the pestilence that walketh in darkness; nor for the destruc-
>   tion that wasteth at noonday.
> A thousand shall fall at thy side, and ten thousand at thy right
>   hand; but it shall not come nigh thee.
>
> —Psalms 91:1–7

This chapter contains an assortment of original documents and tables of data related to information presented elsewhere in this book.

Tables 10.1 and 10.2 contain the most recent lists of nationally and internationally reportable human diseases—that is, the diseases that physicians and other healthcare workers are required to report to state public health agencies. The states, in turn, transmit these reports to the U.S. Centers for Disease Control and Prevention (CDC). Cases of internationally reportable diseases are transmitted to the World Health Organization. Table 10.3 lists the animals most feared by American adults, according to a 2000 poll.

THE DISCOVERY OF VACCINATION

The following account of the work of Lady Montagu and Edward Jenner is reproduced verbatim from *Anomalies and Curiosities of Medicine*, by George M. Gould and Walter L. Pyle (W.B. Saunders, 1896).

Inoculation was known in Europe about 1700, and in 1717 the famous letter of Lady Montagu from Adrianople was issued, containing in part the following statements:—

"The small-pox, so fatal and so general amongst us, is here entirely harmless, by the invention of ingrafting, which is the term they give it. There is a set of old women who make it their business to perform the operation every autumn in the month of September, when the great heat is abated. People send to one another to know if

Table 10.1
Nationally Reportable Human Diseases, United States (as of 2001)

Disease	Mode of Transmission	Cases Reported, 2000
AIDS/HIV	Sex, body fluids, congenital	40,758
Anthrax	Airborne or contact	1
Botulism	Food- or waterborne	138
Brucellosis	Contact, foodborne, airborne	87
Chancroid	Sex	78
Chlamydia trachomatis	Sex or other contact	702,093
Cholera	Waterborne	5
Coccidioidomycosis	Airborne	NR
Cryptosporidiosis	Waterborne	3128
Cyclosporiasis	Waterborne	60
Diphtheria	Contact or foodborne	1
Ehrlichiosis, human granulocytic	Vectorborne (ticks)	351
Ehrlichiosis, human monocytic	Vectorborne (ticks)	200
Ehrlichiosis, human, other	Vectorborne (ticks)	NR
Encephalitis, California	Vectorborne (mosquitoes)	114
Encephalitis, Eastern Equine	Vectorborne (mosquitoes)	3
Encephalitis, Saint Louis	Vectorborne (mosquitoes)	2
Encephalitis, Western Equine	Vectorborne (mosquitoes)	NR
Enterohemorrhagic E. coli	Food- or waterborne	4528
Gonorrhea	Sex	358,995
Haemophilus influenzae, invasive	Contact	1398
Hansen Disease (Leprosy)	Probably contact	91
Hantavirus Pulmonary Syndrome	Airborne	41
Hemolytic Uremic Syndrome, post-diarrheal	Food- or waterborne	249
Hepatitis A	Contact, foodborne, or waterborne	13,997
Hepatitis B	Blood products or contact	8036
Hepatitis B perinatal	Perinatal	NR
Hepatitis C; non A, non B	Blood products or contact	3197
HIV infection, adult (> 13)	Sex, body fluids	NR
HIV Infection, Pediatric	Congenital	NR
Legionellosis	Airborne	1127
Listeriosis	Foodborne	755
Lyme Disease	Vectorborne (ticks)	17,730
Malaria	Vectorborne (mosquitoes)	1560
Measles (Rubeola)	Contact or airborne	86
Meningococcal Disease	Contact or airborne	2256
Mumps	Contact or airborne	338
Pertussis	Contact or airborne	7867
Plague	Vectorborne (fleas)	6
Poliomyelitis, Paralytic	Contact or foodborne (milk)	0
Psittacosis	Airborne or contact	17
Q Fever	Airborne or contact	21

Table 10.1   (Continued)

Disease	Mode of Transmission	Cases Reported, 2000
Rabies, Animal	Animal bites	6934
Rabies, Human	Animal bites	4
Rocky Mountain Spotted Fever	Vectorborne (ticks)	495
Rubella	Contact or airborne droplet	176
Rubella, Congenital Syndrome	Congenital	9
Salmonellosis	Food- or waterborne	39,574
Shigellosis	Contact, waterborne, or foodborne	22,922
Streptococcal Disease, invasive, Group A	Contact	3144
Streptococcal Toxic Shock Synd.	Contact	83
Streptococcus pneumoniae, drug-resistant	Contact or airborne	4533
Streptococcus pneumoniae, invasive in childen <5 years	Airborne or contact	NR
Syphilis	Sex	31,575
Syphilis, Congenital	Congenital	529
Tetanus	Contact	35
Toxic Shock Syndrome	Contact	135
Trichinosis	Foodborne	16
Tuberculosis	Airborne	16,377
Tularemia	Contact, airborne, foodborne	142
Typhoid Fever	Food- or waterborne	377
Varicella*	Contact or airborne	82,455
Yellow Fever	Vectorborne (mosquitoes)	0

*Reporting is mandatory for varicella-related deaths, but reporting of all cases is recommended.

Sources: U.S. Public Health Service, Centers for Disease Control and Prevention, Division of Public Health Surveillance and Informatics; "Final 2000 Reports of Notifiable Diseases" (*Morbidity and Mortality Weekly Report*, August 24, 2001, p. 712).

any of their family has a mind to have the small-pox; they make parties for this purpose, and when they are met, the old woman comes with a nut-shell full of the matter of the best sort of small-pox, and asks what vein you please to have opened. She immediately rips open that you offer her with a large needle, and puts into the vein as much matter as can lie upon the head of her needle, and after that binds up the little wound with a hollow shell, and in this manner opens four or five veins."

Soon after this letter Lady Montagu had her son inoculated in Turkey, and four years later her daughter was to be the first subject inoculated in England. She made rapid progress notwithstanding the opposition of the medical profession, and the ignorance and credulity of the public. The clergy vituperated her for the impiety of seeking to control the designs of Providence. . . .

Despite inoculation, as we have already seen, during the eighteenth century the mortality from small-pox increased. The disadvantage of inoculation was that the person inoculated was affected with a mild form of small-pox, which however, was contagious, and led to a virulent form in uninoculated

Table 10.2
Internationally Reportable Human Diseases (as of 1999)

Diseases Subject to the 1971 International Disease Regulations:
  Cholera
  Plague
  Yellow Fever

Diseases Under Surveillance by the World Health Organization:
  African Trypanosomiasis
  Cholera and Epidemic Dysentery
  Haemorrhagic Fevers
  Hepatitis
  HIV/AIDS
  Influenza
  Leishmaniasis
  Meningococcal Disease
  Plague
  Rickettsial Diseases
  Transmissible Spongiform Encephalopathies (TSE)
  Rabies and Other Zoonotic Diseases
  Other Viral Diseases (Monkeypox, Non-Polio Enteroviruses)

Diseases Requiring Immediate Notification by PAHO Member States:
  Plague
  Cholera
  Yellow Fever
  Smallpox
  Typhus
  "Any other dangerous contagion"

Diseases Reportable by PAHO Member States:
  Plague
  Cholera
  Yellow Fever
  Smallpox
  Typhus
  Epidemic Cerebrospinal Meningitis
  Acute Epidemic Poliomyelitis
  Epidemic Lethargic Encephalitis
  Influenza or Epidemic La Grippe
  Typhoid and Paratyphoid Fevers
  Other diseases that PAHO may add by resolution

Sources: World Health Organization, *International Health Regulations*, 3rd ed., 1983
  (Geneva: WHO, updated 1995); *WHO Recommended Surveillance Standards*, 2nd
  ed. (Geneva: WHO/UNAIDS, 1999).

Table 10.3
Most Feared Animals, 2000

Animal	Percent Declaring It Most Frightening
Snake	34.4
Rat	20.2
Spider	17.1
Cockroach	15.6
Bat	3.5
Worm	0.8
Lizard	0.4
Other	3.3
Undecided	4.8

Source: October 2000 Zogby poll, adult U.S. residents.

persons. As universal inoculation was manifestly impracticable, any half-way measure was decidedly disadvantageous, and it was not until vaccination from cow-pox was instituted that the first decided check on the ravages of small-pox was made.

Vaccination was almost solely due to the persistent efforts of Dr. Edward Jenner, a pupil of the celebrated John Hunter, born May 17, 1749.

In his comments on the life of Edward Jenner, Adams, in "The Healing Art," has graphically described his first efforts to institute vaccination, as follows:

"When Jenner was acting as a surgeon's articled pupil at Sudbury, a young countrywoman applied to him for advice. In her presence some chance allusion was made to the universal disease, on which she remarked: 'I shall never take it, for I have had the cow-pox.' The remark induced him to make inquiries; and he found that a pustular eruption, derived from infection, appeared on the hands of milkers, communicated from the teats of cows similarly disordered; this eruption was regarded as a safeguard against small-pox. . .

"At the meetings of the Alveston and Radborough Medical Clubs, of both of which Jenner was a member, he so frequently enlarged upon his favorite theme, and so repeatedly insisted upon the value of cow-pox as a prophylactic, that he was denounced as a nuisance, and in a jest it was even proposed that if the orator further sinned, he should then and there be expelled.

. . . At last an opportunity occurred of putting his theory to the test. On the 14th day of May, 1796,—the day marks an epoch in the Healing Art, and is not less worthy of being kept as a national thanksgiving than the day of Waterloo—the cow-pox matter or pus was taken from the hand of one Sarah Holmes, who had been infected from her master's cows, and was inserted by two superficial incisions into the arms of James Phipps, a healthy boy of about eight years of age. The cow-pox ran its ordinary course without any injurious effect, and the boy was afterward inoculated for the small-pox,—happily in vain."

This publication produced a great sensation in the medical world, and vaccination spread so rapidly that in the following summer Jenner had the indorsement of the majority of the leading surgeons of London. Vaccination was soon introduced into France, where Napoleon gave another proof of his far-reaching sagacity by his immediate recognition of the importance of vaccination. It was then spread all over the continent; and in 1800 Dr. Benjamin Waterhouse of Boston introduced it into America; in 1801, with his sons-in-law, President Jefferson vaccinated in their own families and those of their friends nearly 200 persons. . . .

After the introduction of vaccination in England the mortality was reduced from nearly 3000 per million inhabitants annually to 310 per million annually. During the small-pox epidemic in London in 1863, Seaton and Buchanan examined over 50,000 school children, and among every thousand without evidences of vaccination they found 360 with the scars of small-pox, while of every thousand presenting some evidence of vaccination, only 1.78 had any such traces of small-pox to exhibit.

U.S. DEPARTMENT OF STATE
WASHINGTON, D.C.

FACT SHEET
Chemical-Biological Agents[1]

The recent terrorist threats and confirmed cases of exposure to anthrax have caused an increase in anxiety over the possibility of attacks using chemical and biological agents (CBA). Currently, the method of delivery of anthrax has been by letter or package. While the risk of such attacks is limited, it cannot be excluded. As always, the Department will promptly share with American citizens overseas any credible information about threats to their safety. Americans should stay informed and be prepared for any eventuality.

In 1999, the Department of Defense announced its intention to commence the Family and Force Protection Initiative (FFPI) in order to provide enhanced protection to the dependents of U.S. military service members and to civilian Department of Defense (DOD) employees and their families. This program was first implemented for U.S. Forces Korea.

The Department of State has had a chemical and biological countermeasure program since 1998, when it began to deploy chemical antidotes and antibiotics to selected posts abroad. While we have no information to indicate there is an imminent threat from use of anthrax or other biological agents as a weapon against our overseas missions at this time, the Department is expanding its countermeasure program. As a precaution, the Department requested our missions overseas to stock a three-day supply of the antibiotic ciprofloxacin for all individuals who work in or frequent the missions.

This small supply of ciprofloxacin is being pre-positioned to ensure rapid access to this protective antibiotic for our employees in case of an anthrax exposure in an overseas USG facility and would allow the mission sufficient time to provide access to care for all individuals exposed while securing additional supplies of antibiotics. Once an exposure is suspected, all individuals who had been exposed in our workplace would be provided antibiotics pending a full investigation of the exposure. This would include any private American citizen present in the facility at the time of exposure.

Again, if the Department becomes aware of any specific and credible threat to the safety and security of American citizens abroad, that information will be provided to them promptly.

Exposures to CBA that occur outside U.S. Government facilities would require the involvement of local public health authorities who would provide information and if necessary, protective antibiotics to the general public. Ciprofloxacin and other antibiotics effective against anthrax, including doxycycline and amoxicillin are available with a prescription in most pharmacies throughout the world.

The Centers for Disease Control and Prevention (CDC) is the lead government agency on infectious diseases, including chemical/biological agents (CBA). *For detailed information on CBA, including anthrax, inquirers are referred to the CDC Internet home page* at http://www.cdc.gov. The CDC's in-

---

[1]U.S. Department of State Fact Sheet, updated October 2001: <http://travel.state.gov/cbw.html>.

ternational travelers hotline telephone number is 1-877-FYI-TRIP (1-877-394-8747); FAX: 1-888-CDC-FAXX (1-888-232-3299).

As always, American citizens should review their own personal security situations and take those precautions they deem appropriate to ensure their well-being.

Some general information on chemical-biological agents (CBA) follows:

A. Biological agents can be dispersed by an aerosol spray which must be inhaled. However, these agents can also be used to contaminate food, water and other products. Attention to basic food hygiene when traveling abroad is very important.

B. Some chemical agents may be volatile—evaporating rapidly to form clouds of agent. Others may be persistent. These agents may act directly on the skin, lungs, eyes, respiratory tract or be absorbed through your skin and lungs causing injury. Choking and nerve agents damage the soft tissue in these organs.

C. When properly used, appropriate masks are effective protection to prevent the inhalation of either biological or chemical agents; however this assumes an adequate warning. Gas masks alone do not protect against agents that act through skin absorption. Those who wish to acquire protective equipment for personal use should contact commercial vendors.

D. There is an incubation period after exposure to biological agents. It is essential that you seek appropriate care for illnesses acquired while traveling abroad to assure prompt diagnosis and treatment.

E. One of the biological agents is the spore-forming bacterium that causes Anthrax, an acute infectious disease. It should be noted, however, that effective dispersal of the Anthrax bacteria is difficult.

— Anthrax is treatable if that treatment is initiated promptly after exposure. The post-exposure treatment consists of certain antibiotics administered in combination with the vaccine.

— An anthrax vaccine that confers protective immunity does exist, but is not readily available to private parties. Efficacy and safety of use of this vaccine for persons under 18 or over 65 and pregnant women have not been determined.

— The anthrax vaccine is produced exclusively by Bioport under contract to the Department of Defense. Virtually all vaccine produced in the United States is under Defense Department contract primarily for military use and a small number of other official government uses.

— For additional information, please consult your health care provider or local health authority.

October 2001

THE BIOLOGICAL AND TOXIN WEAPONS CONVENTION[2]

Convention on the Prohibition of the Development, Production and Stockpiling of Bacteriological (Biological) and Toxin Weapons and on Their Destruction.

Signed at London, Moscow and Washington on 10 April 1972.

Entered into force on 26 March 1975

Depositaries: U.K., U.S. and Soviet governments.

The States Parties to this Convention,

Determined to act with a view to achieving effective progress towards general and complete disarmament, including the prohi-

---

[2]*Source:* University of Bradford, Biological and Toxin Weapons Convention Database.

bition and elimination of all types of weapons of mass destruction, and convinced that the prohibition of the development, production and stockpiling of chemical and bacteriological (biological) weapons and their elimination, through effective measures, will facilitate the achievement of general and complete disarmament under strict and effective international control,

Recognizing the important significance of the Protocol for the Prohibition of the Use in War of Asphyxiating, Poisonous or Other Gases, and of Bacteriological Methods of Warfare, signed at Geneva on June 17, 1925, and conscious also of the contribution which the said Protocol has already made, and continues to make, to mitigating the horrors of war,

Reaffirming their adherence to the principles and objectives of that Protocol and calling upon all States to comply strictly with them,

Recalling that the General Assembly of the United Nations has repeatedly condemned all actions contrary to the principles and objectives of the Geneva Protocol of June 17, 1925,

Desiring to contribute to the strengthening of confidence between peoples and the general improvement of the international atmosphere,

Desiring also to contribute to the realization of the purposes and principles of the United Nations,

Convinced of the importance and urgency of eliminating from the arsenals of States, through effective measures, such dangerous weapons of mass destruction as those using chemical or bacteriological (biological) agents,

Recognizing that an agreement on the prohibition of bacteriological (biological) and toxin weapons represents a first possible step towards the achievement of agreement on effective measures also for the prohibition of the development, production and stockpiling of chemical weapons, and determined to continue negotiations to that end,

Determined for the sake of all mankind, to exclude completely the possibility of bacteriological (biological) agents and toxins being used as weapons,

Convinced that such use would be repugnant to the conscience of mankind and that no effort should be spared to minimize this risk,

Have agreed as follows:

Article I

Each State Party to this Convention undertakes never in any circumstances to develop, produce, stockpile or otherwise acquire or retain:

(1) Microbial or other biological agents, or toxins whatever their origin or method of production, of types and in quantities that have no justification for prophylactic, protective or other peaceful purposes;

(2) Weapons, equipment or means of delivery designed to use such agents or toxins for hostile purposes or in armed conflict.

Article II

Each State Party to this Convention undertakes to destroy, or to divert to peaceful purposes, as soon as possible but not later than nine months after entry into force of the Convention, all agents, toxins, weapons, equipment and means of delivery specified in article I of the Convention, which are in its possession or under its jurisdiction or control. In implementing the provisions of this article all necessary safety precautions shall be observed to protect populations and the environment.

Article III

Each State Party to this Convention undertakes not to transfer to any recipient whatsoever, directly or indirectly, and not in any way to assist, encourage, or induce any State, group of States or international organizations to manufacture or otherwise acquire any of the agents, toxins, weapons, equipment or means of delivery specified in article I of this Convention.

Article IV

Each State Party to this Convention shall, in accordance with its constitutional processes, take any necessary measures to prohibit and prevent the development, production, stockpiling, acquisition, or retention of the agents, toxins, weapons, equipment and means of delivery specified in article I of the Convention, within the territory of such State, under its jurisdiction or under its control anywhere.

Article V

The States Parties to this Convention undertake to consult one another and to cooperate in solving any problems which may arise in relation to the objective of, or in the application of the provisions of, the Convention. Consultation and Cooperation pursuant to this article may also be undertaken through appropriate international procedures within the framework of the United Nations and in accordance with its Charter.

Article VI

(1) Any State Party to this convention which finds that any other State Party is acting in breach of obligations deriving from the provisions of the Convention may lodge a complaint with the Security Council of the United Nations. Such a complaint should include all possible evidence confirming its validity, as well as a request for its consideration by the Security Council.

(2) Each State Party to this Convention undertakes to cooperate in carrying out any investigation which the Security Council may initiate, in accordance with the provisions of the Charter of the United Nations, on the basis of the complaint received by the Council. The Security Council shall inform the States Parties to the Convention of the results of the investigation.

Article VII

Each State Party to this Convention undertakes to provide or support assistance, in accordance with the United Nations Charter, to any Party to the Convention which so requests, if the Security Council decides that such Party has been exposed to danger as a result of violation of the Convention.

Article VIII

Nothing in this Convention shall be interpreted as in any way limiting or detracting from the obligations assumed by any State under the Protocol for the Prohibition of the Use in War of Asphyxiating, Poisonous or Other Gases, and of Bacteriological Methods of Warfare, signed at Geneva on June 17, 1925.

Article IX

Each State Party to this Convention affirms the recognized objective of effective prohibition of chemical weapons and, to this end, undertakes to continue negotiations in good faith with a view to reaching early agreement on effective measures for the prohibition of their development, production and stockpiling and for their destruction, and on appropriate measures concerning equipment and means of delivery specifically designed for the production or use of chemical agents for weapons purposes.

Article X

(1) The States Parties to this Convention undertake to facilitate, and have the right to participate in, the fullest possible exchange of equipment, materials and scientific and technological information for the use of bacteriological (biological) agents and toxins for peaceful purposes. Parties to the Convention in a position to do so shall also cooperate in contributing individually or together with other States or international organizations to the further development and application of scientific discoveries in the field of bacteriology (biology) for prevention of disease, or for other peaceful purposes.

(2) This Convention shall be implemented in a manner designed to avoid hampering the economic or technological development of States Parties to the Convention or international cooperation in the field of peaceful bacteriological (biological) activities, including the international exchange of bacteriological (biological) and toxins and equipment for the processing, use or production of bacteriological (biological) agents and toxins for peaceful purposes in accordance with the provisions of the Convention.

Article XI

Any State Party may propose amendments to this Convention. Amendments shall enter into force for each State Party accepting the amendments upon their acceptance by a majority of the States Parties to the Convention and thereafter for each remaining State Party on the date of acceptance by it.

Article XII

Five years after the entry into force of this Convention, or earlier if it is requested by a majority of Parties to the Convention by submitting a proposal to this effect to the Depositary Governments, a conference of States Parties to the Convention shall be held at Geneva, Switzerland, to review the operation of the Convention, with a view to assuring that the purposes of the preamble and the provisions of the Convention, including the provisions concerning negotiations on chemical weapons, are being realized. Such review shall take into account any new scientific and technological developments relevant to the Convention.

Article XIII

(1) This Convention shall be of unlimited duration.

(2) Each State Party to this Convention shall in exercising its national sovereignty have the right to withdraw from the Convention if it decides that extraordinary events, related to the subject matter of the Convention, have jeopardized the supreme interests of its country. It shall give notice of such withdrawal to all other States Parties to the Convention and to the United Nations Security Council three months in advance. Such notice shall include a statement of the extraordinary events it regards as having jeopardized its supreme interests.

Article XIV

(1) This Convention shall be open to all States for signature. Any State which does not sign the Convention before its entry into force in accordance with paragraph (3) of this Article may accede to it at any time.

(2) This Convention shall be subject to ratification by signatory States. Instruments of ratification and instruments of accession shall be deposited with the Governments of the United States of America, the United Kingdom of Great Britain and Northern Ireland and the Union of Soviet Socialist Republics, which are hereby designated the Depositary Governments.

(3) This Convention shall enter into force after the deposit of instruments of ratification by twenty-two Governments, including the Governments designated as Depositaries of the Convention.

(4) For States whose instruments of ratification or accession are deposited subsequent to the entry into force of this Convention, it shall enter into force on the date of the deposit of their instruments of ratification or accession.

(5) The Depositary Governments shall promptly inform all signatory and acceding States of the date of each signature, the date of deposit or each instrument of ratification or of accession and the date of entry into force of this Convention, and of the receipt of other notices.

(6) This Convention shall be registered by the Depositary Governments pursuant to Article 102 of the Charter of the United Nations.

Article XV

This Convention, the English, Russian, French, Spanish and Chinese texts of which are equally authentic, shall be deposited in the archives of the Depositary Governments. Duly certified copies of the Convention shall be transmitted by the Depositary Governments to the Governments of the signatory and acceding states.

NAVAL FACILITIES ENGINEERING COMMAND
ABSTRACT OF AN ACCIDENT[3]

93–9

ACCIDENT TYPE: Occupational exposure to bacteria/virus

ILLNESS: Leptospirosis

TYPE OF WORK: Refurbishment of sewage pump station

SAFETY EQUIPMENT: Safety glasses, safety shoes and cloth coveralls used. Gloves and Tyvek suit with booties and hood provided but not always worn

DESCRIPTION OF THE ACCIDENT:

A WG-10 Maintenance Mechanic was assigned to completely refurbish an underground sewage pump station that had been flooded with a mixture of fresh water and some waste water. The pump station was drained and all equipment was removed. About 2 weeks prior to becoming ill the employee cleaned out debris and waste water from a clogged sump pump without using gloves. Employee stated he had noticed rodent feces in the area.

On the date of the onset of symptoms the mechanic had to climb the ladder into the station several times. Midday he experienced low back pain, lower leg and neck aches and a headache which he thought were caused by climbing the ladder. He left work and went to the hospital where he was treated for low back strain. Three days later the symptoms had not disappeared and he had difficulty urinating so he returned to the hospital. Tests indicated a high white count and "swollen" liver. Employee was admitted to the hospital with a diagnosis of probable kidney/urinary tract infection and treated with broad spectrum antibiotics. Symptoms disappeared in six days. Tests confirmed leptospirosis.

Approximately one week prior to the mechanic becoming ill, one other co-worker had similar, but less severe, symptoms and was treated for a urinary tract infection with

[3]*Source:* U.S. Department of the Navy, Naval Facilities Engineering Command (downloaded from Internet Web site August 9, 2000).

a broad spectrum antibiotic. Her symptoms disappeared after one week of treatment.

DIRECT CAUSE OF ILLNESS:

Employee failed to wear adequate personal protective equipment to protect him from waste water contamination.

DIRECT CAUSE:

- Employee failed to practice adequate personal hygiene while working in a waste water contaminated area.
- Employees and supervisor failed to recognize a potentially hazardous situation.

LESSONS LEARNED:

- Employees must wear impervious gloves and outer clothing when working in waste water.
- Employees must always practice good personal hygiene especially when working with/around waste water.
- Supervisors and employees must be alert to identify and report unusual illnesses or illness that are affecting several employees within a work center to the appropriate OSH Office or medical clinic for investigation.

FACT SHEET NO. OSHA 92–46 BLOODBORNE PATHOGENS FINAL STANDARD: SUMMARY OF KEY PROVISIONS[4]

PURPOSE: Limits occupational exposure to blood and other potentially infectious materials since any exposure could result in transmission of bloodborne pathogens which could lead to disease or death.

SCOPE: Covers all employees who could be "reasonably anticipated" as the result of performing their job duties to face contact with blood and other potentially infectious materials. OSHA has not attempted to list all occupations where exposures could occur. "Good Samaritan" acts such as assisting a co-worker with a nosebleed would not be considered occupational exposure.

Infectious materials include semen, vaginal secretions, cerebrospinal fluid, synovial fluid, pleural fluid, pericardial fluid, peritoneal fluid, amniotic fluid, saliva in dental procedures, any body fluid visibly contaminated with blood and all body fluids in situations where it is difficult or impossible to differentiate between body fluids. They also include any unfixed tissue or organ other than intact skin from a human (living or dead) and human immunodeficiency virus (HIV)-containing cell or tissue cultures, organ cultures and HIV or hepatitis B (HBV)-containing culture medium or other solutions as well as blood, organs or other tissues from experimental animals infected with HIV or HBV.

EXPOSURE CONTROL PLAN: Requires employers to identify, in writing, tasks and procedures as well as job classifications where occupational exposure to blood occurs—without regard to personal protective clothing and equipment. It must also set forth the schedule for implementing other provisions of the standard and specify the procedure for evaluating circumstances surrounding exposure incidents. The plan must be accessible to employees and available to OSHA. Employers must review and update it at least annually—more often if necessary to accommodate workplace changes.

METHODS OF COMPLIANCE: Mandates universal precautions, (treating body fluids/materials as if infectious) emphasizing engineering and work practice controls. The standard stresses handwashing and requires employers to provide facilities and ensure that employees use them following exposure to blood. It sets forth procedures

[4]U.S. Department of Labor, Occupational Safety and Health Administration, Fact Sheet 92-46, January 1, 1992.

to minimize needlesticks, minimize splashing and spraying of blood, ensure appropriate packaging of specimens and regulated wastes and decontaminate equipment or label it as contaminated before shipping to servicing facilities.

Employers must provide, at no cost, and require employees to use appropriate personal protective equipment such as gloves, gowns, masks, mouthpieces and resuscitation bags and must clean, repair and replace these when necessary. Gloves are not necessarily required for routine phlebotomies in volunteer blood donation centers but must be made available to employees who want them.

The standard requires a written schedule for cleaning, identifying the method of decontamination to be used in addition to cleaning following contact with blood or other potentially infectious materials. It specifies methods for disposing of contaminated sharps and sets forth standards for containers for these items and other regulated waste. Further, the standard includes provisions for handling contaminated laundry to minimize exposures.

HIV AND HBV RESEARCH LABORATORIES AND PRODUCTION FACILITIES: Calls for these facilities to follow standard microbiological practices and specifies additional practices intended to minimize exposures of employees working with concentrated viruses and reduce the risk of accidental exposure for other employees at the facility. These facilities must include required containment equipment and an autoclave for decontamination of regulated waste and must be constructed to limit risks and enable easy clean up. Additional training and experience requirements apply to workers in these facilities.

HEPATITIS B VACCINATION: Requires vaccinations to be made available to all employees who have occupational exposure to blood within 10 working days of assignment, at no cost, at a reasonable time and place, under the supervision of licensed physician/licensed healthcare professional and according to the latest recommendations of the U.S. Public Health Service (USPHS). Prescreening may not be required as a condition of receiving the vaccine. Employees must sign a declination form if they choose not to be vaccinated, but may later opt to receive the vaccine at no cost to the employee. Should booster doses later be recommended by the USPHS, employees must be offered them.

POST-EXPOSURE EVALUATION AND FOLLOW-UP: Specifies procedures to be made available to all employees who have had an exposure incident plus any laboratory tests must be conducted by an accredited laboratory at no cost to the employee. Follow-up must include a confidential medical evaluation documenting the circumstances of exposure, identifying and testing the source individual if feasible, testing the exposed employee's blood if he/she consents, post-exposure prophylaxis, counseling and evaluation of reported illnesses. Healthcare professionals must be provided specified information to facilitate the evaluation and their written opinion on the need for hepatitis B vaccination following the exposure. Information such as the employee's ability to receive the hepatitis B vaccine must be supplied to the employer. All diagnoses must remain confidential.

HAZARD COMMUNICATION: Requires warning labels including the orange or orange-red biohazard symbol affixed to containers of regulated waste, refrigerators and freezers and other containers which are used to store or transport blood or other potentially infectious materials. Red bags or containers may be used instead of labeling. When a facility uses universal precautions in its handling of all specimens, labeling is not required within the facility. Likewise, when all laundry is handled with universal precautions, the laundry need not be labelled. Blood which has been tested and found free of HIV or HBV and released for clinical use, and regulated waste which has been decontaminated, need not be labeled. Signs must be used to identify restricted areas in HIV and HBV research laboratories and production facilities.

INFORMATION AND TRAINING: Mandates training within 90 days of effective date, initially upon assignment and annually—employees who have received appropriate training within the past year need only receive additional training in items not previously covered. Training must include making accessible a copy of the regulatory text of the standard and explanation of its contents, general discussion on bloodborne diseases and their transmission, exposure control plan, engineering and work practice controls, personal protective equipment, hepatitis B vaccine, response to emergencies involving blood, how to handle exposure incidents, the post-exposure evaluation and follow-up program, signs/labels/color-coding. There must be opportunity for questions and answers, and the trainer must be knowledgeable in the subject matter. Laboratory and production facility workers must receive additional specialized initial training.

RECORDKEEPING: Calls for medical records to be kept for each employee with occupational exposure for the duration of employment plus 30 years, must be confidential and must include name and social security number; hepatitis B vaccination status (including dates); results of any examinations, medical testing and follow-up procedures; a copy of the healthcare professional's written opinion; and a copy of information provided to the healthcare professional. Training records must be maintained for three years and must include dates, contents of the training program or a summary, trainer's name and qualifications, names and job titles of all persons attending the sessions. Medical records must be made available to the subject employee, anyone with written consent of the employee, OSHA and NIOSH—they are not available to the employer. Disposal of records must be in accord with OSHA's standard covering access to records.

DATES: Effective date: March 6 1992. Exposure control plan: May 5, 1992. Information and training requirements and recordkeeping: June 4, 1992. And the following other provisions take effect on July 6, 1992: engineering and work practice controls, personal protective equipment, housekeeping, special provisions covering HIV and HBV research laboratories and production facilities, hepatitis B vaccination and post-exposure evaluation and follow-up and labels and signs.

This is one of a series of fact sheets highlighting U.S. Department of Labor programs. It is intended as a general description only and does not carry the force of legal opinion. This information will be made available to sensory impaired individuals upon request. Voice phone: (202) 523-8151. TDD message referral phone: 1-800-326-2577.

THE DURBAN DECLARATION[5]
A DECLARATION BY SCIENTISTS AND PHYSICIANS AFFIRMING HIV IS THE CAUSE OF AIDS

Seventeen years after the discovery of the human immunodeficiency virus (HIV), thousands of people from around the world are gathered in Durban, South

[5]*Source*: <http://www.durbandeclaration.org>, downloaded 2000.

Africa to attend the XIII International AIDS Conference. At the turn of the millennium, an estimated 34 million people worldwide are living with HIV or AIDS, 24 million of them in sub-Saharan Africa (1). Last year alone, 2.6 million people died of AIDS, the highest rate since the start of the epidemic. If current trends continue, Southern and South-East Asia, South America and regions of the former Soviet Union will also bear a heavy burden in the next two decades.

Like many other diseases, such as tuberculosis and malaria that cause illness and death in underprivileged and impoverished communities, AIDS spreads by infection. HIV-1, the retrovirus that is responsible for the AIDS pandemic, is closely related to a simian immunodeficiency virus (SIV) which infects chimpanzees. HIV-2, which is prevalent in West Africa and has spread to Europe and India, is almost indistinguishable from an SIV that infects sooty mangabey monkeys. Although HIV-1 and HIV-2 first arose as infections transmitted from animals to humans, or zoonoses (2), both are now spread among humans through sexual contact, from mother to infant and via contaminated blood.

An animal source for a new infection is not unique to HIV. The plague came from rodents. Influenza and the new Nipah virus in South-East Asia reached humans via pigs. Variant Creutzfeldt-Jakob disease in the United Kingdom came from 'mad cows'. Once HIV became established in humans, it soon followed human habits and movements. Like other viruses, HIV recognizes no social, political or geographic boundaries.

The evidence that AIDS is caused by HIV-1 or HIV-2 is clear-cut, exhaustive and unambiguous. This evidence meets the highest standards of science (3-7). The data fulfill exactly the same criteria as for other viral diseases, such as poliomyelitis, measles and smallpox:

- Patients with acquired immune deficiency syndrome, regardless of where they live, are infected with HIV (3–7).

- If not treated, most people with HIV infection show signs of AIDS within 5–10 years (6, 7). HIV infection is identified in blood by detecting antibodies, gene sequences or viral isolation. These tests are as reliable as any used for detecting other virus infections.

- Persons who received HIV-contaminated blood or blood products develop AIDS, whereas those who received untainted or screened blood do not (6).

- Most children who develop AIDS are born to HIV-infected mothers. The higher the viral load in the mother the greater the risk of the child becoming infected (8).

- In the laboratory HIV infects the exact type of white blood cell (CD4 lymphocytes) that becomes depleted in persons with AIDS (3–5).

- Drugs that block HIV replication in the test tube also reduce viral load and delay progression to AIDS. Where available, treatment has reduced AIDS mortality by more than 80% (9).

- Monkeys inoculated with cloned SIV DNA become infected and develop AIDS (10).

Further compelling data are available (4). HIV causes AIDS (5). It is unfortunate that a few vocal people continue to deny the evidence. This position will cost countless lives.

In different regions of the world HIV/ AIDS shows altered patterns of spread and symptoms. In Africa, for example, HIV-infected persons are 11 times more likely to die within 5 years (7), and over 100 times more likely than uninfected persons to develop Kaposi's sarcoma, a cancer linked to yet another virus (11).

As with any other chronic infection, various co-factors play a role in determining the risk of disease. Persons who are malnourished, who already suffer other infections or who are older, tend to be more susceptible to the rapid development of AIDS following HIV infection. However, none of these factors weaken the scientific evidence that HIV is the sole cause of AIDS.

In this global emergency, prevention of HIV infection must be our greatest worldwide public health priority. The knowledge and tools to prevent infection exist. The sexual spread of HIV can be prevented by monogamy, abstinence or by using condoms. Blood transmission can be stopped by screening blood products and by not re-using needles. Mother-to-child transmission can be reduced by half or more by short courses of antiviral drugs (12,13).

Limited resources and the crushing burden of poverty in many parts of the world constitute formidable challenges to the control of HIV infection. People already infected can be helped by treatment with life-saving drugs, but high cost puts these treatments out of reach for most. It is crucial to develop new antiviral drugs that are easier to take, have fewer side effects and are much less expensive, so that millions more can benefit from them.

There are many ways to communicate the vital information about HIV/AIDS. What works best in one country may not be appropriate in another. But to tackle the disease, everyone must first understand that HIV is the enemy. Research, not myths, will lead to the development of more effective and cheaper treatments, and hopefully a vaccine. But for now, emphasis must be placed on preventing sexual transmission.

There is no end in sight to the AIDS pandemic. By working together, we have the power to reverse the tide of this epidemic. Science will one day triumph over AIDS, just as it did over smallpox. Curbing the spread of HIV will be the first step. Until then, reason, solidarity, political will and courage must be our partners.

References

1. UNAIDS. AIDS epidemic update. December 1999. www.unaids.org/hivaidsinfo/documents.html

2. Hahn, B.H., Shaw, G.M., De Cock, K.M., Sharp, P.M. (2000). AIDS as a zoonosis: scientific and public health implications. Science, 287, 607–614.

3. Weiss R.A. and Jaffe, H.W. (1990). Duesberg, HIV and AIDS. Nature, 345, 659–660.

4. NIAID (1996). HIV as the cause of AIDS. www.niaid.nih.gov/spotlight/hiv00/default.html

5. O'Brien, S.J. and Goedert, J.J. (1996). HIV causes AIDS: Koch's postulates fulfilled. Current Opinion in Immunology, 8, 613–618.

6. Darby, S.C. et al., (1995). Mortality before and after HIV infection in the complete UK population of haemophiliacs. Nature, 377, 79–82.

7. Nunn, A.J. et al., (1997). Mortality associated with HIV-1 infection over five years in a rural Ugandan population: cohort study. BMJ, 315, 767–771.

8. Sperling, R.S. et al., (1996). Maternal viral load, zidovudine treatment, and the risk of transmission of human immunodeficiency virus type 1 from mother to infant. N. Engl. J. Med. 335, 1678–80.

9. Centers for Disease Control and Prevention (CDC). HIV/AIDS Surveillance Report 1999; 11, 1–44.

10. Liska, V. et al., (1999). Viremia and AIDS in rhesus macaques after intramuscular inoculation of plasmid DNA encoding full-length SIVmac239. AIDS Research & Human Retroviruses, 15, 445–450.

11. Sitas, F. et al., (1999). Antibodies against human herpesvirus 8 in black South African patients with cancer. N. Engl. J. Med., 340, 1863–1871.

12. Shaffer, N. et al., (1999). Short course zidovudine for perinatal HIV-1 transmission in Bangkok Thailand: a randomised controlled trial. Lancet, 353, 773–780.

13. Guay, L.A. et al., (1999). Intrapartum and

neonatal single-dose nevirapine compared with zidovudine for prevention of mother-to-child transmission of HIV-1 in Kampala, Uganda: HIVNET 012 randomised trial. Lancet, 354, 795–802.

[Signed by 5,195 physicians and scientists from 83 countries]

EXCERPT FROM A TOBACCO INDUSTRY REPORT[6]

COMPETITIVE ANALYSIS

Background — The Cigarette and the Smoking Experience

Philip Morris USA is a producer of American blend cigarettes. The cigarettes are designed to provide a smoking experience for an adult. Made primarily from tobacco, flavorings and paper, the majority of the products have a cellulose acetate filter to adjust the delivery of the smoke that is emitted when the cigarette is lit. The consumer draws on the cigarette and inhales the smoke or gaseous, vaporous system into his or her lungs, then exhales the smoke into the air. The smoke delivers flavors, carbon monoxide, nicotine and tar to the smoker.

Different people smoke for different reasons. But the primary reason is to deliver nicotine into their bodies. Nicotine is an alkaloid derived from the tobacco plant. It is a physiologically active, nitrogen containing substance. Similar organic chemicals include nicotine, quinine, cocaine, atropine and morphine. While each of these substances can be used to affect human physiology, nicotine has a particularly broad range of influence.

During the smoking act, nicotine is inhaled into the lungs in smoke, enters the bloodstream and travels to the brain in about eight to ten seconds. The nicotine alters the state of the smoker by becoming a neurotransmitter and a stimulant. Nicotine mimics the body's most important neurotransmitter, acetycholine (ACH),which controls heart rate and message sending within the brain.The nicotine is used to change physiological states leading to enhanced mental performance and relaxation. A little nicotine seems to stimulate, while a lot sedates a person. A smoker learns to control the delivery of nicotine through the smoking technique to create the desired mood state. In general, the smoker uses nicotine's control to moderate a mood, arousing attention in boring situations and calming anxiety in tense situations.Smoking enhances the smoker's mental performance and reduces anxiety in a sensorially pleasurable form.

Other reasons for smoking, besides nicotine delivery, include habituation, attachment, personality, culture and genetics. Smoking is many different things to different people, including:

- as an aid to vigilance, rapid information processing and memory
- doing nothing while doing something
- a communication tool
- a sexually alluring act
- a sign of rebelliousness
- something to do with your hands
- an oral gratification device
- a taste experience and other sensory stimulation at back of throat, windpipe and lungs
- a personal statement of image — based on the culture, it is positive or negative
- a sign of a risk-taker
- predisposed in people by genetics

[6]*Source:* Philip Morris Company, circa 1992; cited in A.M. Freedman, "Philip Morris Memo Likens Nicotine to Such Drugs as Cocaine, Morphine" (*Wall Street Journal*, December 8, 1995).

In its broadest sense, the cigarette is a pleasure product. It alters mood states just like the caffeine, alcohol and sugar in other Philip Morris products that affect human physiology and psychology. As with nicotine, these substances become part of an individual's life style and are used as coping mechanisms to help adjust to the environment.

THE WHITE HOUSE
OFFICE OF THE PRESS SECRETARY
FOR IMMEDIATE RELEASE
MAY 16, 1997

REMARKS BY THE PRESIDENT IN APOLOGY FOR STUDY DONE IN TUSKEGEE[7]

The East Room

2:26 P.M. EDT

THE PRESIDENT: Ladies and gentlemen, on Sunday, Mr. Shaw will celebrate his 95th birthday. (Applause.) I would like to recognize the other survivors who are here today and their families: Mr. Charlie Pollard is here. (Applause.) Mr. Carter Howard. (Applause.) Mr. Fred Simmons. (Applause.) Mr. Simmons just took his first airplane ride, and he reckons he's about 110 years old, so I think it's time for him to take a chance or two. (Laughter.) I'm glad he did. And Mr. Frederick Moss, thank you, sir. (Applause.)

I would also like to ask three family representatives who are here — Sam Doner is represented by his daughter, Gwendolyn Cox. Thank you, Gwendolyn. (Applause.) Ernest Hendon, who is watching in Tuskegee, is represented by his brother, North Hendon. Thank you, sir, for being here. (Applause.) And George Key is represented by his grandson, Christopher Monroe. Thank you, Chris. (Applause.)

I also acknowledge the families, community leaders, teachers and students watching today by satellite from Tuskegee. The White House is the people's house; we are glad to have all of you here today. I thank Dr. David Satcher for his role in this. I thank Congresswoman Waters and Congressman Hilliard, Congressman Stokes, the entire Congressional Black Caucus. Dr. Satcher, members of the Cabinet who are here, Secretary Herman, Secretary Slater. A great friend of freedom, Fred Gray, thank you for fighting this long battle all these long years.

The eight men who are survivors of the syphilis study at Tuskegee are a living link to a time not so very long ago that many Americans would prefer not to remember, but we dare not forget. It was a time when our nation failed to live up to its ideals, when our nation broke the trust with our people that is the very foundation of our democracy. It is not only in remembering that shameful past that we can make amends and repair our nation, but it is in remembering that past that we can build a better present and a better future. And without remembering it, we cannot make amends and we cannot go forward.

So today America does remember the hundreds of men used in research without their knowledge and consent. We remember them and their family members. Men who were poor and African American, without resources and with few alternatives, they believed they had found hope when they were offered free medical care by the United States Public Health Service. They were betrayed.

Medical people are supposed to help when we need care, but even once a cure was discovered, they were denied help, and they were lied to by their government. Our government is supposed to protect the rights of its citizens; their rights were

[7]Source: <http://www.pub.whitehouse.gov>, downloaded 1999.

trampled upon. Forty years, hundreds of men betrayed, along with their wives and children, along with the community in Macon County, Alabama, the City of Tuskegee, the fine university there, and the larger African American community.

The United States government did something that was wrong — deeply, profoundly, morally wrong. It was an outrage to our commitment to integrity and equality for all our citizens.

To the survivors, to the wives and family members, the children and the grandchildren, I say what you know: No power on Earth can give you back the lives lost, the pain suffered, the years of internal torment and anguish. What was done cannot be undone. But we can end the silence. We can stop turning our heads away. We can look at you in the eye and finally say on behalf of the American people, what the United States government did was shameful, and I am sorry. (Applause.)

The American people are sorry — for the loss, for the years of hurt. You did nothing wrong, but you were grievously wronged. I apologize and I am sorry that this apology has been so long in coming. (Applause.)

To Macon County, to Tuskegee, to the doctors who have been wrongly associated with the events there, you have our apology, as well. To our African American citizens, I am sorry that your federal government orchestrated a study so clearly racist. That can never be allowed to happen again. It is against everything our country stands for and what we must stand against is what it was.

So let us resolve to hold forever in our hearts and minds the memory of a time not long ago in Macon County, Alabama, so that we can always see how adrift we can become when the rights of any citizens are neglected, ignored and betrayed. And let us resolve here and now to move forward together.

The legacy of the study at Tuskegee has reached far and deep, in ways that hurt our progress and divide our nation. We cannot be one America when a whole segment of our nation has no trust in America. An apology is the first step, and we take it with a commitment to rebuild that broken trust. We can begin by making sure there is never again another episode like this one. We need to do more to ensure that medical research practices are sound and ethical, and that researchers work more closely with communities.

Today I would like to announce several steps to help us achieve these goals. First, we will help to build that lasting memorial at Tuskegee. (Applause.) The school founded by Booker T. Washington, distinguished by the renowned scientist George Washington Carver and so many others who advanced the health and well-being of African Americans and all Americans, is a fitting site. The Department of Health and Human Services will award a planning grant so the school can pursue establishing a center for bioethics in research and health care. The center will serve as a museum of the study and support efforts to address its legacy and strengthen bioethics training.

Second, we commit to increase our community involvement so that we may begin restoring lost trust. The study at Tuskegee served to sow distrust of our medical institutions, especially where research is involved. Since the study was halted, abuses have been checked by making informed consent and local review mandatory in federally-funded and mandated research.

Still, 25 years later, many medical studies have little African American participation and African American organ donors are few. This impedes efforts to conduct promising research and to provide the best health care to all our people, including African Americans. So today, I'm directing the Secretary of Health and Human Services, Donna Shalala,

303

to issue a report in 180 days about how we can best involve communities, especially minority communities, in research and health care. You must — every American group must be involved in medical research in ways that are positive. We have put the curse behind us; now we must bring the benefits to all Americans. (Applause.)

Third, we commit to strengthen researchers' training in bioethics. We are constantly working on making breakthroughs in protecting the health of our people and in vanquishing diseases. But all our people must be assured that their rights and dignity will be respected as new drugs, treatments and therapies are tested and used. So I am directing Secretary Shalala to work in partnership with higher education to prepare training materials for medical researchers. They will be available in a year. They will help researchers build on core ethical principles of respect for individuals, justice and informed consent, and advise them on how to use these principles effectively in diverse populations.

Fourth, to increase and broaden our understanding of ethical issues and clinical research, we commit to providing postgraduate fellowships to train bioethicists especially among African Americans and other minority groups. HHS will offer these fellowships beginning in September of 1998 to promising students enrolled in bioethics graduate programs.

And, finally, by executive order I am also today extending the charter of the National Bioethics Advisory Commission to October of 1999. The need for this commission is clear. We must be able to call on the thoughtful, collective wisdom of experts and community representatives to find ways to further strengthen our protections for subjects in human research.

We face a challenge in our time. Science and technology are rapidly changing our lives with the promise of making us much healthier, much more productive and more prosperous. But with these changes we must work harder to see that as we advance we don't leave behind our conscience. No ground is gained and, indeed, much is lost if we lose our moral bearings in the name of progress.

The people who ran the study at Tuskegee diminished the stature of man by abandoning the most basic ethical precepts. They forgot their pledge to heal and repair. They had the power to heal the survivors and all the others and they did not. Today, all we can do is apologize. But you have the power, for only you — Mr. Shaw, the others who are here, the family members who are with us in Tuskegee — only you have the power to forgive. Your presence here shows us that you have chosen a better path than your government did so long ago. You have not withheld the power to forgive. I hope today and tomorrow every American will remember your lesson and live by it.

Thank you, and God bless you. (Applause.)

INSTRUCTIONS FOR SOLDIERS IN THE SERVICE OF THE UNITED STATES, CONCERNING THE MEANS OF PRESERVING HEALTH

Of CLEANLINESS

Excerpt from: General Orders For the Army under the Command of Brigadier General M'Dougall, 1777, by George Washington[8]

It is extremely difficult to persuade Soldiers that *Cleanliness* is absolutely necessary to the Health of an Army. They can hardly believe that in a military State it becomes

---

[8]*Source:* <http://www.armymedicine.army.mil/history> downloaded 2000.

one of the *Necessaries of Life*. They are either too careless to pay Attention to this Subject, or they deceive themselves by reasoning from Cases, that are by no Means similar. Hitherto they have enjoyed a good State of Health, tho' they paid little or no Attention to such Punctilios; hence they conclude, that, tho' in the Army, they shall continue to enjoy an equal Degree of Health, under the like Degree of Negligence: Such reasoning has proved fatal to thousands. They do not consider the prodigious Difference there is in the Circumstances of five or six People, who live by themselves on a Farm, and of thirty or forty thousand Men, who live together in a Camp. The former chiefly subsist on vegetable Food; they lodge warm and dry, and they breathe in pure Air, which is not contaminated by noxious Vapours: The latter in general subsist too much on animal Food; they sleep frequently on cold and damp Beds, and they breathe foul Air, that is constantly injured by the very Breath of a Multitude; and is frequently rendered much more dangerous by the Stench and Exhalations that arise from putrid Bodies. The Air is injured, as I have just said by the Breath of a Multitude and the perspirable Matter that comes through the Pores of the Skin helps to extend the Disorder. . .

These are some of the reasons why CLEANLINESS of every kind is necessary towards preserving Health in an Army: They are Reasons which every Soldier may understand; but should he neglect to regulate himself accordingly, the Regimental Surgeon will doubtless attend to the Neglect, and his Officers will see that he does his Duty. For every Soldier by his Neglect not only endangers his own Life, but the Lives of his Companions. Nature, or the God of Nature, has commanded, that men who live in Camps should be cleanly: Whoever proves too obstinate, or too slothful to obey this Command, may expect to be punished with Death, or suffer under some dangerous Disease.

CHAPTER 11

Other Print Resources

> I have gathered a posie of other men's flowers, and nothing but the thread that binds them is my own.
>
> —Michel Eyquem de Montaigne, *Essais*, Book III, Chap. 12 (1595)

Chapters 1–9 contain lists of books, articles, and press releases on the topics specific to those chapters. The following lists provide additional resources, such as biomedical reference works, dictionaries, field guides, and handbooks; analyses of the historical significance of disease epidemics, man-eating predators, and other biological hazards; works of fiction with themes related to biological hazards; and relevant periodicals. Nonprint resources, such as Internet Web sites, videotapes, and computer software, appear in Chapter 12.

BOOKS, NONFICTION

Diseases and Microorganisms

Astor, Gerald. 1983. *The Disease Detectives: Deadly Medical Mysteries and the People who Solved Them*. New York: New American Library.

Azevedo, Mario Joaquim, et al., Hartwig, Gerald W., and Patterson, K. David (Editors). 1978. *Disease in African History: An Introductory Survey and Case Studies*. Durham, NC: Duke University Press.

Bagliani, A.P., and Firenze, F.S. (Editors). 1998. *The Regulation of Evil: Social and Cultural Attitudes to Epidemics in the Late Middle Ages*. Micrologus Library. Florence: Sismel.

Bellenir, Karen, and Dresser, Peter D. 1996. *Contagious and Non-Contagious Infectious Diseases Sourcebook*. Detroit, MI: Omnigraphics.

Biddle, Wayne. 1996. *A Field Guide to Germs*. New York: Anchor Books.

Biddle, Wayne. 1998. *A Field Guide to the Invisible*. New York: Henry Holt and Co.

Bollet, Alfred J. 1987. *Plagues and Poxes: The Rise and Fall of Epidemic Disease*. New York: Demos Publications.

Bray, R.S. 1998. *Armies of Pestilence: The Effects of Pandemics on History*. Jersey City, NJ: Parkwest Publications.

Brillman, Judith C., and Quenzer, Ronald W. (Eds.) 1992. *Infectious Disease in Emergency Medicine*. Boston: Little, Brown.

Butman, Alexander M. 1981. *Responding to the Mass Casualty Incident: A Guide for EMS Personnel*. Westport, CT: Emergency Training.

Cartwright, Frederick F., and Biddiss, Michael

D. 1972. *Disease and History*. New York: Crowell.

Champion, J.A.I. 1995. *London's Dreaded Visitation: The Social Geography of the Great Plague in 1665*. Historical Geography Research Series, No. 31. London: Centre for Metropolitan History.

Charles, Edward A. 1980. *Conquest of Epidemic Disease: A Chapter in the History of Ideas*. Madison, WI: University of Wisconsin Press.

Cook, N.D. 1998. *Born to Die: Disease and New World Conquest, 1492–1650*. New York: Cambridge University Press.

Cook, N.D. and Lovell, W.G. 1991. *Secret Judgments of God: Old World Disease in Colonial Spanish America*. Norman, OK: University of Oklahoma Press.

Curson, Peter. 1985. *Times of Crisis: Epidemics in Sydney, 1788–1900*. Sydney: Sydney University Press.

Curson, Peter, and McCracken, Kevin. 1989. *Plague in Sydney: The Anatomy of an Epidemic*. Kensington, NSW, Australia: New South Wales University Press.

Davies, J.N.P. 1979. *Pestilence and Disease in the History of Africa*. Raymond Dart Lectures, No. 14. Johannesburg: Witwatersrand University Press for the Institute for the Study of Man in Africa.

Desalle, Rob (Editor). 1999. *Epidemic!: The World of Infectious Disease*. New York: New Press.

Desowitz, Robert S. 1997. *Who Gave Pinta to the Santa Maria? Torrid Diseases in a Temperate World*. New York: W.W. Norton.

Destaing, Fernand. 1978. *Ces Maladies Qui Ont Changé le Monde*. Paris: Presses de la Cité.

Diamond, Jared. 1999. *Guns, Germs, and Steel: The Fates of Human Societies*. New York: W.W. Norton.

Dick, David. 1998. *The Scourges of Heaven*. Lexington, KY: University Press of Kentucky.

Duffy, John. 1971. *Epidemics in Colonial America*. Baton Rouge: Louisiana State University Press.

Eitzen, E., et al. (Editors). 1998. *Medical Management of Biological Casualties: Handbook*. 3rd ed. Frederick, MD: U.S. Army Medical Research Institute of Infectious Diseases.

Ewald, Paul. 1994. *Evolution of Infectious Disease*. New York: Oxford University Press.

Farrell, Jeanette. 1998. *Invisible Enemies: Stories of Infectious Disease*. New York: Farrar, Straus & Giroux.

Giblin, James. 1995. *When Plague Strikes: The Black Death, Smallpox, AIDS*. New York: Harper Collins.

Gottfried, Robert S. 1978. *Epidemic Disease in Fifteenth Century England: The Medical Response and the Demographic Consequences*. New Brunswick, NJ: Rutgers University Press.

Hays, J.N. 1998. *The Burdens of Disease: Epidemics and Human Response in Western History*. New Brunswick, NJ: Rutgers University Press.

Henig, Robin M. 1994. *A Dancing Matrix: How Science Confronts Emerging Viruses*. New York: Vintage Books.

Herlihy, David, and Cohn, Samuel Kline. 1997. *The Black Death and the Transformation of the West*. Cambridge, MA: Harvard University Press.

Isada, Carlos M., et al. 1997. *Infectious Diseases Handbook*. 2nd ed. Hudson, OH: Lexi-Comp Inc.

Karlen, Arlo. 1995. *Plague's Progress: A Social History of Man and Disease*. London: Gollancz.

Karlen, Arlo. 1996. *Man and Microbes: Disease and Plagues in History and Modern Times*. New York: Touchstone Books.

Kiple, Kenneth F. (Editor). 1997. *Plague, Pox and Pestilence*. London: Weidenfeld & Nicolson.

Kiple, Kenneth F., and Beck, Stephen V. (Editors). 1997. *Biological Consequences of the European Expansion, 1450–1800*. An Expanding World. Vol. 26. Brookfield, VT: Ashgate/ Variorum.

Koch, Robert, and K. Codell Carter. 1987. *Essays of Robert Koch*. Westport, CT: Greenwood Publishing.

Kohn, George C. (Editor). 1998. *Encyclopedia of Plague and Pestilence*. New York: Facts on File.

Last, John M., and Abramson, J.H. 1995. *A Dictionary of Epidemiology*. 3rd ed. New York: Oxford University Press.

Leavitt, Judith W. 1997. *Typhoid Mary: Captive to the Public's Health*. Boston, MA: Beacon Press.

Mack, Arien (Editor). 1991. *In Time of Plague: The*

History and Social Consequences of Lethal Epidemic Disease. New York: New York University Press.

Markel, Howard. 1997. *Quarantine! East European Jewish Immigrants and the New York City Epidemics of 1892*. Baltimore, MD: Johns Hopkins University Press.

Marks, Geoffrey, and Beatty, William K. 1976. *Epidemics*. New York: Scribner's.

McCormick, Joseph, Fisher-Hoch, Susan, and Horvitz, Leslie Alan. 1996. *Level 4: Virus Hunters of the CDC*. Atlanta, GA: Turner Pub.

McNeill, William Hardy. 1989. *Plagues and Peoples*. New York: Anchor Books.

Morse, Stephen S. (Editor) 1996. *Emerging Viruses*. New York: Oxford University Press.

Murray, Christopher J.L., and Lopez, Alan D. (Editors). 1999. *The Global Epidemiology of Infectious Diseases* (Global Burden of Disease and Injury, No 4). Cambridge, MA: Harvard University Press.

Murray, Christopher J.L., and Lopez, Alan D. (Editors). 2000. *The Global Epidemiology of Noncommunicable Diseases: The Epidemiology and Burdens of Cancers, Cardiovascular Diseases, Diabetes Mellitus, Respiratory Disorders, and Other Major Conditions*. Cambridge, MA: Harvard University Press.

Nikiforuk, Andrew. 1996. *The Fourth Horseman: A Short History of Epidemics, Plagues, Famines, and Other Scourges*. Revised ed. Toronto: Penguin Books.

Noah, Norman, and O'Mahony, Mary (Editors). 1998. *Communicable Disease: Epidemiology and Control*. Chichester, NY: John Wiley.

Oldstone, Michael B.A. 1998. *Viruses, Plagues, and History*. New York: Oxford University Press.

Owen, Norman G. (Editor). 1987. *Death and Disease in Southeast Asia: Explorations in Social, Medical, and Demographic History*. New York: Oxford University Press.

Pasteur, Louis, and Lister, Joseph. 1996. *Germ Theory and Its Applications to Medicine, and On the Antiseptic Principle of the Practice of Surgery* (reprint). Amherst, NY: Prometheus Books.

Peters, C.J. 1997. *The Virus Hunter: Thirty Years of Battling Hot Viruses around the World*. New York: Bantam Doubleday Dell Pub.

Preston, Richard. 1994. *The Hot Zone*. New York: Random House.

Prinzing, Friedrich. 1916. *Epidemics Resulting from Wars*. London: H. Milford.

Radetsky, Peter. 1995. *The Invisible Invaders: The Story of the Emerging Age of Viruses*. Boston: Little Brown, and Co.

Ranger, Terence, and Slack, Paul (Editors). 1992. *Epidemics and Ideas: Essays on the Historical Perception of Pestilence*. New York: Cambridge University Press.

Ransford, Oliver. 1983. *Bid the Sickness Cease: Disease in the History of Black Africa*. London: J. Murray.

Regis, Edward. 1996. *Virus Ground Zero: Stalking the Killer Viruses with the Centers for Disease Control*. New York: Pocket Books.

Robins, Joseph. 1995. *The Miasma: Epidemic and Panic in Nineteenth-Century Ireland*. Dublin: Institute of Public Administration.

Rosenburg, Charles E., and Golden, Janet (Editors). 1992. *Framing Disease: Studies in Cultural History* (Health and Medicine in American Society). New Brunswick, NJ: Rutgers University Press.

Rosner, David (Ed.). 1995. *Hives of Sickness: Public Health and Epidemics in New York City*. New Brunswick, NJ: Rutgers University Press.

Ryan, Frank. 1998. *Virus X: Tracking the New Killer Plagues*. Boston: Little Brown and Co.

Scott, Susan, and Duncan, Christopher J. 1998. *Human Demography and Disease*. New York: Cambridge University Press.

Shope, Robert E., Oaks, Stanley C., and Lederberg, Joshua S. (Editors). 1992. *Emerging Infections: Microbial Threats to Human Health in the United States*. Washington, DC: National Academy Press.

Stolley, Paul D., and Lasky, Tamar. 1998. *Investigating Disease Patterns: The Science of Epidemiology*. New York: Scientific American Library.

U.S. Congress, House Committee on International Relations. 1997. *The Threat to the United States from Emerging Infectious Diseases*. Washington, DC: U.S. Government Printing Office, Superintendent of Documents.

U.S. Congress, Senate Committee on Appropriations, Subcommittee on Departments of

Labor, Health and Human Services, Education, and Related Agencies. 1998. *Preparedness for Epidemics and Bioterrorism*. Washington, DC: U.S. Government Printing Office, Superintendent of Documents.

U.S. Congress, Senate Committee on Appropriations, Subcommittee on Foreign Operations, Export Financing, and Related Programs. 1998. *Combating Infectious Diseases*. Washington, DC: U.S. Government Printing Office, Superintendent of Documents.

U.S. Department of the Army. 1996. *Handbook on the Medical Aspects of NBC Defensive Operations*. Army Field Manuel 8–9. Falls Church, VA: HQDA.

U.S. National Research Council. 1999. *Chemical and Biological Terrorism: Research and Development to Improve Civilian Medical Response*. Washington, DC: National Academy Press.

U.S. Public Health Service, National Institutes of Health. 1942. *The Occurrence of Whooping Cough, Chickenpox, Mumps, Measles and German Measles in 200,000 Surveyed Families in 28 Large Cities*. Washington, DC: U.S. Government Printing Office.

Verano, John W., and Ubelaker, Douglas H. 1992. *Disease and Demography in the Americas*. Washington, DC: Smithsonian Institution Press.

Watts, Sheldon. 1998. *Epidemics and History: Disease, Power, and Imperialism*. New Haven, CT: Yale University Press.

Wills, Christopher. 1996. *Plagues: Their Origin, History and Future*. London: Harper Collins.

Wills, Christopher. 1997. *Yellow Fever, Black Goddess: The Coevolution of People and Plagues*. Reading, MA: Perseus Press.

Yancey, Diane. 1994. *The Hunt for Hidden Killers: Ten Cases of Medical Mystery*. Brookfield, CT: Millbrook Press.

Zimmerman, Barry E., and Zimmerman, David J. 1996. *Killer Germs: Microbes and Diseases That Threaten Humanity*. Chicago, IL: NTC/Contemporary Publishing.

Zinsser, Hans. 1935. *Rats, Lice, and History*. Boston: Little, Brown. Reprinted by Bantam Books, 1967.

Dangerous Animals

Agosta, William C. 1996. *Bombardier Beetles and Fever Trees: A Close-Up Look at Chemical Warfare and Signals in Animals and Plants*. Reading, MA: Addison-Wesley.

Fernicola, Richard. 2001. *Twelve Days of Terror: A Definitive Investigation of the 1916 New Jersey Shark Attacks*. New York: Lyons Press.

Halstead, Bruce W. 1995. *Dangerous Marine Animals: That Bite, Sting, Shock, or are Non-Edible*. Cambridge, MA: Cornell Maritime Press.

Herne, Brian. 1999. *White Hunters: The Golden Age of African Safaris*. New York: Henry Holt and Co.

Jenkinson, Michael. 1980. *Beasts Beyond the Fire: True Encounters with Man-Killing Denizens of Land and Sea*. New York: E.P. Dutton.

Levell, J.P. 1998. *A Field Guide to Reptiles and the Law*. Melbourne, FL: Krieger Publishing Co.

Levy, Charles K. 1983. *A Field Guide to Dangerous Animals of North America, Including Central America*. Brattleboro, VT: Stephen Greene Press.

Pearce, Q.L. 1999. *Great Predators of the Land*. Illustrated by Joe Yakovetic. New York: Tor Books.

Pearce, Q.L. 1999. *Great Predators of the Sea*. Illustrated by Joe Yakovetic. New York: Tor Books.

Tilton, Buck. 1995. *How to Die in the Outdoors: 100 Interesting Ways*. Guilford, CT: Globe Pequot Press.

Other Books

Amdur, Mary O., et al. (Editors). 1991. *Casarett and Doull's Toxicology: The Basic Science of Poisons*. New York: McGraw-Hill.

Andrews, M. 1976. *The Life That Lives on Man*. New York: Taplinger Publishing.

Burt, C.W., and Fingerhut, L.A. 1998. *Injury Visits to Hospital Emergency Departments: United States, 1992–95*. National Center for Health Statistics, Vital and Health Statistics 13(131), 86 pp.

Chapman, David. 1994. *Natural Hazards*. New York: Oxford University Press.

Conrad, Barnaby. 1988. *Absinthe: History in a Bottle*. San Francisco: Chronicle Books.

Crosby, Alfred W. 1994. *Germs, Seeds and Animals: Studies in Ecological History*. Sources and Studies in World History Series. Armonk, NY: M. E. Sharpe.

Davis, Lee. 1992. *Natural Disasters: From the Black Plague to the Eruption of Mt. Pinatubo*. New York: Facts on File.

Desowitz, Robert S. 1987. *New Guinea Tapeworms and Jewish Grandmothers: Tales of Parasites and People*. New York: W.W. Norton and Co.

Cloudsley-Thompson, J.L. 1976. *Insects and History*. World Naturalist Series. London: Weidenfeld and Nicolson.

Ebeling, Walter. 1978. *Urban Entomology*. Berkeley: University of California, Division of Agricultural Sciences.

Fumento, Michael. "How to Understand Scientific Studies and Epidemiology." *Consumers' Research Magazine*, June 1993.

Kaplan, David, and Marshall, Andrew. 1996. *The Cult at the End of the World: The Terrifying Story of the Aum Doomsday Cult, from the Subways of Tokyo to the Nuclear Arsenals of Russia*. New York: Crown Publishers.

LaBarre, Weston. 1962. *They Shall Take Up Serpents: Psychology of the Southern Snake-Handling Cult*. Minneapolis: University of Minnesota Press.

Leikin, Jerrold B., et al. 1997. *Poisoning and Toxicology Handbook*. 2nd ed. Hudson, OH: LexiComp Inc.

Noji, Eric K. (Editor). 1996. *The Public Health Consequences of Disasters*. New York: Oxford University Press.

U.S. Department of the Army. *U.S. Army Survival Manual* (FM 21–76). Reprinted 1992 by Dorset Press, New York.

Wald, P., and Stave, G. 1994. *Physical and Biological Hazards in the Workplace*. New York: John Wiley.

FICTION

All the novels and short stories in the following list contain themes related to one or more of the biological hazards in this book. The short stories are literary classics, but the novels vary considerably in quality. (*Note*: Several novels with "virus" in the title are missing from this list because they are about computer viruses, not biological ones.)

Bailey, Kathleen C. 1995. *Death for Cause*. Livermore, CA: Meerkat Publishing Co.

Baird, Thomas. 1988. *Where Time Ends*. New York: Harper & Row.

Beatty, Robert. 1996. *Sapo*. Corvallis, OR: Ecopress.

Benchley, Peter. 1974. *Jaws*. Garden City, NY: Doubleday.

Benchley, Peter. 1992. *The Beast*. New York: Random House.

Benson, Ann. 1997. *The Plague Tales*. New York: Delacorte Press.

Benson, Ann. 1999. *The Burning Road*. New York: Delacorte Press.

Borden, William. 1968. *Superstoe*. New York: Harper & Row.

Brouwer, Sigmund. 1995. *Double Helix*. Cincinnati, OH: Word Press.

Caine, Peter. 1989. *Virus*. New York: NAL Onyx.

Camus, Albert. 1948. *The Plague*. New York: Modern Library, Random House.

Carpenter, William. 1994. *A Keeper of Sheep*. Minneapolis, MN: Milkweed Editions.

Case, John F. 1998. *The First Horseman*. New York: Fawcett Books.

Clancy, Tom. 1998. *Rainbow Six*. New York: Putnam Publishing Group.

Close, William T. 1995. *Ebola: A Documentary Novel of Its First Explosion*. New York: Ivy Books.

Cook, Robin. 1994. *Acceptable Risk*. New York: Putnam.

Cook, Robin. 1999. *Toxin*. New York: Berkley.

Cook, Robin. 1999. *Vector*. New York: Putnam.

Cook, Robin. 2000. *Contagion*. New York: Berkley.

Crane, Leonard. 2000. *Ninth Day of Creation*. Pasadena, CA: Connection Books.

de Maupassant, Guy. 1902. "Bed No. 29 [Le Lit 29]," in *The Complete Short Stories of Guy de Maupassant*. New York: W.J. Black.

Defoe, Daniel. 1722. *Journal of the Plague Year*. Reprinted 1974. New York: AMS Press.

Other Print Resources

Desai, Ketan. 1999. *Germs of War*. London: Minerva Press.

Deutermann, Peter T. 1998. *Zero Option*. New York: St. Martin's Press.

Drabek, Jan. 1980. *The Lister Legacy*. North York, Ontario: General Publishing Co. Ltd.

Federspiel, J.E. 1983. *The Ballad of Typhoid Mary*. New York: E.P. Dutton.

Fitzhugh, Bill. 1997. *Pest Control*. New York: Avon Books.

Fleischman, Paul. 1983. *The Path of the Pale Horse*. New York: Harper & Row.

Gerritsen, Tess. 1998. *Bloodstream*. New York: Pocket Books.

Goliszek, Andrew. 1998. *World Order*. New York: Forge Books.

Grant, Charles L. 1996. *Symphony*. New York: Tor Books.

Grant, Charles L. 1998. *Chariot*. New York: Forge Books.

Grant, Charles L. 1998. *In the Mood*. New York: Forge Books.

Grant, Charles L. 1999. *Riders in the Sky*. New York: Forge Books.

Guibert, Herve. 1991. *To the Friend Who Did Not Save My Life*. English translation by L. Coverdale. New York: Atheneum.

Harrington, William. 1991. *Virus*. New York: W. Morrow.

Hemingway, Ernest. 1932. *Death in the Afternoon*. New York: Scribner's.

Hemingway, Ernest. 1952. *The Old Man and the Sea*. New York: Scribner's.

Herbert, Frank. 1982. *The White Plague*. New York: Putnam.

Herbert, James. 1997. *'48*. New York: Harper-Prism.

Hey, Stan. 1999. *Scare Story*. London: Hodder & Stoughton.

Hillerman, Tony. 1998. *The First Eagle*. New York: HarperCollins Publishers.

Hogan, Chuck. 1999. *The Blood Artists*. New York: Avon/Eos.

Hudson, Jan. 1984. *Sweetgrass*. Edmonton: Tree Frog Press.

Johnson, Stanley. 1982. *Marburg Virus*. London: Heinemann.

King, Stephen. 1980. *The Stand*. New York: New American Library.

Kipling, Rudyard. 1894. "Rikki-Tikki-Tavi," in *The Jungle Book*. Reprinted 1997. New York: Morrow Junior Books.

Leslie, Peter. 1992. *The Melbourne Virus*. Hampton, NH: Severn House.

Lewitt, Shariann. 1995. *Memento Mori*. New York: Tor Books.

Lindgren, Torgny. 1992. *Light*. English translation by Tom Geddes. London: Harvill.

Litman, Robert B. 1991. *The Treblinka Virus*. New York: Ivy League Press.

London, Jack. 1912. "Koolau the Leper," in *The House of Pride and Other Tales of Hawaii*. New York: Macmillan.

Lutzeier, Elizabeth. 1990. *Coldest Winter*. New York: Oxford University Press.

Lynch, Patrick. 1995. *Carriers*. New York: Villard Books.

Lynch, Patrick. 1997. *Omega*. New York: E.P. Dutton.

Marr, John S., and Baldwin, John. 1998. *The Eleventh Plague: A Novel of Medical Terror*. New York: Cliff Street Books.

McGrath, Eamonn. 1990. *The Charnel House*. Belfast: Blackstaff.

Melville, Herman. 1981. *Moby Dick*. New York: Bantam Books.

Moler, Lee. 1999. *Bone Music*. New York: Simon & Schuster.

Monjo, F.N. 1971. *The Jezebel Wolf*. New York: Simon & Schuster.

Nance, John J. 1995. *Pandora's Clock*. New York: St. Martin's.

Newth, Mette. 1998. *The Dark Light*. English translation by Faith Ingwersen. New York: Farrar Straux & Giroux.

O'Nan, Stewart. 1999. *A Prayer for the Dying: A Novel*. New York: Holt.

Parry, Ric. 1992. *Venom Virus*. New York: Pocket Books.

Porter, Katherine Anne. 1939. *Pale Horse, Pale Rider: Three Short Novels*. New York: Modern Library.

Preston, Richard. 1997. *The Cobra Event*. New York: Random House.

Querry, Ron. 1999. *Bad Medicine*. New York: Bantam Books.

Randall, John D. 1991. *The Tojo Virus*. New York: Zebra.

Romkey, Michael. 1998. *The Vampire Virus*. New York: Fawcett Books.

Rovin, Jeff. 2000. *Fatalis*. New York: St. Martin's Press.

Savage, Douglas. 1994. *Incident in Mona Passage*. Conshohocken, PA: Combined Books.

Schonberg, Leonard A. 1997. *Deadly Indian Summer*. Santa Fe, NM: Sunstone Press.

Shelley, Mary Wollstonecraft. 1826. *The Last Man*. Reprinted 1993. Lincoln: University of Nebraska Press.

Smith, Martin Cruz. 1991. *Nightwing*. New York: Ballantine Books.

Strongman, Phil. 1997. *Cocaine*. London: Abacus.

Stewart, Chris. 1998. *The Kill Box*. New York: M. Evans and Co.

Taylor, Barry. 1990. *The Deadfall Trap*. New York: Walker and Co.

Taylor, Sheila Ortiz. 1998. *Coachella*. Albuquerque: University of New Mexico Press.

Zimmerman, R.D. 1998. *Hostage*. New York: Dell Books.

PERIODICALS

The titles of the following periodicals are largely self-explanatory. Most are available at university libraries, and a few have electronic versions that are searchable online.

Diseases and Microorganisms

AIDS Weekly. Atlanta, GA: C.W. Henderson.

American Journal of Public Health. Washington, DC: American Public Health Association.

Annals of Tropical Medicine and Parasitology. London: Academic Press.

Annual Progress Report, U.S. Army Medical Research Institute of Infectious Diseases. Frederick, MD: USAMRIID.

Biodefense Quarterly. Baltimore, MD: Johns Hopkins University, Center for Civilian Biodefense Strategies.

Canadian Journal of Infectious Diseases. Oakville, Ontario, Canada: Pulsus Group Inc.

Clinical Infectious Diseases. Chicago: University of Chicago Press.

Emerging Infectious Diseases. Washington, DC: U.S. National Center for Infectious Diseases. Online at <http://www.cdc.gov/ncidod/eid/index.htm>.

Epidemiology and Infection. New York: Cambridge University Press.

Foodborne and Waterborne Disease Outbreaks: Annual Summary. Atlanta, GA: U.S. Centers for Disease Control and Prevention.

Hepatitis Weekly. Atlanta, GA: Charles W. Henderson.

Infectious Disease News. Thorofare, NJ: Slack, Inc.

Journal of Applied Toxicology. New York: John Wiley.

Journal of Infectious Diseases. Chicago: University of Chicago Press.

Journal of Parasitology. Lawrence, KS: American Society of Parasitologists.

Journal of Spirochetal and Tick-borne Diseases. Hartford, CT: Lyme Disease Foundation, Inc.

Morbidity and Mortality Weekly Report. Atlanta, GA: U.S. Department of Health and Human Services, Public Health Service, Centers for Disease Control and Prevention. Online at <http://www.cdc.gov/mmwr>.

Parasitology Today. Amsterdam: Elsevier Science Publishers.

Reported Tuberculosis in the United States. Atlanta, GA: U.S. Department of Health and Human Services, Public Health Service, Centers for Disease Control and Prevention.

Summary of Health Information for International Travel. Atlanta, GA: U.S. Centers for Disease Control and Prevention. Online at <http://www.cdc.gov/travel/blusheet.htm>.

TB and Outbreaks Weekly (formerly *Tuberculosis and Airborne Diseases Weekly*). Atlanta, GA: C.W. Henderson.

Virus Weekly (formerly *Antiviral Weekly*). Atlanta, GA: C.W. Henderson.

Weekly Epidemiological Record. Geneva: World Health Organization. Online at <http://www.who.int/wer>.

World Disease Weekly Plus (formerly *Malaria and*

Other Print Resources

Tropical Disease Weekly). Atlanta, GA: C.W. Henderson.

World Health Statistics Annual. Geneva: World Health Organization. English and French.

World Health Statistics Report. Geneva: World Health Organization. English and French.

World Health Statistics Quarterly. Geneva: World Health Organization. English and French.

Other Periodicals

Allergy. Copenhagen, Denmark: Munksgaard.

Allergy and Immunology Week. Atlanta, GA: C.W. Henderson.

American Journal of Aerosol Research. Cincinnati, OH: American Association for Aerosol Research.

American Journal of Epidemiology. Cary, NC: Oxford University Press.

Annals of Allergy, Asthma, and Immunology. Palatine, IL: American College of Allergy, Asthma, and Immunology.

Annals of Emergency Medicine. St. Louis, MO: Mosby-Year Book, Inc.

Disaster Recovery Journal. St. Louis, MO: Disaster Recovery Institute.

Environmental Hazards. Columbia: University of South Carolina, Department of Geography.

Epidemiology and Infection. New York: Cambridge University Press.

Foodborne and Waterborne Disease in Canada. Ottawa: Health and Welfare Canada.

Handbook of Natural Toxins. Published since 1983 (not at regular intervals) by Marcel Dekker, New York.

Jane's NBC [nuclear-biological-chemical] *Protection Equipment*. Alexandria, VA: Jane's Information Group.

Journal of Environmental Health. Denver, CO: National Environmental Health Association.

Journal of Natural Toxins. Fort Collins, CO: Alaken, Inc. Published semiannually, 1992 to present.

Journal of Venomous Animals and Toxins. Botucatu, Brazil: Center for the Study of Venoms and Venomous Animals, São Paulo State University. Published biannually since 1995; available in the United States through Chemical Abstracts.

Medicine and Global Survival. Brookline, MA: BMJ Publishing Group. Online at <http://www2.healthnet.org/MGS/>.

Mushroom Journal. London: Mushroom Grower's Association. Published monthly.

SIPRI [Stockholm International Peace Research Institute] *Chemical and Biological Warfare Studies*. Philadelphia: Taylor & Francis.

The Shark Line. Sarasota, FL: Center for Shark Research at Mote Marine Laboratory.

Vaccine Weekly. Atlanta, GA: C. W. Henderson.

Wilderness and Environmental Medicine. The Wilderness Medical Society. New York: Chapman & Hall.

Wing Beats. Brunswick, NJ: American Mosquito Control Association.

CHAPTER 12

Nonprint Resources

Everything is dangerous, my dear fellow. If it wasn't so, life wouldn't be worth living.
—Oscar Wilde, *An Ideal Husband* (1895)

This chapter contains an assortment of resources that the reader may find useful or entertaining, including Internet Web sites, motion pictures, and other films available on videocassette, computer games and other software, and miscellaneous items. For lists of books and periodicals related to biological hazards, see Chapter 11.

INTERNET WEB SITES

General Reference

American Council on Science and Health:
http://www.acsh.org/publications/index.html

American Red Cross, Talking about Disaster:
http://www.redcross.org/disaster/safety/guide.html

Chemical Abstracts Service:
http://www.cas.org

Combined Health Information Database (CHID):
http://www.chid.nih.gov/

Public Health Reports, Oxford University Press:
http://www3.oup.co.uk/publhr/contents/

PubMed (medical literature databases):
http://www.ncbi.nlm.nih.gov/PubMed/

TOXNET (toxicology and hazardous chemical databases):
http://toxnet.nlm.nih.gov/index.html

University of North Carolina School of Public Health, webcasts:
http://www.sph.unc.edu/about/webcasts

Infectious Disease (Human) and Vaccination

Anti-Immunization Activists (critique by Dr. Ed Friedlander):
http://www.pathguy.com/antiimmu.htm

The Big Picture Book of Viruses:
http://www.tulane.edu/~dmsander/Big_Virology/BVHomePage.html

Communicable Disease Surveillance and Response (CSR), Disease News:
http://www.who.int/emc/diseases/

Nonprint Resources

Council of State and Territorial Epidemiologists:
http://www.cste.org/

Discovery Online, Epidemic Site:
http://www.discovery.com/exp/epidemic/epidemic.html

eMedicine, Infectious Diseases:
http://www.emedicine.com/med/INFECTIOUS_DISEASES.htm

Emerging Infectious Diseases (electronic journal):
http://www.cdc.gov/ncidod/eid/index.htm

Federation of American Scientists, Animal Health/Emerging Animal Disease:
http://www.fas.org/ahead/

History of Diseases:
http://www.mic.ki.se/HistDis.html

Influenza News:
http://www.who.int/emc/diseases/flu/country.html

Lincolnshire Post-Polio Network:
http://www.ott.zynet.co.uk/polio/lincolnshire/index1.html

Lyme Foundation (advocacy group):
http://www.lymenet.org

Morbidity and Mortality Weekly Report:
http://www2.cdc.gov/mmwr

National Necrotizing Fasciitis Foundation:
http://www.nnff.org/

National Vaccine Information Center (anti-vaccination):
http://www.909shot.com/

Outbreak News, World Health Organization:
http://www.who.int/disease-outbreak-news/

Parasite Links, American Society of Parasitologists:
http://www-museum.unl.edu/asp/asp_image/links4.html

U.S. Centers for Disease Control, Health Topics:
http://www.cdc.gov/health/diseases.htm

Vaccination Questions and Answers (pro-vaccination):
http://www.caringforkids.cps.ca/immunization/Questions.htm

Wonderful World of Diseases Bookstore:
http://www.diseaseworld.com/books.htm

Zoonosis Web Site, Texas Department of Health:
http://www.tdh.state.tx.us/zoonosis/

Livestock and Crop Pests and Diseases

Africanized "Killer" Bees:
http://agnews.tamu.edu/bees/home.html

American Phytopathological Society:
http://www.apsnet.org/

Federal Noxious Weed List:
http://www.aphis.usda.gov/ppq/weeds/

Integrated Pest Management (IPM) Access:
http://www.efn.org/~ipmpa/

International Plant Protection Convention:
http://www.fao.org/WAICENT/FaoInfo/Agricult/AGP/AGPP/PQ/

Mad Cow Disease References (Sperling Biomedical Foundation):
http://www.mad-cow.org/

Plant Viruses Online:
http://image.fs.uidaho.edu/vide/
http://biology.anu.edu.au/Groups/MES/vide/

USDA Agricultural Research Service:
http://www.ars.usda.gov/

USDA National Biological Control Institute Store (free publications and videos):
http://www.aphis.usda.gov/nbci/nbcistor.html

Biological Warfare and Terrorism

Biodefense Quarterly, Johns Hopkins University:
http://www.hopkins-biodefense.org/pages/news/quarter.html

Biological Weapons and Warfare site, Tulane University:
http://www.tulane.edu/~dmsander/garryfavwebbw.html

Bioterrorism Links:
http://www.qis.net/~edwardmc/docs/bioterror.htm

eMedicine, Biological Warfare Agents:
http://www.emedicine.com/emerg/topic853.htm

Federation of American Scientists, Biological (and Chemical) Weapons:
http://www.fas.org/bwc/index.html

Food Safety

Arizona Food Safety Page:
http://www.ag.arizona.edu/pubs/health/foodsafety

Bad Bug Book, Center for Food Safety and Applied Nutrition:
http://vm.cfsan.fda.gov/~mow/intro.html

Guide to Plant Relationships (food intolerance and allergy information):
http://www.purr.demon.co.uk/Food/RelatedPlantList.html

International Food Information Council:
http://ificinfo.health.org/

MeatNet (an excellent European Web site, mostly in English):
http://www.meatnet.nl/

National Food Safety Database:
http://www.foodsafety.ifas.ufl.edu/search.htm

Animals

Bear-Human Conflicts:
http://www.mala.bc.ca/www/discover/rmot/project.htm

Bird Strike Committee USA:
http://www.birdstrike.org/

Dangerous and Venomous Marine Organisms, Hawaii:
http://www.aloha.com/~lifeguards/critters.html

Dog Bites, National Center for Injury Prevention and Control:

http://www.cdc.gov/ncipc/duip/dogbites.htm

Herpdigest (weekly e-magazine on reptiles and amphibians):
http://www.herpdigest.org

Herp Forum International:
http://www.kingsnake.com/forum/index2.html

International Shark Attack File:
http://www.flmnh.ufl.edu/fish/Sharks/ISAF/ISAF.htm

Medical Herpetology (snakebite and related topics):
http://www.xmission.com/~gastown/herpmed/med.htm

Mountain Lion Attacks:
http://tchester.org/sgm/lists/lion_attacks.htm

Shark Research Committee:
http://www.sharkresearchcommittee.com

Transport Canada Bird Hazard Web Site:
http://www.tc.gc.ca/aviation/wildlife.htm

Venoms, Toxins, and Allergens

American Academy of Allergy, Asthma and Immunology Online:
http://www.aaaai.org/

American Association of Poison Control Centers:
http://www.aapcc.org/

Botanical Dermatology Database (BoDD):
http://bodd.cf.ac.uk/index.html

eMedicine, Environmental (bites, stings, envenomations):
http://emedicine.com/emerg/ENVIRONMENTAL.htm

Herbal Products and Alternative Medicines:
http://www.ny2aap.org/npsherbs.html

Poisonous Plant Bibliography:
http://vm.cfsan.fda.gov/~djw/readme.html

Pollen Counts, United States:
http://www.pollen.com/Pollen.com.asp

Substances Toxiques [most links are in English]:
http://pages.infinet.net/chimtic/
substances_toxiques.htm

VENOMS Database (Atheris Laboratories):
http://www.atheris.ch/venoms.html

Occupational Health and Safety

Bio-Hazards to Cavers Page:
http://www.texascavers.com/tsa/
biohaz.htm

Canadian Centre for Occupational Health and
Safety:
http://www.ccohs.ca/oshanswers/

Needlestick Injuries:
http://www.nursingworld.org/
needlestick/nshome.htm

U.S. Department of Labor, OSHA, Bloodborne
Pathogens:
http://www.osha-slc.gov/SLTC/
bloodbornepathogens/index.html

U.S. Department of Labor, OSHA, Other
Biological Hazards:
http://www.osha-slc.gov/SLTC/index.html

Substance Abuse

American Cancer Society (tobacco and cancer):
http://www.cancer.org/eprise/main/
docroot/ped/ped_10

National Clearinghouse for Alcohol and Drug
Information:
http://www.nsawi.health.org/

National Institute on Drug Abuse (NIDA):
http://www.nida.nih.gov/

MOTION PICTURES

All of the following motion pictures—old and new, excellent and rotten alike—are about one or more biological hazards. (The list excludes some movies with seemingly obvious titles; *Virus*, for example, was about a computer virus.)

Alien, 1979; *Aliens*, 1986; *Alien 3*, 1992; *Alien Resurrection*, 1997 (all rated R, starring Sigourney Weaver). Just as the motion picture *Apollo 13* brought to life the real dangers of space travel, the *Alien* series dragged the imaginary ones out from under the bed. Relevant themes: parasitism, quarantine, and biological warfare.

Alligator, 1980 (R, Robin Forster). A fine combination of horror and comedy, based on the urban legend of alligators in the sewers of New York. The 1990 sequel (*Alligator II*) resorts to the standard one-star theme of a town threatened by a large animal.

Anaconda, 1997 (PG-13, Eric Stoltz). The biggest, baddest, fakest-looking snake ever seen in the Amazon rain forest.

And the Band Played On, 1993 (PG-13, Matthew Modine). The story of the scientific team that discovered the AIDS virus. Made for cable; available on videocassette.

The Andromeda Strain, 1971 (G, Arthur Hill). A satellite contaminated with an alien microorganism crashes to Earth and infects a town. The bug contains no amino acids and can instantly convert blood to a dry powder. There are dark hints that the Army is responsible—but just when all seems lost, the bug mutates to a harmless form and falls into the ocean.

Arachnophobia, 1990 (PG-13, Jeff Daniels). A deadly South American spider, imported by accident, infests a small California town.

Bats, 1999 (R, Lou Diamond Phillips). Possibly the worst motion picture of its type ever made. We recommend it to anyone who has ever looked up into the night sky and wondered why the science achievement scores of American students are so low.

The Beast, 1996 (not rated, William L. Petersen). A big octopus, rarely seen, and lots of slow-moving dialog. The novel is better. Made for TV; available on videocassette.

The Birds, 1963 (PG-13, Rod Taylor). Hitchcock classic about ordinary birds suddenly attacking a town for no apparent reason. Dated, but scary.

Black Death, 1992 (not rated, Kate Jackson). A physician races against time to find a cure for a fatal virus that threatens the population of New York City.

The Black Scorpion, 1957 (not rated, Richard Denning). Giant scorpions pop out of a volcano in Mexico and terrorize a city. A minor cult classic; much better than it sounds.

Casual Sex?, 1988 (R, Victoria Jackson). Two disease-conscious women take their vacation at a health spa, hoping to find safe sex partners and/or committed relationships. A comedy for the AIDS generation.

Contagious, 1997 (PG-13, Lindsay Wagner). An epidemiologist combats a cholera outbreak in the United States (and traces it to airline food obtained in South America).

Cujo, 1983 (R, Dee Wallace Stone). Stephen King classic about a big dog with rabies.

Deep Blue Sea, 1999 (R, Samuel L. Jackson). Scientists working on a cure for Alzheimer's disease meddle unwisely with Mother Nature, somehow creating smart, violent sharks instead.

Deep Rising, 1998 (R, Treat Williams). Squidlike things invade a luxury cruise ship.

An Early Frost, 1985 (not rated, Aidan Quinn). A gay man with AIDS confronts his family.

Epidemic, 1988 (not rated, Lars Von Trier). In Danish. Writers develop a script about a nationwide disease epidemic, but then the story becomes reality.

The Fly, 1986 (R, Jeff Goldblum). Excellent, despite the all-too-familiar theme of scientists tampering with forces that are best left alone. When Goldblum began tearing off parts of his face, however, we nearly ran for the toilet. The 1958 Vincent Price version is less graphic.

Freaked, 1993 (PG-13, Alex Winter). Exposure to a mysterious toxic chemical transforms a television celebrity into a, well, you know.

Frogs, 1972 (PG, Ray Milland). Giant frogs attack the owners of an island who have shown no respect for Mother Nature.

The Ghost and the Darkness, 1996 (R, Michael Douglas/Val Kilmer). As the title suggests, this may be the first predator movie that does not even pretend to be about predators. The most frightening aspect of the two lions is not their tendency to eat people, but the fact that their behavior defies our understanding.

The Giant Gila Monster, 1959 (not rated, Don Sullivan). This low-budget production may be the best giant-lizard movie ever made. (To our knowledge, there have been only two; dinosaurs are not lizards.) It also features a polio victim with leg braces, a familiar sight in the 1950s, but more shocking to modern audiences than the monster.

Grizzly, 1976 (PG, Christopher George). A giant grizzly bear goes on a rampage in a national park.

The Island of Dr. Moreau, 1996 (PG-13, Marlon Brando). Long before people knew about DNA, they distrusted any scientist who might presume to tinker with the fundamental processes of life. Compare this movie with the 1977 version and with the original H.G. Wells novel, both written in the days before genetic engineering.

It Came from Beneath the Sea, 1955 (not rated, Faith Domergue). Your typical big octopus, this time rescued from oblivion by the special effects of Ray Harryhausen.

Jaws, 1975 (PG, Robert Shaw). Steven Spielberg's immortal classic based on the Peter Benchley novel. The sequels have been less successful.

Jeffrey, 1995 (R, Patrick Stewart). A critically acclaimed comedy about the AIDS epidemic of the late twentieth century and its impact on the gay male community of New York City.

Lake Placid, 1999 (R, Bill Pullman). The computer-generated crocodile is superb, if a bit large. The people get a few good lines, but for the most part we rooted for the crocodile.

Longtime Companion, 1990 (R, Bruce Davison). A sensitive depiction of gay life in Manhattan in the early 1980s, focusing on the impact of the AIDS epidemic.

The Lost World, 1997 (PG-13, Jeff Goldblum). Don't confuse it with Sir Arthur Conan Doyle's unrelated classic. This sequel to *Jurassic Park* offers fine special effects and a wealth of misinformation on many subjects (conotoxin, genetic engineering, paleontology).

Mimic, 1997 (R, Mira Sorvino). An entomologist creates a mutant insect to kill cockroaches that are spreading a disease, but the bug escapes and becomes a monster—more deadly than the epidemic, and capable of mimicking a human being, at least in dim light. A vivid parable of the dangers of biotechnology; the bug looks like us because it *is* us.

Mission of the Shark, 1991 (not rated, Stacy Keach). After a Japanese submarine sank the USS *Indianapolis* in 1945, hundreds of its crew members were eaten by sharks before rescuers arrived. School classes might watch this one on Memorial Day.

Moby Dick, 1998 (PG, Patrick Stewart). An excellent retelling of the classic novel of obsession and revenge, focusing on the human need to personalize the destructive forces of nature. If Stewart's interpretation of Captain Ahab seems a bit shrill, try the 1956 version starring Gregory Peck.

Mosquito, 1995 (R, Gunnar Hansen). Alien-infected mosquitoes turn into blood-sucking monsters.

Mutant Species, 1995 (R, Leo Rossi). Modified DNA transforms a soldier into a predatory beast. Not an artistic triumph, but a good example of this increasingly popular theme.

The Naked Jungle, 1954 (not rated, Charleton Heston). A plantation owner in South America has a problem with army ants.

Out of Africa, 1985 (PG, Meryl Streep). A Danish writer with an estate in Kenya catches syphilis from her boyfriend, long before the discovery of antibiotics.

Outbreak, 1995 (R, Dustin Hoffman). Civilization intrudes on the African rain forest, bringing humans into contact with a terrifying new plague. The acting is good, the medical science so-so. Audiences may tend to avoid pet stores after seeing this one.

Panic in the Streets, 1950 (not rated, Richard Widmark). Old but excellent suspense thriller about New Orleans police hunting criminals infected with plague.

Philadelphia, 1993 (PG-13, Tom Hanks). A young attorney with AIDS fights discrimination.

Piranha, 1996 (R, Soleil Moon Frye). A remake of the 1978 cult classic about killer mutant fish invading a river. Not strictly accurate, but entertaining.

The Plague, 1993 (R, William Hurt). Doctors fight a deadly plague in a South American city; a critically non-acclaimed adaptation of the classic Albert Camus novel.

Predator, 1987 (R, Arnold Schwarzenegger) and *Predator II*, 1990 (R, Danny Glover). It's scary enough when a familiar bear or alligator turns the tables and starts hunting us, but at least we can call a game warden. In the *Predator* movies, the situation is considerably worse.

Quarantine, 2000 (not rated, Harry Hamlin). A terrorist group creates a genetically engineered virus that finds its way to the United States. Highly unrealistic and inaccurate, except for the basic premise that biological terrorism could happen. Made for TV.

The Savage Bees, 1976 (not rated, Ben Johnson). This made-for-TV classic, available on videotape, features African killer bees attacking an orange Volkswagen at Mardis Gras.

Shark Attack, 1998 (R, Casper Van Dien). The protagonist is a hammerhead shark, rather than the usual great white.

Silent Predators, 1999 (not rated, Harry Hamlin). Aggressive but normal-sized hybrid rattlesnakes threaten a community. Made for TV.

Stephen King's The Stand, 1994 (not rated, Gary Sinise). Survivors of a worldwide disease epidemic confront an evil telepath. Available on videotape (360 minutes total).

The Swarm, 1978 (PG, Michael Caine). Killer bees attack Houston, Texas.

Tentacles, 1977 (PG, John Huston). A giant octopus attacks a coastal town. The usual.

Them!, 1954 (not rated, James Whitmore). Giant ants, unleashed by atomic radiation, invade the Southwest. Superior acting, script, and special effects for the time and genre.

The Third Man, 1949 (not rated, Orson Welles). The Graham Greene classic about the moral dilemma of a black market drug dealer in postwar Vienna, who sells a watered-down version of a valuable new drug called penicillin.

Ticks [originally called *Infested*], 1994 (R, Peter Scolari). A marijuana farmer, trying to enhance his crop, releases chemicals that make local ticks grow to the size of dinner plates. They kill him and then go after a group of troubled youths on an outing in the woods—but one of the kids is on steroids, and the tick that bites him ends up five feet long.

Trainspotting, 1996 (R, Ewan McGregor). A Scottish heroin addict tries to kick the habit. Good reviews.

Tremors, 1989 (PG-13, Kevin Bacon). This wonderful movie pokes fun at scientists, survivalists, rednecks, monsters, group dynamics, and the human heart, without once resorting to cheap cynicism. The sequel was less successful.

Twelve Monkeys, 1995 (R, Bruce Willis). The hero travels back in time to stop the release of a biological warfare agent and rescue humanity from a post-apocalyptic future.

White Hunter, Black Heart, 1990 (PG, Clint Eastwood). An arrogant, self-destructive movie director goes to Africa to kill an elephant. An uncomplimentary portrayal of hunters.

The X-Files (Movie), 1998 (PG-13, David Duchovny). We did not entirely understand the plot, but it has something to do with alien parasites and genetically engineered viruses.

VIDEOTAPES (OTHER THAN MOVIES)

Some of these documentaries and educational films are more suitable than others for young audiences. Teachers and parents should review them before showing them to children.

Diseases and Allergies

AIDS. 1994. Important information for grades 7-12. Wynnewood, PA: Schlessinger Teen Health Video Series, 40 min.

AIDS: The Plague of the Century. 1997. The history of the AIDS pandemic, and the efforts of researchers to stop it. Princeton, NJ: Films for the Humanities, 96 min.

Asthma and Allergies. 1992. Cause, treatment, and prevention. Princeton, NJ: Films for the Humanities, 28 min.

Asthma, Asthma, You Can't Stop Me. 1998. Chino, CA: Kidsafety of America, 17 min.

Banished: Living with Leprosy. 1999. Bethesda, MD: Discovery, 52 min.

Body Story: Body Snatchers. 1999. A detailed investigation of the effects on the human body of two tiny visitors—a human embryo, and an influenza virus. Bethesda, MD: Discovery, 52 min.

Breathing Lessons. 1996. The story of poet-journalist Mark O'Brien, who contracted polio in childhood and has spent most of his life in an iron lung. Boston, MA: Fanlight Productions, 35 min.

British Beef in Chains. 1997. A documentary on the British beef industry's response to the BSE (mad cow disease) and *E. coli* crises. Saskatoon, Canada: University of Saskatchewan, Extension Division, 28 min.

Case Studies in Clinical Infection: Urinary Tract Infection, Enteric Infection, and Endocarditis. 1997. A documentary on three types of bacterial infection. Princeton, NJ: Films for the Humanities, 31 min.

Chicken Pox: Vaccinate and Prevent. 1996. The facts about chickenpox and the benefits of immunization. Princeton, NJ: Films for the Humanities, 22 min.

Chlamydia: The Hidden Disease. 1995. Information about the most often reported infectious disease in the United States, with an estimated 4 million new cases per year. Princeton, NJ: Films for the Humanities, 22 min.

Cholera. 1997. The resurgence of cholera in South America and its relationship to poverty. Princeton, NJ: Films for the Humanities, 29 min.

Coping with Allergies. 1995. Award-winning guide to the causes and treatment of allergies. Boston, MA: Xenejenex, 34 min.

Core Evidence: E. coli and Apple Juice. 1999. How apple juice became contaminated with deadly bacteria. Princeton, NJ: Films for the Humanities, 26 min.

Deadly Meat: When a Hamburger Can Kill. 1994. ABC News *Turning Point* program on *E. coli* outbreaks, including the role of the USDA and other agencies in preventing them. Princeton, NJ: Films for the Humanities, 43 min.

Deadly Parasites. 1998. The discovery of *Crypto-*

sporidium in the drinking water supply in Milwaukee, Wisconsin. Princeton, NJ: Films for the Humanities, 24 min.

E. coli: Case of the Mysterious Microbe. 1997. The evolution of the deadly 0157 strain and its relationship to other diseases including flu and tuberculosis. Princeton, NJ: Films for the Humanities, 26 min.

Ear Infections: Too Serious to Ignore. 1996. Why middle-ear infections in children are increasing, and what to do about it. Princeton, NJ: Films for the Humanities, 22 min.

Ebola: Diary of a Killer. 1996. The 1995 ebola outbreak in Zaire and its aftermath. Princeton, NJ: Films for the Humanities, 61 min.

The Elusive Illness. 1980. Nova segment on the development of a Hepatitis B vaccine; dated, but informative. Boston: WGBH Education Foundation, 52 min.

Epidemics and the Environment. 1997. Plague, cholera, Lyme disease, and other epidemics. Princeton, NJ: Films for the Humanities, 29 min.

Fatal Fungus. 1997. A 1994 outbreak of lung hemorrhage in infants in Cleveland, Ohio, caused by the fungus *Stachybotrys atra*. (As noted in Chapter 7, the CDC later retracted its conclusions regarding the cause of this outbreak.) Princeton, NJ: Films for the Humanities, 24 min.

Foreign Body: Mad Cow Disease. 1998. A documentary on the human and animal encephalopathies. Princeton, NJ: Films for the Humanities, 24 min.

Genital Herpes. 1997. Transmission, treatment, and coping. Princeton, NJ: Films for the Humanities, 20 min.

Guardian of Africa: The Tsetse Fly. 1994. The presence of the tsetse fly in East Africa's woodlands protects wildlife by preventing cattle from grazing there. Princeton, NJ: Films for the Humanities, 45 min.

Guinea Worm: The End of the Road. 1992. Efforts to eradicate the Guinea worm parasite in Africa and Asia. New York: First Run/Icarus Films, 29 min.

Hepatitis A. 1996. U.S. outbreaks, symptoms, prevention, and treatment. Princeton, NJ: Films for the Humanities, 20 min.

Hepatitis B: The Enemy Within. 1996. Current medical knowledge and treatment. Princeton, NJ: Films for the Humanities, 22 min.

Hepatitis C: The Silent Scourge. 1995. Causes, prevention, and treatment. Princeton, NJ: Films for the Humanities, 23 min.

HPV: Issues and Answers. 1998. Human papillomavirus and its link to genital warts and cervical cancer. Princeton, NJ: Films for the Humanities, 24 min.

Immunizations. 1997. Information on the DPT, hepatitis B, polio, HIB, and MMR vaccines. Princeton, NJ: Films for the Humanities, 20 min.

Influenza 1918. 1998. The story of the worst disease epidemic in American history. Alexandria, VA: PBS Home Video, 60 min.

The Kuru Mystery. 1984. Nobel laureate Carleton Gajdusek searches for the cause of kuru in New Guinea. Alexandria, VA: PBS Home Video, 57 min.

The Last Outcasts. 1984. Doctors treating leprosy in Nepal must also fight superstition and prejudice regarding the disease. Alexandria, VA: PBS Home Video, 60 min.

The Last Wild Virus. 1984. The WHO eliminates smallpox from its last stronghold in Bangladesh. Alexandria, VA: PBS Home Video, 60 min.

Legionnaires' Disease. 1996. The first Legionnaires' outbreak and the discovery of its cause. Princeton, NJ: Films for the Humanities, 24 min.

Lyme Disease in Our Own Backyard. 1991. Dated but excellent documentary on the discovery and impact of Lyme disease. Princeton, NJ: Films for the Humanities, 56 min.

Malaria: Battle of the Merozoites. 1992. A BBC production on malaria. Princeton, NJ: Films for the Humanities, 50 min.

Meningitis: The Urgent Diagnosis. 1993. Three children with meningitis fight for their lives. Princeton, NJ: Films for the Humanities, 52 min.

Modern Marvels: Polio Vaccine. 1993. The history of polio and the search for a cure. New York: A&E Entertainment, 46 min.

The Origin of AIDS: Mystery of the Chimps. 1999. The hypothesis that the HIV-1 virus came from an endangered subspecies of chimpanzees in sub-Saharan Africa. Princeton, NJ: Films for the Humanities, 22 min.

Panama Canal. 1994. Documentary about the construction of the Panama Canal, including the role of yellow fever and malaria in delaying its completion. New York: A&E Home Video, 50 min.

Paralyzing Fear: The Story of Polio in America. 1997. Award-winning documentary on the arrival of polio in the U.S. in 1916, the epidemics of the 1940s and 1950s, the impact on victims and on American society, and the development of a successful vaccine. Alexandria, VA: PBS Home Video, 89 min.

Plagued. 1992. Four parts: (1) The Origins of Disease, (2) Epidemics, (3) Invisible Armies, (4) Will We Ever Learn? A documentary that examines the relationships between disease, epidemics, medical science, history, and the environment. New York: Filmakers Library, 240 min.

Plagues. 1987. Nobel laureate Baruch S. Blumberg examines the mysteries of epidemics including cholera in mid-nineteenth-century London, and influenza, legionnaire's disease, myxomatosis, and malaria in the 20th century. Alexandria, VA: PBS Home Video, 59 min.

Pneumonia: All You Need to Know. 1997. Prevention and treatment of the various forms of pneumonia. Princeton, NJ: Films for the Humanities, 20 min.

Poison in Paradise: Guam Disease. 1996. BBC documentary on a neurological disease of unknown cause, found only on Guam. Princeton, NJ: Films for the Humanities, 50 min.

Polio and Postpolio Syndrome. 1993. Many of those who survived polio in the first half of the twentieth century later developed pain and disability. Princeton, NJ: Films for the Humanities, 28 min.

Polio: The Last Word. 1996. Award-winning documentary. Budapest: Adam Csillag, 60 min.

Post-Polio Syndrome. 1990. Another documentary on the delayed effects of polio. Largo, FL: Suncoast Media, 29 min.

A Practical Guide to Sexually Transmitted Diseases. 1990. AIDS, gonorrhea, chlamydia, herpes, venereal warts, and others. Princeton, NJ: Films for the Humanities, 23 min.

Preventing Hantavirus Disease. 1994. Award-winning educational videotape, available in English and Spanish. Atlanta, GA: Centers for Disease Control and Prevention, Office of Planning and Health Communications, 27 min.

Sinusitis. 1997. Causes and treatment. Princeton, NJ: Films for the Humanities, 21 min.

Something for Nothing. 1994. Topics include a cholera epidemic and its effects on history, by James Burke. Connections2 series. Bethesda, MD: Discovery, 25 min.

STDs (Sexually Transmitted Diseases). 1994. Important information for grades 7-12. Wynnewood, PA: Schlessinger Teen Health Video Series, 30 min.

The Three Valleys of St. Lucia. 1984. Researchers study schistosomiasis, a parasitic disease, on the Caribbean island of Santa Lucia. Alexandria, VA: PBS Home Video, 60 min.

Tracking Post-Polio Syndrome. 2000. Neurobiologists from the Salk Institute and UCLA discuss the syndrome and recent advances. San Diego, CA: Post Polio Group of San Diego, 145 min. (PPSVideos@mail.com).

The Trouble with Malaria. 1997. The efforts of health agencies to combat malaria. Princeton, NJ: Films for the Humanities, 46 min.

Tuberculosis: The Forgotten Plague. 1993. An examination of TB outbreaks and treatment on three continents. Princeton, NJ: Films for the Humanities, 50 min.

Tuberculosis 2000: A Satellite Course. 1997. A three-part course for medical professionals. San Francisco: Francis J. Curry National Tuberculosis Center, 180 min.

Ulcer Wars. 1995. The efforts of Dr. Barry Marshall to prove his theory that bacteria cause stomach ulcers. Princeton, NJ: Films for the Humanities, 50 min.

Viruses, the Mysterious Enemy. 1985. A somewhat dated overview of the biology of viruses and the efforts of medical researchers to eliminate viral diseases. Pleasantville, NY: Human Relations Media, 39 min.

Whooping Cough. 1997. The causes, symptoms, and treatment of pertussis. Princeton, NJ: Films for the Humanities, 21 min.

With Every Breath: The Hanta Virus. 1999. The discovery of the hanta virus in the American southwest. Princeton, NJ: Films for the Humanities, 26 min.

Dangerous Animals

Crocodile Territory. 1997. About the saltwater crocodiles of Australia. Bethesda, MD: Discovery, 50 min.

Crocodiles with David Attenborough (Nova). 1998. The life of crocodiles; good photography. Alexandria, VA: PBS Home Video, 60 min.

Crocodiles: Here Be Dragons. 1990. An excellent documentary on crocodiles in Tanzania. Washington, DC: National Geographic, 50 min.

Deadly Bugs. 1999. An introduction to dangerous insects, spiders, and parasites. Bethesda, MD: Discovery, 52 min.

Demons of the Deep. 1997. Sharks and barracudas. Bethesda, MD: Discovery, 51 min.

Dragons of Komodo. 1997. The world's largest lizard in action. Wild Discovery. Bethesda, MD: Discovery, 56 min.

Forbidden Video, Vol. II: Animal Attacks. 1999. Scenes of people being attacked by (mostly captive) animals including elephants, polar bears, and sharks. Real Entertainment, 50 min.

The Great Siberian Grizzly. 1997. The grizzly bears of the Kamchatka peninsula. Bethesda, MD: Discovery, 52 min.

Great White. 1997. The famous predatory shark. Bethesda, MD: Discovery, 90 min.

Grizzly Diaries. 1999. The life of the grizzly bear. Bethesda, MD: Discovery, 52 min.

Hunters. 1997. A series of four videos on the larger mammalian predators. Bethesda, MD: Discovery, 240 min.

Killer Bees? 1999. The origins and behavior of Africanized honey bees, hosted by Don Collier. Alexandria, VA: PBS Video, 30 min.

Killer Bees, Wasps and Spiders. 1996. How employees can protect themselves. Durham, NC: Long Island Productions, 37 min.

Last Charge of the Rhino. 1996. The efforts of two American scientists to save the African black rhinoceros from extinction. Bethesda, MD: Discovery, 48 min.

Leopards of the Night. 1998. The behavior of the leopard. Alexandria, VA: PBS Home Video, 60 min.

Little Killers: Power of Venom. 2000. Venomous snakes, spiders, insects, scorpions, and ticks. Bethesda, MD: Discovery, 52 min.

Little Killers: Sea Stingers. 2000. Venomous marine animals, including the blue-ringed octopus, sea snakes, stone fish, jellyfish, zebra fish, stingrays, and cone snails. Bethesda, MD: Discovery, 52 min.

The Portuguese Man-of-War. 1986. A brief glimpse of the dangerous jellyfish. Princeton, NJ: Films for the Humanities, 11 min.

Project Grizzly. 1999. After surviving a grizzly bear attack, Canadian Troy Hurtubise designs a preposterous suit of bear-fighting armor, and beta-tests it by allowing himself to be thrown off a cliff and rammed by a pickup truck. New York: First Run Features, 72 min.

Quest for the Giant Squid. 2000. Biologists from Woods Hole Oceanographic Institute search for giant squid in the Sea of Cortez. Bethesda, MD: Discovery, 52 min.

The Secret Leopard. 1988. Wild leopards in Africa. Washington, DC: National Geographic. 60 min.

Shark Attack Files. 1997. The recent increase in shark attacks on human beings, and how to prevent them. Bethesda, MD: Discovery Video Library Series, 60 min.

Shark Bait. 1997. Misconceptions about sharks; increasing numbers of shark attacks. Bethesda, MD: Discovery, 45 min.

The Ultimate Guide: Snakes. 1997. Spectacular footage of snakes, including a 29-foot anaconda swallowing a caiman (alligator-like reptile). Bethesda, MD: Discovery, 52 min.

Wild Discovery 6-Pack. 1997. Three of the volumes deal with grizzly bears, crocodiles, and Komodo dragons, respectively. Bethesda, MD: Discovery, 300 min.

Substance Abuse

The Addicted Brain. 1987. Recent developments in the biochemistry of addiction and addictive behavior. Princeton, NJ: Films for the Humanities, 26 min.

Alcohol Addiction. 1987. A visit to the Rutgers University Alcohol Research Lab. Princeton, NJ: Films for the Humanities, 23 min.

Alcohol and Alcoholism. 1991. Grades 7 and up. Wynnewood, PA: Schlessinger Media, Video Encyclopedia of Psychoactive Drugs Series, 30 min.

Alcohol: Brain under the Influence. 1999. The effects of alcohol on various parts of the brain. Scottsdale, AZ: Amethyst Technologies, 45 min.

Coca. 1994. The history of the coca plant and cocaine. Princeton, NJ: Films for the Humanities, 29 min.

Cocaine and Crack: The New Epidemic. 1991. Grades 7 and up. Wynnewood, PA: Schlessinger Media, Video Encyclopedia of Psychoactive Drugs Series, 30 min.

The Forbidden Plant: Hemp. 1999. The history and legal status of marijuana worldwide. New York: Filmaker's Library, 56 min.

From Nowhere to Somewhere: Street Drugs and Your Rehabilitation. 1988. Houston, TX: Institute for Rehabilitation and Research, 15 min.

The Hijacked Brain. 1998. The chemistry of addiction and its possible genetic components. Princeton, NJ: Films for the Humanities, 57 min.

LSD and Ergot. 1993. The ergot fungus and its derivatives. Princeton, NJ: Films for the Humanities, 28 min.

Marijuana: Its Effects on Mind and Body. 1991. Grades 7 and up. Wynnewood, PA: Schlessinger Media, Video Encyclopedia of Psychoactive Drugs Series, 30 min.

Nicotine: An Old-Fashioned Addiction. 1991. Grades 7 and up. Wynnewood, PA: Schlessinger Media, Video Encyclopedia of Psychoactive Drugs Series, 30 min.

Nicotine War (PBS Frontline). 1995. The FDA's attempts to regulate tobacco. Alexandria, VA: PBS Home Video, 57 min.

The Opium Poppy. 1993. The origin and addictiveness of opium, morphine, and heroin. Princeton, NJ: Films for the Humanities, 28 min.

Smoke and Mirrors: A History of Denial. 1999. An expose of the tobacco industry. New York: American Lung Association, 75 min.

Smokeless Tobacco: Breaking Free. 1996. The health hazards of smokeless tobacco, and advice on how to quit. Princeton, NJ: Films for the Humanities, 17 min.

Superbugs: When Antibiotics Don't Work. 1998. The problem of antibiotic resistance in bacteria. Princeton, NJ: Films for the Humanities, 44 min.

Tobacco Blues. 1998. The culture and ethics of tobacco farming, from the farmer's perspective. New York: Filmaker's Library, 58 min.

Tobacco Road: A Dead End. 1997. Award-winning documentary on the dangers of tobacco, including shock footage of lung surgery and interviews with victims of tobacco-related illnesses. Princeton, NJ: Films for the Humanities, 30 min.

Other

Alliance of Shame. 1985. Japan's use of American prisoners as experimental subjects for biological warfare research during World War II. New York: American Broadcasting Companies, 20 min.

Animal Awareness Driving. 1990. A brief video that tells drivers how they can safety avoid collisions with animals on the road. Chesterfield, MO: Safety Times, 15 min.

Belladonna and Mandragola. 1993. Belladonna and related poisonous plants. Princeton, NJ: Films for the Humanities and Sciences, 26 min.

Biological Control: A Natural Alternative. 1989. Biological control as a pest control option. Riverdale, MD: USDA National Biological Control Institute, 28 min.

Disarming Iraq: Controlling Biological Weapons. 1998. Documentary on United Nations weapons inspections in Iraq. Princeton, NJ: Films for the Humanities and Sciences, 29 min.

Edible Wild Plants. 1988. A botanist explains how to identify both edible and poisonous wild plants commonly found in North America. Edwardsburg, MI: Media Methods, 60 min.

Frontline: Plague War. 1998. An investigation of the threat of biological warfare. Alexandria, VA: PBS Video, 60 min.

Fruit of the Gods. 1986. A comprehensive survey of mushrooms, including poisonous species. Pensacola, FL: Florida Mycology Research Center, 83 min.

Jellies and Other Ocean Drifters. 1996. Jellyfishes and related marine animals. Monterey, CA: Monterey Bay Aquarium Foundation, 35 min.

Louis Pasteur. 1997. A profile of the scientist who proved that microorganisms cause fermentation and disease, and who created the first vaccines against rabies, anthrax, and chicken cholera. Princeton, NJ: Films for the Humanities, 10 min.

Mosquito Control and Biology Videotape. [Undated] Mosquitoborne diseases, control and prevention measures, and research agencies. New Brunswick, NJ: American Mosquito Control Association, 27 minutes.

Myths and Monsters. 1986. The role of animals in mythology, rituals, and phobias. Princeton, NJ: Films for the Humanities, 27 min.

Our Nation's Blood Supply: The Next Threshold for Safe Blood. 1995. Blood safety and related issues. Princeton, NJ: Films for the Humanities, 22 min.

The Passionate Statistician: Florence Nightingale. 1995. The famous nurse uses statistics from the Crimean War to prove that most soldiers died of diseases contracted in unsanitary Army hospitals, not in battle as reported. Princeton, NJ: Films for the Humanities, 25 min.

Poisonous Plants. 1989. A brief instructional video on common poisonous and allergenic plants, both wild and domesticated. Chesterfield, MO: Safety Times, 12 min.

Scare Me. 1999. Why people seek out frightening situations. Bethesda, MD: Discovery, 47 min.

Too Much Medicine? The Need for Clinical Evidence. 1997. Explores the possibility that the pharmaceutical industry exploits the public by redefining normal aspects of the aging process as "diseases." Princeton, NJ: Films for the Humanities, 51 min.

Transgenesis: Agricultural Biotechnology. 1995. A documentary on genetically modified crop plants and livestock. Princeton, NJ: Films for the Humanities, 51 min.

Trappin' Snappers. 1998. How to catch, butcher, and eat snapping turtles. (We are not advising readers to do any such thing, but the video is informative.) Available at <http://www.sunjess.com/turtles/>, 105 min.

Up Close and Personal: Our Secret Ecology. 2000. The bacteria, fungi, and mites (mostly harmless) that occupy our bodies and homes. Canadian Broadcasting Corporation. New York: Filmakers Library, 48 min.

Vaccines: Separating Fact from Fear. 2001. Answers parents' questions about the relative risks of various diseases and the vaccines that can prevent them. Philadelphia: Children's Hospital of Philadelphia, 27 minutes.

COMPUTER SOFTWARE

All the following computer games and other programs are for an IBM PC platform unless otherwise specified.

Games

3D Hunting Extreme. This game does not limit players to the usual quarry, such as lions, crocodiles, and elephants. You can even hunt extinct animals, such as dinosaurs or saber-toothed cats. Available weapons range from an AK-47 to a bow and arrows. Macmillan Digital Publishing U.S.A.

3D Hunting Grizzly. Choose your terrain and weapons, bring along a virtual buddy and dog— sorry, no virtual beer—and go git you a b'ar! In "Maneater Mode," you can even participate in a rescue mission. Bears will attack only if they see you as a threat, but just as in real life, it's hard to say how the bear might interpret all that gear you are carrying. Macmillan Digital Publishing U.S.A.

3D Hunting Shark. An underwater shark hunt, complete with scuba gear, weapons, a shark cage, sound effects, and dazzling scenery. The marketing blurb reflects some prevalent shark mythology: "True-to-life prey, kill or be killed!" Macmillan Digital Publishing U.S.A.

Abomination: The Nemesis Project. Romp through a future world of genetically altered soldiers, plague survivors, evil mutants, and something described as a "slithering, gibbering nightmare." Yum. Available from Eidos Games at <http://www.nemesisproject.com>.

Biohazard/Resident Evil 2. A viral epidemic has swept through a city and transformed nearly everyone into flesh-eating zombies. You need to find the uninfected survivors. Available from CapCom for IBM and other platforms.

The Blackout Syndrome. A stressful game in which you must quickly identify the disease that is causing a child to bleed uncontrollably. Download from Access Excellence at <http://www.accessexcellence.org/AE/mspot/>.

Deer Avenger. In this game you are the deer, luring the human hunter with your "beer call" and then blowing him away with your M-16. Being a predator has never been easy. Published by Simon & Schuster Interactive.

Dr. Goo 2: The Plague. The title character, who is sticky enough to hang from walls, is trying to develop a vaccine to save the world from a germ unleashed by foolish scientists. Appropriately priced (free) at <http://www.drgoo.8m.com>.

LateBlight Version 3.1, a Plant Disease Management Game. Originally developed at Cornell University in 1990 and later adapted for Windows, this simulation is downloadable at <http://www.apsnet.org/online/feature/lateblit/Software.htm>.

River of Venom. Killer bees on the rampage; another science mystery from Access Excellence. Download at <http://www.accessexcellence.org/AE/mspot/>.

Savage. In this unusual computer game, the player is the lion, not the human being. You can eat a zebra, defend your hunting grounds, escape from poachers, or die. You can even mark your territory (we didn't ask how). Available on CD-ROM at <http://www.discoverystore.com>.

Snake. According to the instructions, the player's goals are to "eat the black dots, don't hit the walls, and don't bite your tail." This sounds straightforward enough. Play it online at <http://www.nokia.com/snake/game.html>.

Syphon Filter and Syphon Filter 2. Save Washington, DC from a deadly virus deployed by terrorists. At present, this game apparently is available only for Sony PlayStation.

X-COM: Apocalypse. Have you always wanted to hire your own defense contractor to develop weapons of mass destruction? Have you longed to experience the benefits of biological warfare without the drawbacks? Then try this strategy combat game from MicroProse, Inc. <http://www.microprose.com>

Other Software

APHIS Video Clips. The USDA Animal and Plant Health Inspection Service has downloadable short video clips on classical swine fever, the Asian long-horned beetle, quarantine services, and other topics. <http://www.aphis.usda.gov/lpa/video/index.html>.

Biological Hazards Overview. This OSHA-oriented training course covers not only the usual infectious waste and pathogens, but some additional biological hazards such as insects, spiders, and plant toxins. (It skips things like alligators, which do not occur in most offices or factories.) Available at <http://www.firstnetlearning.com>.

Biotech Version 1.02: Veterinary Biotechnology Database. Veterinary applications of biotechnology research for animal disease prevention and diagnosis. Download at <http://www.oie.int/software/A_downld.htm>.

Doctor Disk. This online application was designed to help small businesses develop the workplace health and safety policies and documents required by OSHA. Available at: http://www.aiha-rms.org/smallbusiness/doctor/start.htm

Epi Info. A series of programs for epidemiological data management and analysis, developed by the U.S. Centers for Disease Control and prevention. Free download at: <http://www.cdc.gov/epo/pub_sw.htm>.

The Fifth Kingdom. A comprehensive reference on fungi, with over 800 pictures and animations. Sold on CD-ROM by Mycologue Publications, Sidney, British Columbia, Canada.

Food-Borne Illness and Prevention Techniques. The most common food-related pathogens and how to avoid transmitting them. Sold on CD-ROM by Films for the Humanities, Princeton, NJ.

Hepatitis A to E Slideshow. An informative presentation on the clinical and epidemiological features of the various forms of hepatitis. Downloadable from: <http://www.cdc.gov/ncidod/diseases/hepatitis/slideset/httoc.htm>.

Integrated Pest Management Information System (IPMIS). Developed by the U.S. Armed Forces Pest Management Board. The program, a software patch, and the manual are at: <http://www.afpmb.org/ipmis.htm>.

Lassa Online Video Documentary. The story of Lassa fever, filmed in Sierra Leone. Requires Windows Media Player. Available at: <http://www.cdc.doc/ncidod/dvrd/spb/mnpages/lassavideo.htm>.

Latex Allergy. A CD-ROM for health-care professionals who are latex sensitive; also includes self-tests for continuing education. Medical College of Wisconsin, 1999.

Mortality Data, Multiple Cause-of-Death Public-Use Data Files. Useful for research purposes, or for anyone who wishes to confirm the rarity of biological hazard-related deaths in the United States. Data for 1968-1997 are available on tape or CD-ROM from the Government Printing Office or NTIS. Ordering information is on the NCHS Web site: <http://www.cdc.gov/nchs/products/catalogs/subject/mortmcd/mortmcd.htm>.

Patty's Industrial Hygiene/Toxicology. Provides data on toxic chemicals and worker exposure; includes the NIOSH Manual of Analytical Methods. Available from <http://www.scientificsoftware.com>.

Pests In and Around the Home. Available on CD-ROM from the University of Florida Extension, Institute of Food and Agricultural Science, Gainesville, FL.

Physical and Biological Hazards in the Workplace. Available on CD-ROM from John Wiley & Sons, New York.

Pigs on the Internet. Everything you always wanted to know about pigs, including their diseases. Available from the Pig Disease Information Centre Ltd. <www.pighealth.com>.

Preventing Emerging Infectious Diseases. Slide set to accompany text. Available at: <http://www.cdc.doc/ncidod/emergplan/index.htm>.

Preventing Hantavirus Disease. A multimedia presentation, based on the award-winning CDC videotape of the same title. Download files at: <http://icb.usp.br/~mlracz/animations/hantavirus/hanta94.htm>.

RAPID (Random Access Plant IDentification) for Windows. Developed by the University of Idaho College of Agriculture for identification of weeds and poisonous plants found in North America. Information available at <http://sdg.ag.uidaho.edu/rapid/>.

Rinderpest, Foot-and-Mouth Disease, and Poultry Diseases. Three multimedia presentations on these major livestock diseases, downloadable at: <http://www.fao.org/waicent/FaoInfo/Agricult/AGA/AGAH/EMPRES/down2.htm>.

Rusty. This program was developed by Kansas State University's Plant Pathology Department to predict wheat rust severity based on soil moisture, rust inoculum survival, and other factors. For information, see <http://www.ars.usda.gov/is/pr/1997/rusty0597.htm>.

STD*MIS v. 4.0. A program used by many state and local health departments to manage their data on sexually transmitted diseases (STDs). Available from the CDC Division of Sexually Transmitted Diseases at <http://www.cdc.gov/nchstp/dstd/STD-MIS.htm>.

Tuberculosis: An Interactive CD-ROM for Clinicians. Available from the Francis J. Curry National Tuberculosis Center <http://www.nationaltbcenter.edu/distance.html>.

VACMAN. A database management system used by many state and local government agencies to manage their vaccination programs. Available from the U.S. National Immunization Program at <http://www.cdc.doc/nip/vacman/about.htm>.

Youth97. Five years of Youth Risk Behavior Survey data on CD-ROM. Available from the U.S. Centers for Disease Control and Prevention at <http://www.cdc.gov/nccdphp/dash/yrbs/youth97.htm>.

OTHER RESOURCES

Anatomical Chart Company. Their catalog contains a wide range of gift items that might appeal to readers of this book, including various disease posters, eyeball-shaped drinking mugs, and a gelatin mold in the shape of a human brain (add marshmallows to simulate a spongiform encephalopathy). <http://www.anatomical.com>.

Datura, Visions for the Celestial. Okay, so it's just the name of the band, but this death metal/doom rock CD is a safer alternative to the plant itself. Waikato, New Zealand: Cranium Music, 1999.

The Ebola Song. The file ebola.wav is available at several Web sites, including <http://www.bergen.org/ACADEMY/Bio/advbiot2.html>. Sample lyrics:

> Well, I caught it in Zaire and it made me ill
> Now there ain't no cure and there ain't no pill
> For Ebola.

Germs True Type Font. A hand-drawn font with each capital letter in the form of a monster with teeth. Surprise your boss or publisher. Available at: <http://members.aol.com/vroomfonde/ttf/index.html>.

Infectious Awareables Collection, Health Media International. This company markets neckties, scarves, boxer shorts, and other items with images of disease organisms and related themes. Motifs include AIDS, anthrax, breast cancer, cholera, chlamydia, dental plaque, dust mites, E. coli, giardia, gonorrhea, herpes, influenza, plague, staphylococcus, and tuberculosis. The company donates a portion of its proceeds to various charitable and research organizations. Contact them at (800) 388-1237 or (818) 990-6264.

PHIL (Public Health Image Library). A collection of still images, image sets, and multimedia files related to public health. Searchable at <http://phil.cdc.gov/Phil/default.asp>.

Pop Defect, Live in Big Bear: Drinking Poison, Handling Serpents, Speaking in Tongues. The band performs several songs that seem to fit here. US Flipside, 1995.

Real Goods (catalog and Web site). Real Goods sells some relevant items, but we won't promise that any of them work. Examples: an air purifier that you wear around your neck, to remove allergens and viruses; an insect trap that lets mosquitoes and other pests "end their lives in nontoxic sugary bliss" (in other words, it drowns them in syrup); and a device that allegedly repels mosquitoes with high-frequency sound. <http://www.realgoods.com>.

Safety Syringe Movie File. Health-care workers suffer an estimated 800,000 needle-stick injuries each year. In an effort to solve this problem, a company called Retractable Technologies is marketing a new type of syringe with a retractable needle. The demo is downloadable at <http://www.vanishpoint.com/>.

SBBCOM Nuclear, Biological and Chemical Defense Clothing. Is your attic full of hantavirus-laden mouse droppings? Is your kitchen overgrown with toxic fungi? Wait no longer— buy your very own NBC suit today, and grab a mop. Natick offers a full catalog at <http://www.sbccom.army.mil/products/nbc.htm>.

Skunk Spray, The Movie. This QuickTime file is exactly what it sounds like. Links for downloading both video and animated versions of this small classic are accessible from <http://granicus.if.org/~firmiss/m-d.html>.

Snakeproof Leggings, Chaps, and Boots. Forestry Suppliers Inc. (800-647-5368) sells a full range of high-quality products designed to protect hikers and outdoor workers from venomous snakebites. The same catalog contains many other useful items, such as gas masks, snakebite kits, bugproof shirts, and creams to treat or prevent the rash of poison ivy.

Toxic Bean Soup. If it were literally toxic, we would not recommend it to our readers. Despite the name, it is basically an extreme soup with red beans, chipotles, and garlic. Hint: Serve it to old friends, not new ones. The recipe is available at <http://user.sfcc.net/jyawn/beansoup.htm>.

CHAPTER 13

Organizations

Evils draw men together.

—Aristotle, *Rhetoric*

For those readers who have skipped directly to this chapter, the definitions of hazard, risk, and disaster bear repeating. A hazard is something with the potential to cause harm; a risk is a measure of the probability that the hazard *will* cause harm, combined with its severity; and a disaster is a sudden event that causes major, widespread harm. Agencies and organizations that study hazards also tend to analyze risk, but disaster management usually is a separate issue.

Rattlesnakes, for example, represent a biological hazard. Herpetological organizations and wildlife agencies study their behavior and distribution, while medical researchers work to develop better antivenoms. But the individual risk is low—few people are bitten—and it is hard to imagine how rattlesnakes could cause a disaster. As silly examples, perhaps hundreds of rattlers might emerge from a hibernaculum under the basement of a school, enter the building through a crack in the foundation, and start biting students; or perhaps a truckful of rattlers might overturn on a free-

way (on the way to a Hollywood movie set or a Texas roundup), causing slick pavement and multiple traffic accidents. The agencies responding to these disasters might include the local animal control department and an ambulance service.

There are better examples of biological disasters, such as natural disease epidemics and major crop failures, but disaster management agencies per se are not the ones that usually deal with them. The University of Colorado Natural Hazards Center, for example, focuses on nonbiological events. The American Red Cross publication *Talking about Disaster*, an excellent guide for families who wish to prepare themselves for various emergencies, refers to biological hazards only indirectly (boil water after a flood). It covers everything else in great detail, including geological and meteorological events, nonbiological hazardous materials spills, and fires.

There are two main reasons for excluding biological disasters from the usual definition. First, biological problems tend to be complicated. Anyone can grab a shovel and dig someone out of a mud slide, but not everyone knows how to help a victim of bubonic plague. In the latter case, simplified instructions might be worse than nothing, and too many eager volunteers might start an epidemic. Second, disease outbreaks and other biological disasters often occur more or less predictably on the heels of other natural disasters or wars. Thus, they are secondary emergencies that less often take us by surprise.

But there are exceptional cases in which a biological emergency arrives independently and without fanfare. An act of biological terrorism, for example, might cause thousands of infectious disease casualties in a short time. At least two agencies in the United States, the Federal Emergency Management Agency (FEMA) and the Centers for Disease Control and Prevention (CDC), partially fulfill the role of a clearinghouse for such emergencies. The CDC and state and local health departments would identify and treat the victims, with FEMA most likely providing emergency relief to the devastated communities.

Unfortunately, several incidents—such as the response of U.S. hospitals to a minor 1999 influenza outbreak—suggest that a biological emergency might quickly overload available facilities. A May 2001 study showed that fewer than 20 percent of hospital emergency departments had plans or equipment for handling a major biological weapons incident. The confusion that may follow such events became apparent in November 2001, when several hundred children at a school in Manassas, Virginia suddenly developed an unexplained fever and rash. The outbreak was particularly alarming because of the recent anthrax deaths; but as of March 2002, the CDC and Virginia Department of Health had not yet identified the illness, which fortunately was not life-threatening. Several agencies and manufacturers are working to develop more effective technologies for rapid identification of pathogens, while others are developing bioterrorism training programs, better surveillance systems, improved vaccines and antibiotics, and other countermeasures.

In Tables 13.1 and 13.2, organizations and agencies appear in alphabetical sequence, followed by the numbers of chapters in this book where their areas of interest appear. As thousands of different entities deal with some aspect of biological hazards, the table provides only a sample, and any omissions are unintentional.

Table 13.1
Some Organizations and Agencies that Deal with Specific Biological Hazards

Name and Address	Chapter Reference
Advisory Committee on Immunization Practices (ACIP) U.S. Public Health Service Centers for Disease Control and Prevention 4770 Buford Highway Atlanta, GA 30341	4, 5, 9
AIDS Action Council 1875 Connecticut Avenue NW, Suite 700 Washington, DC 20009	5
Alligator Snapper Foundation 6879 North Farm Road Strafford, MO 65757	8
American Association of Poison Control Centers 3201 New Mexico Avenue, Suite 310 Washington, DC 20016	7
American Council on Science and Health 1995 Broadway, Second Floor New York, NY 10023-5860	7, 9
American Dietetic Association 216 West Jackson Boulevard Chicago, IL 60606-6995	3
American Foundation for AIDS Research 120 Wall Street, 13th Floor New York, NY 10005-3902	5
American Lung Association 1740 Broadway New York, NY 10019	4
American Mosquito Control Association 2200 E. Prien Lake Road Lake Charles, LA 70601-7975	5
American Phytopathological Society 3340 Pilot Knob Road St. Paul, MN 55121-2097	6
American Society of Agricultural Engineers 2950 Niles Road St. Joseph, MI 49085	3, 6
American Society of Agronomy 677 South Segoe Road Madison, WI 53711	3, 6

(continued)

Table 13.1 (Continued)

Name and Address	Chapter Reference
American Society of Ichthyologists and Herpetologists Grice Marine Laboratory University of Charleston 205 Fort Johnson Road Charleston, SC 29412	7, 8
American Society of Parasitologists Department of Biological Sciences University of Iowa Iowa City, IA 52242	2, 3, 5, 6
American Tarantula Society P.O. Box 756 Carlsbad, NM 88221	7
American Water Resources Association 950 Herndon Parkway, Suite 300 Herndon, VA 20170-5531	2
Anaphylaxis Campaign P.O. Box 275 Farnborough, Hampshire, GU146XS, UK	7
Bird Strike Committee USA Richard Dolbeer, Chair 6100 Columbus Avenue Sandusky, OH 44870	8
Border Collie Rescue Birdstrike Control Program 886 State Road 26 Melrose, FL 32666	8
Chemical and Biological Arms Control Institute 1747 Pennsylvania Avenue, NW, 7th Floor Washington, DC 20006	9
Consortium for International Plant Protection Cornell University, NYSAES Geneva, NY 14456-0462	6
Council of State and Territorial Epidemiologists 2872 Woodcock Boulevard, Suite 303 Atlanta, GA 30341	2, 3, 4, 5
Gay Men's Health Crisis 119 West 24th Street New York, NY 10011	5

Table 13.1   (Continued)

Name and Address	Chapter Reference
Infectious Diseases Society of America 99 Canal Center Plaza, Suite 210 Alexandria, VA 22314	2, 3, 4, 5
Institute of Food Science and Engineering (IFSE) Center for Food Safety Texas A&M University College Station, TX 77843	3
Integrated Pest Management Practitioners Association P.O. Box 10313 Eugene, OR 97440	6
International Coalition on AIDS and Development 180 Argyle Avenue Ottawa, Ontario K2P 1B7, Canada	5
International Food Information Council Foundation 1100 Connecticut Avenue NW, Suite 230 Washington, DC 20036	3, 7, 9
International Laboratory for Tropical Agricultural Biotechnology Scripps Research Institute 10550 North Torrey Pines Road La Jolla, CA 92037	6, 9
International Polio Network 4207 Lindell Boulevard, Suite 110 St. Louis, MO 63108	5
International Varanid Association John Hogston, Editor 1740 Norfolk Avenue, Suite 14 Saint Paul, MN 55116	8
International Venomous Snake Society Thomas Marcellino P.O. Box 4498 Apache Junction, AZ 85278-4498	7
National Center for Infectious Diseases Centers for Disease Control and Prevention Mail Stop C-14 1600 Clifton Road Atlanta, GA 30333	2,3,4,5

(*continued*)

Table 13.1   (Continued)

Name and Address	Chapter Reference
National Clearinghouse for Alcohol and Drug Information P.O. Box 2345 Rockville, MD 20847	7
National Council Against Health Fraud P.O. Box 1276 Loma Linda, CA 92354-1276	9
National Council on Alcoholism and Drug Dependence 12 West 21st Street New York, NY 10010	7
National Environmental Health Association 720 South Colorado Boulevard Denver, CO 80246	2, 3, 4, 7
National Highway Traffic Safety Administration 400 7th Street SW Washington, DC 20590	8
National Institute of Allergy and Infectious Disease Office of Communications Building 31, Room 7A-50 31 Center Drive MSC 2520 Bethesda, MD 20892-2520	2, 3, 4, 5, 6, 7
National Institute on Alcohol Abuse and Alcoholism 6000 Executive Boulevard Willco Building Bethesda, MD 20892-7003	7
National Institute on Drug Abuse 6001 Executive Boulevard Bethesda, MD 20892-9561	7
National Minority AIDS Council 1931 13th Street NW Washington, DC 20009	5
National Pest Management Association 8100 Oak Street Dunn Loring, VA 22027	4, 5, 6
National Safety Council 1121 Spring Lake Drive Itasca, IL 60143-3201	7, 8
Office International des Epizooties (OIE) 12 rue de Prony 75017 Paris, France	6

Table 13.1   (Continued)

Name and Address	Chapter Reference
Pan American Health Organization 525 23rd Street, NW Washington, DC 20037	2, 3, 4, 5
Polio Connection of America P.O. Box 182 Howard Beach, NY 11414	5
Society of Environmental Toxicology and Chemistry 1010 North 12th Avenue Pensacola, FL 32501	7
Society for the Study of Amphibians and Reptiles Department of Biology, Saint Louis University St. Louis, MO 63103-2010	7, 8
Society of Nematologists P.O. Box 1897 Lawrence, KS 66044	2, 3, 5, 6
Society of Toxicology 1767 Business Center Drive, Suite 302 Reston, VA 20190	7
U.S. Air Force BASH Program Air Force Safety Center 9700 G Avenue SE Kirtland AFB, NM 87117	8
United States Animal Health Association P.O. Box K227 Richmond, VA 23288	6
U.S. Army Medical Research Institute of Infectious Disease (USAMRIID) Fort Detrick Frederick, MD 21702	4, 9
U.S. Consumer Product Safety Commission 4330 East-West Highway Bethesda, MD 20814-4408	3, 9
U.S. Department of Agriculture Animal and Plant Health Inspection Service (APHIS) National Biological Control Institute (NBCI) 4700 River Road, Unit 5 Riverdale, MD 20737-1229	6

(continued)

Table 13.1   (Continued)

Name and Address	Chapter Reference
U.S. Department of Agriculture Food Safety Inspection Service (FSIS) Washington, DC 20250	3, 9
U.S. Department of Agriculture Wildlife Services 1201 Oakridge Drive Fort Collins, CO 80525	8
U.S. Food and Drug Administration Center for Food Safety and Applied Nutrition 200 C Street SW Washington, DC 20204	3, 9
U.S. Public Health Service Centers for Disease Control and Prevention Health Studies Branch Disaster Assessment and Epidemiology Division of Environmental Hazards and Health Effects NCEH/CDC 4770 Buford Highway Atlanta, GA 30341	2, 3, 4, 5
Water Quality Association 4151 Napierville Road Lisle, IL 60532	2
World Health Organization Avenue Appia 20 1211 Geneva 27 Switzerland	2, 3, 4, 5

Table 13.2
Some Disaster Management and Safety Organizations

American Academy on Veterinary Disaster
    Medicine
P.O. Box 34
West River, MD 20778

American College of Emergency Physicians
Section on Disaster Medicine
P.O. Box 619911
Dallas, TX 75261-9911

American Red Cross
National Headquarters
Disaster Services Department
431 18th Street NW
Washington, DC 20006

Association of Contingency Planners
7044 South 13th Street
Oak Creek, WI 53154

Canadian Center for Emergency Preparedness
P.O. Box 2911
Hamilton, Ontario, Canada L8N 3R5

Center for Civilian Biodefense Strategies
Johns Hopkins University
Candler Building, Suite 850, 111 Market Place
Baltimore, MD 21202

Center for the Study of Emergency
    Management
112 N. Harvard Avenue, Suite 30
Claremont, CA 91711

Center of Excellence in Disaster Management
    and Humanitarian Assistance
Tripler Army Medical Center
1 Jarrett White Road (MCPA-DM)
Tripler AMC, HI 96859-5000

Centre for Research on Epidemiology of
    Disasters
Unit of Epidemiology
School of Public Health
Catholic University of Louvain
30.94 Clos Chappelle-aux-Champs
1200 Brussels, Belgium

Chemical and Biological Information Analysis
    Center
Battelle Memorial Institute
Aberdeen Proving Ground
P.O. Box 196
Gunpowder, MD 21010-0196

Disaster Recovery Institute International
1810 Craig Road, Suite 125
St. Louis, MO

European Centre for Disaster Medicine
Ministry of Public Health, State Hospital
47893 Republic of San Marino

Federal Emergency Management Agency
500 C Street, SW
Washington, DC 20472

Harvard Center for Risk Analysis
Harvard School of Public Health
718 Huntington Avenue
Boston, MA 02115

Hazardous Materials Advisory Council
1101 Vermont Avenue NW, Suite 301
Washington, DC 20005

Institute for Business and Home Safety
175 Federal Street, Suite 500
Boston, MA 02110-2222

Institute for Crisis, Disaster, and Risk
    Management
George Washington University
20101 Academic Way, Room 220
Ashburn, VA 22011

International Association of Emergency
    Managers
111 Park Place
Falls Church, VA 22046-4513

International Federation of Red Cross and Red
    Crescent Societies (IFRC)
P.O. Box 372
CH-1211 Geneva 19, Switzerland

(continued)

Table 13.2   (Continued)

International Medical Corps
11500 W. Olympic Boulevard, Suite 506
Los Angeles, CA 90064

Medicins Sans Frontieres
[Doctors Without Borders]
International Office
Rue de la Tourelle, 39
Brussels, Belgium 1040

National Academy of Sciences/National
  Research Council
Board on Natural Disasters
2101 Constitution Avenue, NW, HA 468E
Washington, DC 20418

National Emergency Management Association
P.O. Box 11910
Lexington, KY 40578-1910

National Emergency Training Center
16825 South Seton Avenue
Emmitsburg, MD 21727

National Response Center
2100 Second Street, SW, Room 2611
Washington, DC 20593

Natural Hazards Center
Campus Box 482
University of Colorado
Boulder, CO 80309

Pacific Disaster Center
590 Lipoa Parkway, Suite 259
Kihei, Maui, HI 96753

Society for Risk Analysis
1313 Dolley Madison Boulevard, Suite 402
McLean, VA 22101

Special Medical Agencies Response Teams
P.O. Box 874
New Albany, IN 47151-0874

United Nations Development Programme
  (UNDP)
Emergency Response Division (ERD)
1 UN Plaza
New York, NY 10017

United Nations Food and Agriculture
  Organization (FAO)
Emergency Prevention System (EMPRES)
Rome, Italy

United Nations Industrial Development
  Organization (UNIDO)
Biosafety Information Network and Advisory
  Service
1 UN Plaza
New York, NY 10017

U.S. Agency for International Development
  (USAID)
Office of Foreign Disaster Assistance (OFDA)
Ronald Reagan Building
Washington, DC 20523-0016

U.S. Environmental Protection Agency
Chemical Emergency Preparedness and
  Prevention Office
Office of Solid Waste and Emergency
  Response
401 M Street, SW
Washington, DC 20460

U.S. Geological Survey
Center for Integration of Natural Disaster
  Information
MS-500, National Center
Reston, VA 20192

U.S. Public Health Service
Office of Emergency Preparedness
National Disaster Medical System
12300 Twinbrook Parkway, Suite 360
Rockville, MD 20852

Glossary

When a torrent sweeps a man against a boulder, you must expect
him to scream, and you need not be surprised if the scream is
sometimes a theory.
—Robert Louis Stevenson, *Virginibus Puerisque*

absinthe. (1) A highly toxic herb (*Artemisia*). (2)
A liqueur that contains absinthe. (3) An anise-
flavored liqueur that contains no absinthe.

acaricide. Any chemical used to kill mites.

acetylcholine. A chemical that transmits nerve
impulses in the body.

aconitine. A toxin produced by monkshood (*Ac-
onitum*) and related plants.

active immunity. *See* immunity.

acute. Having a sudden onset, sharp rise, and
short course.

acute idiopathic polyneuritis. *See* Guillain-Barré
syndrome.

adenovirus. Any of a group of DNA viruses that
cause acute respiratory infections and other
diseases in humans.

aerosol. Tiny particles (droplet nuclei, dust,
spores, etc.) suspended in air.

aflatoxin. Any of a group of cancer-causing toxins produced by the fungus *Aspergillus flavus*.

African sleeping sickness. An infectious disease
caused by the protozoans *Trypanosoma
gambiense* and *T. rhodesiense*, transmitted by
the tsetse fly.

African swine fever (ASF). An infectious disease of swine caused by a DNA virus.

ague. Old term for the fever and chills of malaria.

AIDS. Acquired immune deficiency syndrome;
a T-cell deficiency disease caused by infection with the human immunodeficiency
virus (HIV).

airborne transmission. Transmission of an infectious agent to a susceptible host by inhalation of an aerosol. (The inhalation of larger
droplets, such as those produced by a sneeze
at close range, is regarded as direct contact
transmission.)

algae. A group that includes various unicellular and multicellular photosynthetic organisms; all were formerly regarded as plants,
but many are now classified as Protista. *See*
cyanobacteria.

alkaloid. Any of a diverse group of plant chemicals with pharmacological activity.

allergen. A substance to which an individual is
hypersensitive; can cause a local inflammatory reaction or, in some cases, severe shock.
See anaphylactic shock; anaphylaxis.

Glossary

allergy. An immunologically mediated adverse reaction to a chemical, resulting from previous sensitization to that chemical or a similar one; examples are hay fever or contact dermatitis.

alveolar hydatid disease (AHD). *See* echinococcosis.

alpha-hemolytic streptococcus. Any of a group of *Streptococcus* bacteria with certain enzymes that break down red blood cells.

amanitin. A highly toxic peptide produced by the death cap mushroom (*Amanita phalloides*).

amatoxin. Any of a group of toxins produced by mushrooms in the genus *Amanita*.

ameba (or **amoeba**). Any of a group of protozoans.

amebiasis. Infection with an ameba.

American trypanosomiasis. *See* Chagas' disease.

amnesic shellfish poisoning. An illness caused by ingestion of shellfish contaminated with domoic acid.

amygdalin. A plant toxin that releases cyanide when digested.

anaerobic. Occurring in the absence of oxygen.

anaphylactic shock. Severe, sometimes fatal shock symptoms resulting from exposure to an antigen to which an individual is hypersensitive (allergic).

anaphylactoid reaction. A syndrome resembling an anaphylactic reaction, but dose dependent and reversible by removal of the antigen.

anaphylaxis. A rapid hypersensitive response arising on second exposure to a foreign antigen.

anatoxin. A neurotoxin produced by *Anabaena flos-aquae*, a cyanobacterium.

angel's trumpet. Any of several highly toxic ornamental plants in the genus *Datura* or *Brugmansia*.

anisakiasis. Infestation with nematodes in the family Anisakidae.

antagonism (in toxicology). The situation in which two chemicals administered together interfere with each other's actions.

anthrax. An infectious disease of livestock and humans, caused by the bacterium *Bacillus anthracis*.

antibiotic. Any of a number of organic compounds, either produced by microorganisms or synthesized in the laboratory, that can kill or inhibit the growth of other microorganisms.

antibiotic resistance. The ability of certain microorganisms to resist antibiotics. *See* plasmid.

antibody. A protein that acts against a specific antigen in the body.

antigen. Any substance (usually a foreign protein) that provokes an immune response and is capable of specific binding to an antibody or a T-cell receptor.

antigenic shift. The appearance of a new strain of a pathogen, such as influenza A.

antihistamine. Any of various chemical compounds that counteract histamine in the body; used to treat allergic reactions and symptoms of the common cold.

antiseptic. A chemical that prevents the growth of microorganisms.

antiserum. A serum containing antibodies.

antitoxin. An antibody that is capable of neutralizing a specific toxin in the body, or a serum containing such antibodies.

antivenin or **antivenom**. An antitoxin to a venom, or a serum containing such antitoxins.

apiary. A collection of hives in a beekeeping establishment.

arbovirus. An arthropod-borne virus; not a taxonomic group.

ARC. AIDS-related complex.

arenavirus. Any of a group of RNA viruses that cause diseases such as Lassa fever and lymphocytic choriomeningitis.

Argentinian hemorrhagic fever. An infectious disease caused by the Junin virus.

arthritis. Inflammation of joints.

arthropod. Any of a group of invertebrate animals with a segmented body, jointed appendages, and usually a hard exoskeleton; includes the insects, spiders, mites, scorpions, crustaceans, and others.

ascariasis. Infestation with parasitic worms, especially roundworms (*Ascaris*).

asepsis. The condition of being aseptic.

aseptic. (1) Preventing infection. (2) Free of pathogenic microorganisms.

aseptic meningitis. *See* viral meningitis.

ASP. Amnesic shellfish poisoning.

aspergillosis. Infection with the fungus *Aspergillus*.

aspergillus. A fungus (genus *Aspergillus*) that can grow on stored grains, legumes, and nuts.

asthma. A condition characterized by labored breathing, wheezing, coughing, and a sense of constriction in the chest.

astrovirus. An RNA virus in the family Astroviridae.

atropine. An alkaloid produced by a number of plants in the family Solanaceae, such as jimson weed and nightshade.

Aujeszky's disease. *See* pseudorabies.

avian influenza. An infectious disease of birds, caused by an avian strain of influenza virus.

B cell or B lymphocyte. A lymphocyte that differentiates to become an antibody-producing plasma cell after encountering an antigen.

babesiosis. An infectious disease of domestic animals and humans, caused by the protozoan *Babesia microti* and transmitted by ticks.

bacillary dysentery. *See* shigellosis.

bacteria. Microscopic, single-celled organisms that lack a nucleus.

bacterial meningitis. Meningitis caused by a bacterial infection (often due to group B streptococcus, Hib, the meningococcus, or *Listeria monocytogenes*).

bacterial pneumonia. Pneumonia caused by a bacterial infection.

bacteriological warfare. *See* biological warfare.

bacteriophage. A virus that infects bacteria.

balantidiasis. A waterborne or foodborne disease of the human colon, caused by the protozoan *Balantidium coli*.

bark scorpion. Any of several venomous scorpions in the genus *Centruroides*.

batrachotoxin. A potent neurotoxin produced by certain South African frogs.

BCG vaccine. A vaccine that provides immunity from mycobacterial infection, made from a weakened strain of *Mycobacterium tuberculosis*, var. *bovis*.

bejel. A nonvenereal infectious disease similar to syphilis.

belladonna. (1) Nightshade. (2) Atropine or a similar medicinal extract obtained from nightshade and related plants.

benign lymphoreticulosis. *See* cat-scratch fever.

benign tertian malaria. A relatively mild form of malaria caused by the protozoan *Plasmodium vivax*.

beta-hemolytic streptococcus. Any of a group of *Streptococcus* bacteria with certain enzymes that break down red blood cells, forming a clear zone around the colony on a blood agar medium.

bilharzia. *See* schistosomiasis.

bilious. Showing signs of jaundice.

biohazard. *See* biological hazard.

biological disaster. As defined in this book, a disaster with a biological cause.

biological hazard. (1) Any hazard of biological origin. (2) Infectious or cytotoxic waste. (3) Any hazard that affects living organisms.

biological warfare. Warfare in which the weapons are living organisms (usually pathogenic bacteria) or toxins of biological origin.

biological weapon. An organism (usually microscopic) or biological toxin used as an instrument of warfare or terrorism.

bioterrorism. Terrorist activity involving the use of biological weapons.

Black Death. A series of major plague epidemics that started in 1347 and killed about half the population of England and continental Europe.

black water fever. In malignant tertiary malaria, the presence of hemoglobin in the urine.

black widow. A venomous spider (*Latrodectus*).

blastomycosis. (1) An airborne disease of the lungs caused by any of several fungi. (2) European blastomycosis, another name for cryptococcosis.

blight. Any of several plant diseases.

blue-green algae. *See* cyanobacteria.

bluetongue. An infectious disease of cattle, caused by a reovirus.

Bolivian hemorrhagic fever. An infectious disease caused by the Machupo virus.

Borna disease. An infectious encephalomyelitis of cats, horses, and other animals, caused by a bornavirus.

bornavirus. A member of a newly recognized family of RNA viruses.

borreliosis. Any of several diseases caused by bacteria in the genus *Borrelia*, such as Lyme disease.

botulin. A neurotoxin produced by the anaerobic bacterium *Clostridium botulinum*.

botulism. An acute paralytic foodborne or waterborne disease caused by botulin.

bovine respiratory disease. *See* pneumonic pasteurellosis.

bovine spongiform encephalopathy (BSE). An infectious foodborne disease of cattle, caused by a prion.

Brainerd diarrhea. A syndrome of acute onset of watery diarrhea lasting four weeks or longer; the agent is unknown.

breakbone fever. *See* dengue fever.

breakthrough infection. An infectious disease acquired after vaccination for that disease.

brevetoxin. A neurotoxin produced by the marine dinoflagellate *Gymnodinium breve*.

brown spider. *See* recluse.

brucellosis. An infectious disease of livestock and humans, caused by bacteria in the genus *Brucella*.

BSE. Bovine spongiform encephalopathy.

bubo. An inflammatory swelling of a lymph node.

bubonic plague. The most common presentation of plague in humans; the name refers to the presence of swollen lymph nodes (buboes).

bufotenine. A psychedelic chemical derived from secretions of certain toads.

bufotoxin. A toxin produced by cells in the skin of toads.

bunyavirus. Any of a group of RNA viruses that cause Rift Valley fever and some forms of encephalitis; related viruses also infect plants.

Buruli ulcer. A skin ulcer caused by a toxin produced by *Mycobacterium ulcerans*.

cable mites and **paper mites**. Invisible or nonexistent mites that cause otherwise unexplained itching; both have figured prominently in delusional parasitosis and urban folklore.

calicivirus. Any of a group of RNA viruses that cause various diseases in humans and livestock; an example is the hepatitis E virus.

California encephalitis. A form of encephalitis caused by a bunyavirus and transmitted by mosquitoes.

camp fever. *See* epidemic typhus.

camphor. (1) A tree (*Cinnamomum camphora*) that contains chemicals used as insecticides and pharmaceuticals. (2) Paradichlorobenzene or moth crystals, a synthetic insecticide.

campylobacteriosis. Infection with bacteria in the genus *Campylobacter*.

cancer. Any of numerous diseases caused by abnormal changes in cells that lead to the growth of invasive tumors in the body.

candidiasis. Infection with a fungus of the genus *Candida*.

candirú. A small South American catfish (*Vandellia cirrhosa*) that can lodge in the human urethra.

canine distemper. An infectious disease of dogs and other mammals, caused by a paramixovirus.

cantharidin. A toxic chemical found in blister beetles.

carcinogen. A chemical, virus, or other agent that causes cancer.

cardiotoxin. A toxin that acts primarily on the cardiovascular system.

carrier. An individual infected with a disease but showing no symptoms.

case. An individual animal or person with an infectious or parasitic disease.

case-control study. A study design in which the investigators compare two groups of subjects, one group with a given disease (cases) and the other without the disease (controls), to assess the role of exposure to a possible causal factor.

cat-scratch fever. An infectious disease caused by the bacterium *Bartonella henselae* and possibly other bacteria.

catarrh. Inflammation of a mucous membrane, as from the common cold or allergic rhinitis.

CBW. Chemical and biological warfare.

CDC. The U.S. Public Health Service Centers for Disease Control and Prevention.

cephalotoxin. A toxin found in the salivary glands of octopi.

cestodes. Tapeworms.

Chagas' disease. An infectious disease caused by the protozoan *Trypanosoma cruzi*, transmitted by cone-nosed bugs or kissing bugs (Reduviidae).

chancre. An ulcer that appears in primary syphilis.

chancroid. A sexually transmitted disease caused by the bacterium *Haemophilus ducreyi*.

chemical idiosyncrasy. A genetically determined abnormal reaction to a chemical.

chickenpox. An infectious disease caused by the varicella-zoster virus (HHV-3).

chigger. A parasitic mite larva.

Chikungunya virus. A mosquito-borne togavirus that causes hemorrhagic fever.

chlamydia. A sexually transmitted disease caused by the bacterium *Chlamydia trachomatis*.

cholera. An infectious waterborne or foodborne disease caused by the bacterium *Vibrio cholerae*.

choriomeningitis. Meningitis with cellular infiltration of the meninges.

chronic. Marked by long duration or frequent recurrence.

ciguatera. A form of poisoning that results from eating certain marine fishes that have fed on dinoflagellates.

ciguatoxin. A neurotoxin produced by the marine dinoflagellate *Gambierdiscus toxicus*.

CJD. Creutzfeldt-Jakob disease.

clap. Slang term for gonorrhea.

Class 1 reportable disease. A disease that is subject to the International Health Regulations and/or under surveillance by the World Health Organization.

Class 2 reportable disease. A disease for which a case report is regularly required wherever the disease occurs.

Class 3 reportable disease. A disease that is selectively reportable in recognized endemic areas.

Class 4 reportable disease. A disease for which only epidemics must be reported.

Class 5 reportable disease. A disease for which an official report is not ordinarily justifiable.

classical swine fever. *See* hog cholera.

cocaine. An alkaloid derived from leaves of the coca plant (*Erythroxylon coca*).

coccidian. A parasitic protozoan of the order Coccidia.

coccidioidomycosis. An infectious airborne disease caused by the fungus *Coccidioides immitis*.

coccidiosis. Infestation with coccidian protozoa.

coccus (plural, cocci). A spherical bacterium.

cohort. A defined population that is followed in an epidemiological study.

Colorado tick fever. An infectious disease caused by a reovirus and transmitted by ticks.

colostrum. The first milk secreted by the mammary glands at the end of pregnancy, containing antibodies that give the infant temporary passive immunity to some diseases.

common cold. An upper respiratory infection caused by many different viruses.

communicable disease. A disease that results when an infectious agent is transmitted directly or indirectly from a reservoir to a susceptible host.

cone-nose bug. Any of several blood-sucking insects in the genus *Triatoma*.

Congo fever. A tickborne hemorrhagic fever caused by a bunyavirus.

conjunctivitis. An inflammation of the mucous membrane that lines the inner surface of the eyelids; caused by various bacteria and viruses.

conotoxin. A toxin produced by several marine snails in the genus *Conus*.

consumption. Old name for tuberculosis.

contact. (1) Association with an infected person or animal or with a contaminated environment. (2) A person or animal that has been in such association.

contagious disease. A disease that one susceptible host can transmit to another.

contamination. The presence of an infectious agent or other unwanted material.

coronavirus. Any of a group of RNA viruses that cause respiratory diseases such as the common cold.

cowpox. A mild infectious disease of cattle; humans who contract this disease become immune to smallpox.

coxiellosis. *See* Q fever.

coxsackievirus. Any of a group of picornaviruses that cause diseases such as pharyngotonsillitis and the common cold.

crack. A highly purified form of cocaine.

Creutzfeldt-Jakob disease (CJD). A spongiform encephalopathy in human beings, caused by a prion.

Crimean hemorrhagic fever. *See* Congo fever.

crotalid. Any of a family of snakes (Crotalidae) that includes the rattlesnakes and other pit vipers.

croup. An upper respiratory disease of children, caused by any of several viruses.

cryptococcosis. An airborne infectious disease caused by the fungus *Cryptococcus neoformans*.

cryptosporidiosis. A waterborne or foodborne infectious disease of humans and various herd animals, caused by the protozoan *Cryptosporidium parvum*.

cyanobacteria. A group of primitive, photosynthetic bacteria; also called blue-green algae.

cyanosis. A bluish coloration of the skin caused by oxygen deficiency.

cyclosporosis. A waterborne or foodborne infectious disease caused by coccidian protozoa in the genus *Cyclospora*.

cysticercosis. Infestation with the larval stage of the pork tapeworm.

cytomegalovirus (CMV). A common herpesvirus, potentially fatal to infants if transmitted during pregnancy.

cytotoxic. Toxic to cells.

cytotoxic T cell. A T lymphocyte that recognizes and kills body cells that have been altered, usually as a result of virus infection.

death cap. A highly toxic mushroom (*Amanita phalloides* and related species).

delta agent. The hepatitis D virus (HDV).

delusional parasitosis. The belief that one is infested by numerous external or internal parasites, often of types unknown to science.

dengue fever. An infectious disease caused by a flavivirus and transmitted by mosquitoes.

dermatitis. Inflammation of the skin.

dermatophytosis. A skin infection caused by a fungus.

devil's grip. *See* pleurodynia.

diarrhea. Abnormally frequent bowel movements with more or less liquid stool.

dinoflagellate. Any of a group of unicellular, mostly marine planktonic organisms.

diphtheria. An infectious disease caused by a toxin that is produced by the bacterium *Corynebacterium diphtheriae* when it contains a prophage.

direct transmission. Transmission of an infectious agent directly from an infected person or animal to a susceptible host.

disaster. A sudden event bringing great damage, loss, or destruction.

disease. A condition of a living organism that impairs normal functioning.

disinfection. Procedures intended to destroy the infectious or parasitic agents of diseases.

DNA virus. A virus in which the genetic material consists of deoxyribonucleic acid (DNA).

domoic acid. A toxin produced by certain marine diatoms; causes amnesic shellfish poisoning.

dope. A slang term for almost any street drug.

dose. (1) A measured quantity of a therapeutic agent. (2) A slang term for gonorrhea.

dose-response relationship. A graph or equation describing the response of an individual or population of a given species to varying doses of a given chemical.

DPT or **DTP**. A vaccine that protects children against diphtheria, pertussis, and tetanus.

dracontiasis or **dracunculiasis**. Infestation with the nematode worm *Dracunculus medinensis*.

droplet nuclei. Residues released into the air when fluid from an infected host evaporates.

Durban Declaration. A statement signed by several thousand physicians and researchers in 2000, affirming that HIV is the cause of AIDS.

dust mite. Any of a group of mites (Pyroglyphidae) that live in beds, carpets, and upholstery.

dysentery. Severe diarrhea with passage of mucus and blood.

E. coli. The common name for bacteria of the species *Escherichia coli*.

eastern equine encephalitis (EEE). A form of encephalitis caused by a group A togavirus and transmitted by mosquitoes.

Ebola hemorrhagic fever. An infectious disease caused by a filovirus.

echinococcosis. An infestation with the tapeworm *Echinococcus granulosus*.

echovirus or **ECHO** (enteric cytopathogenic human orphan) **virus**. A picornavirus associated with fever, aseptic meningitis, and respiratory disease.

ectoparasite. A parasite that lives on the exterior of its host.

ehrlichiosis. An infectious disease of humans, domestic animals, and wildlife, caused by bacteria in the genus *Ehrlichia* and transmitted by ticks.

elapid. Any of a family of snakes (Elapidae) that includes the coral snakes and cobras.

elephantiasis. (1) Massive swelling of a body part due to filariasis. (2) Massive enlargement of a body part due to any disease or disorder.

emerging disease. A disease whose incidence in humans has increased within the past two decades, or threatens to increase in the near future.

emetic. An agent that causes vomiting.

encephalitis. Inflammation of the brain.

encephalopathy. A disease of the brain, especially one that involves changes in brain structure. **endemic**. (1) Of a disease: always present in a given geographic area, but not unique to that area. (2) Of an animal or plant species: uniquely present in a given geographic area.

endemic typhus. An infectious disease caused by *Rickettsia mooseri* and transmitted by flea-bites.

endocarditis. Inflammation of the lining and valves of the heart.

endoparasite. A parasite that lives inside its host.

endotoxin. A bacterial toxin that is an integral component of the cell and remains within or attached to the cell.

enteritis. Inflammation of the intestine.

enterobiasis. Infestation with pinworms.

enterococcus. Any of several species of bacteria normally found in the human intestinal tract.

enterotoxin. A bacterial toxin that affects the intestines.

enterovirus. Any of a group of viruses that includes the polioviruses, coxsackieviruses, echoviruses, and others.

enzootic. Describes an animal disease that is always present within a given geographic area.

enzyme. A protein that catalyzes a biological reaction.

ephedra. A toxic herbal preparation sold by health-food dealers; studies have linked its use to adverse effects including kidney stone formation, vasculitis, and hypersensitivity myocarditis.

epidemic. The occurrence of a higher-than-expected number of cases of a given human illness, often derived from a common source.

epidemic typhus. An infectious disease caused by *Rickettsia prowazekii* and transmitted by lice.

epidemiology. (1) The science that deals with the incidence, distribution, and control of disease in a population. (2) The factors controlling the presence or absence of a disease or pathogen.

epizootic. An outbreak of disease affecting many animals of the same species.

Epstein-Barr virus (EBV). A herpesvirus that causes infectious mononucleosis and other diseases such as pharyngotonsillitis.

ergot. A fungus that grows on rye.

ergotin. A mycotoxin produced by ergot.

ergotism. A toxic condition produced by ergotin or by an ergot drug.

erysipelas. An acute infectious disease caused by hemolytic streptococci.

eschar. A crusted or necrosed area on the skin.

eukaryote. An organism composed of one or more cells that contain a membrane-bounded nucleus and organelles.

exanthem subitum. *See* roseola.

exotic. Foreign; not native to the place where found.

exotoxin. A toxin secreted by bacteria.

exposure. An opportunity to contract a disease.

falciparum malaria. *See* malignant tertian malaria.

FAO. United Nations Food and Agriculture Organization.

fasciolopsiasis. Infestation with the trematode *Fasciolopsis buski*.

fatality rate. The percentage of persons with a given illness who die as a result of that illness.

favism. A form of anemia that can occur in persons who eat undercooked beans and also have a hereditary enzyme deficiency.

fecal-oral route. A route of disease transmission in which fecal contamination is transferred to the mouth, often by a food preparer with inadequately washed hands.

fifth disease. A usually mild rash illness caused by the human parvovirus B19.

filariasis. Infestation with any of several nematode worms that release microfilariae (larvae) into the bloodstream.

filovirus. Any of a group of RNA viruses that can cause severe hemorrhagic fevers in humans and non-human primates.

flavivirus. Any of a group of RNA viruses that cause diseases such as dengue and yellow fever.

flesh-eating bacteria. *See* necrotizing fasciitis.

flu. *See* influenza.

flux. An obsolete term for dysentery.

fomite. An inanimate object contaminated with an infectious agent.

food poisoning. (1) Gastrointestinal illness caused by toxins produced by foodborne bacteria. (2) Any gastrointestinal illness caused by a foodborne infectious agent.

foodborne disease. A disease caused by an infectious agent ingested with food.

foot-and-mouth disease. An infectious disease of livestock, caused by a picornavirus.

fowl cholera. An infectious disease of birds caused by the bacterium *Pasteurella multocida*.

fowl plague. *See* avian influenza.

fugu poison. *See* tetrodotoxin.

fulminant. Occurring suddenly, with great intensity or severity (of a disease).

fungicide. Any chemical used for the destruction of fungi.

fungus. Any of a group of organisms of organisms including yeasts, molds, and mushrooms; most taxonomists now treat the fungi as a separate kingdom.

gamma globulin. *See* human gamma globulin.

gas gangrene. Tissue necrosis caused by anaerobic bacteria in the genus *Clostridium*.

gastroenteritis. Inflammation of the lining of the stomach and intestines.

genetic toxicology. The branch of toxicology that deals with the effects of chemicals on DNA in living cells.

genital herpes. Herpesvirus lesions on the genitalia; caused by HSV-1 or HSV-2.

germ warfare. *See* biological warfare.

German measles. *See* rubella.

giardiasis. A waterborne disease caused by the protozoan *Giardia lamblia*.

glanders. An infectious disease of horses and donkeys, caused by bacteria in the genus *Pseudomonas*; occasionally transmitted to humans.

gonorrhea. A sexually transmitted disease caused by the bacterium *Neisseria gonorrhoeae*.

gonyautoxin. A component of paralytic shellfish poison, produced by dinoflagellates.

gram negative. A term describing bacteria that appear light red after a standard staining procedure.

gram positive. A term describing bacteria that appear dark blue-violet after a standard staining procedure.

grayanotoxin. A toxin found in some plants of the family Ericaceae; honey made from the nectar of these plants can be toxic to humans.

green monkey virus. The Marburg filovirus, the agent of Marburg hemorrhagic fever.

grippe. *See* influenza.

grocer's itch. A skin disease caused by mites (*Glycophagus*) in sugar or flour.

group A streptococcus (GAS). Any of a group of *Streptococcus* bacteria that cause many human diseases such as endocarditis, "strep" throat, impetigo, and necrotizing fasciitis; most are beta-hemolytic.

group B streptococcus (GBS). Any of a group of *Streptococcus* bacteria that cause many human diseases including severe neonatal pneumonia and meningitis; many are alpha-hemolytic.

Guillain-Barré syndrome. Paralysis or muscular weakness that may occur after certain viral infections.

guinea worm disease. *See* dracontiasis.

hand, foot and mouth disease. An infectious disease of children caused by a coxsackievirus. It is not related to foot-and-mouth disease of livestock.

Hansen's disease. An infectious disease caused by the bacterium *Mycobacterium* leprae.

hantavirus. Any of a group of bunyaviruses that cause various human diseases, including hemorrhagic fever with renal syndrome (HFRS) and hantavirus pulmonary syndrome (HPS).

hantavirus pulmonary syndrome (HPS). A New World infectious disease caused by any of several hantaviruses, including the Sin Nombre, Bayou, Black Creek Canal, Monongahela, and New York viruses.

hashish. The concentrated resin of the female hemp plant (*Cannabis sativa*).

hazard. A potential source of danger.

helminth. Any of a number of parasitic worms.

helper T cell. A T lymphocyte that is activated by foreign antigen on a cell surface and, in turn, activates B cells.

hemolytic uremic syndrome. A form of kidney failure that can occur for various reasons, especially after food poisoning with *Escherichia coli* O157.

hemorrhagic fever. A syndrome of high fever with severe internal and/or external bleeding; can occur in any of several infectious diseases, many of them caused by arboviruses.

hemorrhagic jaundice. *See* leptospirosis.

hemotoxin. A toxin that causes destruction of red blood cells.

hemp. A widely cultivated plant (*Cannabis sativa*) whose fibers are used for making rope; also the source of marijuana and hashish.

Hendra virus. A paramyxovirus that infects livestock and humans, causing a form of encephalitis.

hepadnavirus. A DNA virus that causes hepatitis B.

hepatitis. Any of several diseases marked by inflammation of the liver.

hepatitis A virus (HAV). A foodborne or waterborne picornavirus that can cause acute or subacute hepatitis, with recovery usual.

hepatitis B virus (HBV). A hepadnavirus that can cause chronic hepatitis with permanent liver damage and an increased risk of liver cancer; transmitted by blood products or sexual activity.

hepatitis C virus (HCV). An RNA virus that can cause acute or chronic hepatitis with permanent liver damaged and an increased risk of liver cancer; transmitted by blood products, sexual activity, or unknown means.

hepatitis D virus (HDV). A defective virus (similar to a plant viroid) that is often associated with HBV; infection with both HBV and HDV can cause severe acute or chronic hepatitis.

hepatitis E virus (HEV). A waterborne, calicivirus-like RNA virus or virion that has caused large epidemics of hepatitis in India, Africa, and Mexico.

hepatitis F virus (HFV). A little-known virus that apparently causes some sporadic cases of human hepatitis.

hepatitis G virus (HGV or GBV-C). A recently discovered, apparently harmless hepatitis virus that has been reported to interfere with HIV infection.

herbicide. Any chemical used for the destruction of plants.

herd immunity. Immunity (to a given disease) in a high enough percentage of a population that spread of the disease is unlikely.

heroin. An addictive narcotic drug derived from morphine.

herpes labialis. Cold sores or fever blisters.

herpes simplex. An infectious disease that takes various forms, ranging from fever blisters or genital lesions to a generalized infection or encephalitis; caused by the herpes simplex viruses. *See* HSV-1; HSV-2.

herpes zoster. *See* chickenpox.

herpesvirus. Any of a group of DNA viruses that cause various diseases, ranging in severity from fever blisters to some cancers.

HFRS. Hemorrhagic fever with renal syndrome.

HHV. *See* human herpesvirus and HSV headings.

Hib. *Haemophilus influenzae* serotype B.

Hib conjugate vaccine. A vaccine used to protect children against Hib disease.

Hib disease. An infectious disease, often presenting as pneumonia or meningitis, caused by the bacterium *Haemophilus influenzae* serotype B.

histamine. A compound released by the body during allergic reactions, causing dilatation of capillaries and contraction of smooth muscle.

histamine poisoning. *See* scombroid poisoning.

histoplasmosis. An infectious disease caused by the fungus *Histoplasma capsulatum*.

HIV. The human immunodeficiency virus, a retrovirus that causes AIDS.

hog cholera. An infectious disease of swine, caused by an RNA virus.

hoof-and-mouth disease. An incorrect name for foot-and-mouth disease.

hookworm. Any of several parasitic nematode worms that infest humans and domestic animals.

host. A person (or other animal) used by an infectious agent for subsistence or lodgment.

HPS. *See* hantavirus pulmonary syndrome.

HSV-1 (herpes simplex virus type 1). A herpesvirus that causes fever blisters, genital sores, and some forms of encephalitis.

HSV-2 (herpes simplex virus type 2). A herpesvirus that causes primarily genital lesions.

HTLV-I (human T-cell lymphotropic virus type I). A retrovirus associated with two human diseases, adult T-cell leukemia and tropical spastic paraparesis.

human gamma globulin. A preparation of human plasma containing the antibodies of normal adults.

human herpesvirus 1 (HHV-1). *See* HSV-1.

human herpesvirus 2 (HHV-2). *See* HSV-2.

human herpesvirus 3 (HHV-3). *See* varicella-zoster virus.

human herpesvirus 4 (HHV-4). *See* Epstein-Barr virus.

human herpesvirus 5 (HHV-5). *See* cytomegalovirus.

human herpesvirus 6 (HHV-6). A herpesvirus that causes roseola and may be associated with the development of multiple sclerosis.

human herpesvirus 7 (HHV-7). Another herpesvirus that causes roseola.

human herpesvirus 8 (HHV-8). A herpesvirus associated with Kaposi's sarcoma in AIDS patients.

human parainfluenza viruses (HPIVs). Any of a group of viruses that cause respiratory tract illness in humans.

humoral immunity. Immunity associated with circulating antibodies, and thus restricted to the blood.

HUS. Hemolytic uremic syndrome.

hydatid disease or hydatidosis. *See* echinococcosis.

hydrophobia. *See* rabies.

hypersensitivity. *See* allergy.

ichthyotoxism. Poisoning that results from eating toxic fish.

Ig. *See* immunoglobulin.

IHR. International Health Regulations.

immune. Having protective antibodies or cellular immunity to a given disease as a result of prior exposure or immunization.

immunity. Resistance to an infectious agent, usually associated with possession of antibodies. Short-term passive immunity results from maternal transfer or inoculation with antibodies. Active immunity is present when the immune system produces its own antibodies following exposure.

immunization. The injection of an antigen, or a serum containing antibodies, to render a person or animal immune to a specific disease.

immunoglobulin (Ig). Any of a class of proteins that includes antibodies. Ig classes based on structure and antigenicity include IgG, IgA, IgM, IgD, and IgE.

impetigo. An infectious disease caused by group A streptococci.

inapparent infection. An infection that produces no noticeable symptoms.

incidence rate. The number of cases of a disease diagnosed or reported during a given time period, divided by the total number of persons or animals in the affected population; may be expressed as the rate for a specific age group, gender, or other subpopulation.

incubation period. The time interval between exposure to an infectious agent and the appearance of the first sign or symptom of the disease.

indirect transmission. Transmission of an infectious agent from an infected person or animal to a susceptible host by way of (1) the host's air, water, or food; (2) biological products, such as a transfusion of contaminated blood; (3) an insect or other vector; or (4) a contaminated object or surface.

infantile paralysis. *See* poliomyelitis.

infection. The entry and development or multiplication of an infectious agent in the body.

infectious agent. An organism that is capable of producing infection or infectious disease.

infectious disease. A disease resulting either from an infection or from overgrowth of a host's normal microbes.

infectious mononucleosis. An infectious disease caused by the Epstein-Barr virus. Some studies have suggested an association between this disease and multiple sclerosis.

infectious parotitis. *See* mumps.

infective dose. The dose (number of organisms) of a given pathogen necessary to contract the disease.

infective period. The longest period during which an affected animal or person can be a source of infection.

infestation. (1) The lodgment, development, and reproduction of arthropods on the body surface of or in clothing. (2) The presence of any parasite in or on a host.

influenza. An acute infectious respiratory disease caused by any of three main orthomyxoviruses, designated as type A (usually the most severe), type B, and type C.

insecticide. Any chemical used to kill insects or other arthropods.

intoxication. (1) An abnormal physiological state induced by a toxin or other poison. (2) The state of being incapacitated by alcohol or drugs.

invasive group A streptococcal disease. *See* group A streptococcus; necrotizing fasciitis; streptococcal toxic shock syndrome.

invasive group B streptococcal disease. *See* group B streptococcus.

IPPC. International Plant Protection Convention.

IPV. Inactivated polio vaccine.

jail fever. *See* epidemic typhus.

jaundice. (1) Yellowish pigmentation of the skin caused by liver disease. (2) Hepatitis.

Jesuit's bark. An old name for the bark of the cinchona tree, which contains quinine.

jimson weed. A toxic plant (*Datura stramonium*).

Junin virus. An arenavirus that causes Argentinian hemorrhagic fever.

kala-azar. *See* leishmaniasis.

Kaposi's sarcoma. A connective tissue tumor seen primarily in AIDS patients.

kava. An intoxicating beverage made from the root of an Australasian plant (*Piper methysticum*).

kissing bug. *See* cone-nose bug.

Koch's postulates. A standard test for determining causality of infectious disease: (1) The specific organism should be present in all animals with a specific disease, but not in other animals; (2) the organism should be isolated from the diseased animal and grown in pure culture on artificial media; (3) the isolated organism, when inoculated into a healthy animal, should cause the same disease seen in the original animal; (4) the organism should be reisolated in pure culture from the experimental infection.

kuru. An infectious disease endemic to the highlands of New Guinea, caused by a prion.

LaCrosse (LAC) encephalitis. A form of encephalitis caused by a bunyavirus and transmitted by tree-hole mosquitoes.

lambliasis. *See* giardiasis.

larva migrans. Any of several diseases caused by wandering of a larval worm (usually a nematode) in the host tissues.

Lassa fever. A hemorrhagic fever caused by an arenavirus.

latrodectism. The effects of the bite of the black widow and related spiders.

LD$_{50}$. The dose of a given poison required to kill 50 percent of exposed subjects.

leech. Any of a group of freshwater worms with a segmented body and a sucker at each end.

legionellosis or **Legionnaires' disease**. An infectious disease caused by *Legionella pneumophila* and related bacteria.

leishmaniasis. An infectious disease caused by protozoa in the genus *Leishmania*.

lentivirus. Any of a group of retroviruses that includes HIV and the maedi-visna virus.

leprosy. *See* Hansen's disease.

leptospirosis. An infectious disease of humans and domestic animals, caused by spirochetes in the genus *Leptospira*.

lesion. A wound, injury, or pathological change in a tissue.

lethality. Ability to cause death.

List A disease. A transmissible animal disease that has the potential for very serious, rapid international spread.

List B disease. A transmissible animal disease that has socioeconomic or public health importance within a country and that is significant in international trade.

listeriosis. An infectious disease caused by the bacterium *Listeria monocytogenes*.

lockjaw. *See* tetanus.

loco weed or **locoweed**. (1) Any of several North American plants in the genus *Astragalus* that can cause chronic poisoning in livestock or humans. (2) Jimson weed or datura.

locoism or **loco**. Intoxication by loco weed.

loxoscelism. The effects of the bite of the recluse and related violin spiders.

LSD. (1) Lumpy skin disease of cattle. (2) Lysergic acid diethylamide, a synthetic hallucinogen that is chemically related to mescaline and psilocybin.

lumpy skin disease. An infectious disease of cattle, caused by a poxvirus.

Lyme disease. An infectious disease caused by the spirochete *Borrelia burgdorferi* and transmitted by ticks.

lymphocyte. Any of several types of white blood cell involved in immune reactions. *See* B cell; T cell; natural killer cell.

lymphocytic choriomeningitis. An infection found primarily in mice and other laboratory animals, but transmissible to humans; caused by an arenavirus.

lyssavirus. A rhabdovirus similar to the rabies virus.

ma-huang. *See* ephedra.

MAC. *Mycobacterium avium* complex (the bacteria *M. avium* and *M. intracellulare*); associated with pulmonary disease, especially in persons with weakened immune systems.

Machupo virus. An arenavirus that causes Bolivian hemorrhagic fever.

maculotoxin. A toxin produced by the blue-ringed octopus (*Hapalochlaena maculosa*), which injects it as a venom; chemically similar or identical to tetrodotoxin.

mad cow disease. *See* bovine spongiform encephalopathy.

maedi. An infectious disease of sheep, caused by the maedi-visna retrovirus.

maggot. A fly larva.

malaria. (1) Any of four infectious diseases caused by protozoa in the genus *Plasmodium* and transmitted by mosquitoes. (2) *See* malignant tertian malaria.

malignant tertian malaria. The most severe form of malaria, caused by the protozoan *Plasmodium falciparum*.

Malta fever. *See* brucellosis.

MAP. *Mycobacterium avium paratuberculosis* or *Mycobacterium paratuberculosis*. A bacterium that causes illness in cattle and possibly also Crohn's disease in humans.

Marburg hemorrhagic fever. An infectious disease caused by a filovirus.

marijuana. The dried leaves and flowering tops of the female hemp plant (*Cannabis sativa*).

MDRTB. Multi-drug-resistant tuberculosis.

measles or **red measles**. An infectious disease caused by a paramyxovirus.

melioidosis. An infectious disease caused by the bacterium *Pseudomonas pseudomallei*.

meningitis. Inflammation of the meninges (membranes surrounding the brain and spinal cord).

meningococcal disease. A form of meningitis caused by the bacterium *Neisseria meningitidis*.

meningococcus. The bacterium *Neisseria meningitidis*.

methicillin. A form of penicillin that is resistant to an enzyme produced by staphylococci.

mescal bean. A shrub (*Sophora secundiflora*) that contains toxic and psychoactive chemicals.

mescaline. A hallucinogen found in the mescal cactus (*Lophophora williamsii*) and certain other plants.

microcystin. A liver toxin produced by certain cyanobacteria.

microorganism. An organism that is too small to observe in detail without a microscope, such as the bacteria and single-celled algae.

mildew. A whitish growth or discoloration on organic matter, caused by various fungi.

milk sickness. (1) An intoxication caused by drinking milk from cows that have eaten the white snakeroot plant (*Eupatorium rugosum*). (2) Diphasic milk fever, a form of viral encephalitis that can be transmitted in raw milk. (3) A slight fever in humans after parturition, not associated with infection. (4) A severe paralytic disease of dairy cattle after parturition. (5) Lactose intolerance in humans. (6) A name once applied to almost any illness in a young infant.

mitotic poison. One that interferes with cell division.

MMR. A vaccine that protects children against measles, mumps, and rubella.

monkeypox. An acute infectious disease similar to smallpox and caused by a related poxvirus.

mononucleosis. *See* infectious mononucleosis.

morbidity rate. The incidence rate, with reference to an entire population.

morbilli. *See* measles.

morphine. An addictive narcotic drug derived from opium, used as an analgesic and sedative.

mortality rate. The number of deaths occurring in a population during a given time period, divided by the total number of persons or animals in the affected population. Total or crude mortality refers to deaths from all causes, whereas a disease-specific mortality rate is limited to deaths from one disease.

mosaic virus. Any of several viruses that cause plant diseases.

MSRA. Methicillin-resistant *Staphylococcus aureus*.

mud fever. *See* leptospirosis.

mumps. An infectious disease caused by a paramyxovirus.

muscarine. A neurotoxin produced by any of several mushrooms.

mussel poisoning. *See* saxitoxin.

mutagen. Any agent that causes mutations (changes in cellular DNA).

myiasis. Infestation with fly larvae.

mycobacteriosis. Infection with bacteria in the genus *Mycobacteria*.

mycoplasma. Any of a group of small bacteria without a cell wall.

mycosis. An infection or disease caused by a fungus.

mycotoxin. A toxin produced by a fungus.

myotoxin. A toxin that acts primarily on the muscles.

mytilotoxin. *See* saxitoxin.

myxovirus. An old name for the orthomyxoviruses and paramyxoviruses.

nagana. The equivalent of African sleeping sickness in cattle.

natural killer cell or **NK cell**. A large, granular lymphocyte that recognizes and kills certain types of tumor cells and cells infected with some viruses.

NBC. Nuclear, biological and chemical warfare.

necrotic arachnidism. *See* loxoscelism.

necrotizing fasciitis. A severe invasive disease caused by group A streptococci.

nematocyst. A stinging structure found in jellyfish.

nematode. Any of a group of elongated, cylindrical worms, some of them parasitic and others free-living.

neonatal herpes. A severe disease of infants who contract HSV during or soon after birth.

nephropathia epidemica. An infectious disease caused by the Puumala virus, a hantavirus.

nettle. Any of several plants (*Urtica* and related genera) with hollow stinging hairs that inject irritating chemicals.

neurotoxicant. Any poison that acts on the nervous system.

neurotoxin. A toxin that acts on the nervous system.

Newcastle disease. An infectious disease of chickens, caused by a paramyxovirus.

NGU. Nongonococcal urethritis; inflammation of the urethra, not caused by gonorrhea.

nicotine. A poisonous alkaloid found in tobacco and other plants.

nightmare weke. A tropical goatfish (*Upeneus arge*), which produces a toxin that can cause violent nightmares and hallucinations in persons who eat its flesh.

nightshade. Any of a group of toxic plants in the family Solanaceae.

Nipah virus. A paramyxovirus that infects livestock and humans, causing a form of encephalitis.

nocardiosis. A chronic infectious disease caused by the bacterium *Nocardia asteroides*.

non-A non-B hepatitis. Old name for hepatitis C.

Norwalk virus. A foodborne calicivirus that causes gastroenteritis.

nosocomial infection. An infection that originates in a medical facility.

notifiable disease. A disease that must be brought to the attention of a health agency (such as the CDC or OIE), once detected or suspected.

ocular herpes. A herpesvirus infection of the eye (the site of about 3% of all primary HSV infections).

OIE. The Office International des Epizootie in Paris, France.

onchocerciasis. A chronic infectious disease caused by the nematode *Onchocerca volvulus*.

o'nyong-nyong fever. A mosquito-borne hemorrhagic fever caused by a togavirus.

opium. An addictive narcotic drug made from the opium poppy (*Papaver somniferum*).

OPV. Oral polio vaccine.

orthomixovirus. Any of a group of RNA viruses that cause influenza in humans.

otitis media. Inflammation of the middle ear.

outbreak. A sudden rise in the incidence of a disease or the numbers of a harmful organism within a given area. Compare epidemic.

ovale malaria. A relatively mild form of malaria caused by the protozoan *Plasmodium ovale*.

PAHO. Pan American Health Organization.

palytoxin. A toxin produced by a type of coral.

pandemic. A major outbreak of a disease over a wide geographic area.

papillomavirus. Any of a group of papovaviruses associated with human diseases such as warts and cervical cancer.

papovavirus. Any of a group of DNA viruses that cause warts and various types of tumors.

pappataci fever. *See* sandfly fever.

paramyxovirus. Any of a group of RNA viruses that cause diseases such as mumps and measles.

parasite. Any organism that lives in or on the body of a larger organism of a different species, called the host, on which the parasite depends for food.

parasitic disease. A disease caused by infestation with a parasite.

paratrachoma. *See* conjunctivitis.

paratyphoid fever. An infectious disease caused by several species of bacteria in the genus *Salmonella*.

parrot fever. *See* psittacosis.

passive immunity. *See* immunity.

pasteurization. Partial sterilization of a substance (such as milk) by heat or radiation.

pathogen. A bacterium, virus, or other agent that causes disease.

pathogenicity. The capability of an infectious agent to cause disease in a susceptible host.

patient zero. The first known patient with a disease under investigation.

pediculosis. Infestation with lice.

PEP. Postexposure prophylaxis.

peptide. A molecule consisting of two or more amino acids; a component of a protein.

pertussis. *See* whooping cough.

pest. (1) Any organism that causes economic harm to humans by damaging crops, livestock, or their stored products. (2) An old name for plague.

pesticide. Any chemical used to kill any unwanted lower organisms.

peyote. A hallucinogenic drug made from the mescal cactus (*Lophophora williamsii*).

pharyngotonsillitis. Inflammation of the throat and tonsils, caused by any of a number of different viruses and bacteria.

phlebotomus fever. *See* sandfly fever.

phthisis. Old name for tuberculosis.

picornavirus. Any of a group of RNA viruses that cause diseases such as poliomyelitis, hepatitis A, and foot-and-mouth disease.

pinkeye. *See* conjunctivitis.

pinta. An infectious disease caused by the spirochete *Treponema carateum*.

pinworm. The parasitic roundworm *Enterobius vermicularis*.

pit viper. Any of a group of snakes with a sensory pit on each side of the head.

placental transfer. Transfer (of an infectious agent, toxin, or other entity) from a female mammal to a fetus via the placenta.

plague. (1) An infectious disease caused by the bacterium *Yersinia pestis*. (2) Any major disease epidemic. *See* bubonic plague; pneumonic plague; sylvatic plague.

plasmid. A small, circular DNA molecule that can be transferred from one bacterium to another, conferring characteristics such as antibiotic resistance.

pleurodynia. An infectious disease caused by the Coxsackie B virus.

pneumocystis pneumonia. Pneumonia caused by the bacterium *Pneumocystis carinii*.

pneumonia. An inflammatory disease of the lungs, caused by any of a variety of bacteria, fungi, viruses, or chemicals.

pneumonic pasteurellosis. An infectious disease of cattle, caused by the bacterium *Pasteurella haemolytica*.

pneumonic plague. (1) A secondary pneumonia in patients with bubonic plague. (2) A highly infectious, usually fatal primary pneumonia resulting from inhalation of the agent of plague.

poison. Any chemical agent that kills or harms an organism.

poison oak and **poison ivy**. Plants in the genus *Toxicodendron* that cause dermatitis as a result of delayed contact sensitivity in about 80 percent of people.

poisonous. Having the properties or effects of a poison.

poliomyelitis or **polio**. An infectious disease caused by a picornavirus.

poliovirus. The picornavirus that causes poliomyelitis in humans.

pollinosis. Hay fever caused by pollen.

polypeptide. A chain of amino acids; a component of a protein.

Pontiac fever. *See* legionellosis.

postherpetic neuralgia (PHN). A complication of shingles (herpes zoster) in which the patient continues to feel pain after the skin lesions have crusted.

potentiation. A situation in which a chemical is not toxic in itself, but increases the toxicity of another chemical when the two are administered together.

poxvirus. Any of a group of DNA viruses that cause diseases such as smallpox and cowpox.

predator. An animal that obtains food by killing other animals.

prevalence rate. The percentage of persons or animals in a population having a certain disease or condition at a given time.

prion. An infectious particle composed entirely of protein.

progressive rubella panencephalitis. A progressive neurological disorder occurring in a child with congenital rubella (German measles).

prokaryote. A single-celled organism that lacks a distinct nucleus.

prophage. Viral DNA that has become integrated into a bacterial chromosome.

prophylaxis. The prevention of disease.

protist. An organism in the kingdom Protista, which includes the protozoa and some of the algae. Some taxonomists also include the bacteria and fungi in the Protista, whereas others place these organisms in separate kingdoms, the Monera and Fungi, respectively.

provirus. Viral DNA that has become integrated into a host cell's chromosomes.

pruritis. Itching.

pseudorabies. An infectious disease of swine and other livestock, caused by a herpesvirus.

psilocybin. A hallucinogen produced by the fungus *Psilocybe mexicana*.

psittacosis. An infectious disease of birds that can be transmitted to humans; caused by the bacterium *Chlamydia psittaci*.

PSP. Paralytic shellfish poisoning; see saxitoxin.

ptomaine. An indefinite term applied to poisonous substances (such as toxic amines) formed during bacterial decomposition of protein.

puerperal fever. Infection that occurs after childbirth, caused by various microorganisms including E. coli and group A streptococci.

purpura. Purple patches from bleeding under the skin or mucous membranes.

pustule. A small elevation of the skin that contains pus.

Q fever. An infectious disease caused by the rickettsia *Coxiella burneti*.

quarantine. A state of enforced isolation, usually to prevent the spread of a disease.

quartan malaria. A mild form of malaria caused by the protozoan *Plasmodium malariae*.

quinine. An antimalarial drug made from the bark of the cinchona tree.

quinsy. An abscess near a tonsil, usually caused by a bacterial infection.

rabbit fever. *See* tularemia.

rabies. An infectious disease caused by the rabies virus, one of the rhabdoviruses.

rat-bite fever. An infectious disease, transmitted as the name implies; caused by the bacteria *Streptobacillus moniliformis* and *Spirillum minor*.

recluse. Any of several venomous spiders (*Loxosceles*).

red measles. *See* measles.

red tide. A proliferation of certain types of ocean plankton that produce toxins.

relapsing fever. Either of two infectious diseases caused by spirochetes in the genus *Borrelia*, transmitted by ticks and lice, respectively.

reovirus. Any of a group of RNA viruses that cause diseases such as Colorado tick fever; some related viruses infect plants and invertebrates.

reservoir. (1) Any human beings, wild or domestic animals, plants, soil, or inanimate matter in which an infectious agent normally lives and multiplies. (2) A supply of drinking water.

resistance. The total effect of the body's mechanisms for resisting the invasion or multiplication of infectious agents or damage by their toxic products; includes the various forms of acquired immunity plus inherent resistance. *See* immunity.

respiratory syncytial virus (RSV). A paramyxovirus that causes upper and lower respiratory tract disease in humans.

Reston virus. A filovirus similar to the Ebola virus.

retrovirus. Any of a group of RNA viruses that possess the reverse transcriptase enzyme, which enables them to copy their RNA into

DNA that enters a host cell chromosome. Some retroviruses cause serious diseases such as AIDS and cancer, whereas others appear harmless.

reverse zoonosis. An infection or infectious disease that is transmissible from human beings to livestock or other vertebrate animals.

Reye syndrome. An acute, potentially fatal metabolic disease seen primarily in children, often following an infectious disease such as chickenpox.

rhabdovirus. Any of a group of RNA viruses that cause diseases such as rabies in humans and vesicular stomatitis in cattle.

rheumatic fever. A group A streptococcal infection that may cause damage to the heart valves.

rhinitis. Inflammation of the mucous membrane of the nose.

rhinovirus. A picornavirus that may cause the majority of cases of the common cold in humans, as well as foot-and-mouth disease in cattle.

ricin. A toxin produced by the castor bean plant (*Ricinus communis*).

rickettsia. Any of a group of bacteria that can live only as parasites inside cells.

rickettsialpox. An infectious vectorborne disease caused by *Rickettsia akari*.

Rift Valley fever (RVF). A vectorborne hemorrhagic fever of livestock that can be transmitted to humans; caused by a bunyavirus.

rinderpest. An infectious disease of livestock and wildlife that has caused major epidemics; caused by a paramyxovirus related to the human measles virus.

ringworm. Not a worm, but a common disease of the skin or nails caused by several species of fungi (*Microsporum* and *Trichophyton*).

risk. The probability of exposure to a given hazard, combined with the probability of being harmed by that exposure.

risk assessment. The process of identifying hazards and measuring and prioritizing their associated risks.

river blindness. *See* onchocerciasis.

RNA virus. A virus in which the genetic material consists of ribonucleic acid (RNA).

Rocky Mountain spotted fever. An infectious disease caused by *Rickettsia rickettsi* and transmitted by ticks.

rodenticide. Any chemical used to kill rodents.

roseola. An infectious disease of young children, caused by the HHV-6 and HHV-7 herpesviruses.

rotavirus. A reovirus that causes severe diarrhea in children.

roundworm. *See* nematode.

rubella. A usually mild infectious disease caused by a togavirus; can cause severe birth defects if contracted by a pregnant woman in the first trimester.

rubeola. *See* measles.

rust. Any of several plant diseases caused by fungi.

sad horse disease. *See* Borna disease.

Saint Anthony's fire. *See* ergotism.

Saint Louis encephalitis (SLE). A form of encephalitis caused by a togavirus and transmitted by mosquitoes.

salmonellosis. Infection with bacteria of the genus *Salmonella*.

sandfly fever. (1) An infectious disease caused by any of several bunyaviruses transmitted by the sandfly (*Phlebotomus* and other genera). (2) *See* also leishmaniasis.

saponin. Any of a group of chemicals found in certain plants; most are toxic and produce a soapy lather.

saxitoxin. A toxin produced by the dinoflagellate *Gonyaulax* and other plankton; sometimes concentrated in the tissues of clams, mussels, oysters, and scallops, which then become poisonous. The result of ingesting the toxin is called paralytic shellfish poisoning (PSP).

scabies. Infestation with the mite *Sarcoptes scabiei*.

scarlet fever or **scarlatina**. A group A streptococcal disease characterized by a skin rash and high fever.

schistosomiasis. Infestation with blood flukes (trematodes) in the genus *Schistosoma*.

scombroid poisoning. A type of food poisoning that results from ingestion of inadequately preserved scombroid (tuna and mackerel) or other fish containing high levels of histamine produced by the action of normally present bacteria.

scombrotoxin. Histamine and other amines produced in dead fish by certain bacteria.

scrapie. An infectious disease of sheep, caused by a prion.

screwworm. The parasitic larva of either of two fly species: New World screwworm, *Cochliomyia hominivorax*, or Old World screwworm, *Chrysomya bezziana*.

scrofula. Tuberculosis of the lymph nodes of the neck.

selective toxicity. Toxicity to one type of living matter but not to another (e.g., a the ability of a pesticide to kill pests but not crops).

sensitization. The process of becoming sensitized (allergic) to an antigen.

sepsis. A toxic condition resulting from the spread of bacteria or their products form a focus of infection.

septicemia. Invasion of the bloodstream by virulent microorganisms from a local seat of infection.

seroconversion. The appearance of an antibody in the blood.

seroprevalence. The percentage of a population whose blood tests positive for a given pathogen.

serotype or **serovar**. A group of closely related microorganisms with a common set of antigens.

Shiga toxin. A toxin produced by bacteria in the genus *Shigella*.

shigellosis. An infectious disease caused by any of several bacteria in the genus *Shigella*.

shingles. A disease that occurs when the dormant varicella virus becomes reactivated many years after a chickenpox infection.

ship fever. *See* epidemic typhus.

shipping fever. *See* pneumonic pasteurellosis.

shock. A state of profound physical and mental depression that may result from severe injury, infection, or anaphylaxis.

sick building syndrome or **sick house syndrome**. A situation in which occupants of a building report symptoms such as fatigue, headaches, or difficulty in concentrating; variously attributed to fungi, unidentified chemicals, or psychological factors.

sin nombre virus (SNV). The bunyavirus that causes hantavirus pulmonary syndrome.

Sindbis fever. A mosquito-borne infectious disease caused by a group A togavirus.

slow viral disease. A chronic degenerative disease with a prolonged incubation, such as subacute sclerosing panencephalitis (rubeola virus) and progressive rubella panencephalitis (rubella virus).

slow virus. A virus or virus-like agent associated with a slow viral disease.

smallpox. An infectious disease caused by the variola poxvirus; now eradicated worldwide, except for laboratory specimens.

sodoku. *See* rat-bite fever.

source (of infection). The person, animal, object, or substance from which an infectious agent passes directly to a susceptible host.

Spanish influenza. The strain of influenza virus that caused the pandemic of 1918-1919.

spirochete. Any of a group of gram-negative bacteria that are helically coiled; several are responsible for human diseases.

spoilage. Any disagreeable change in a food that can be detected with the senses.

sporadic. Occurring singly rather than in groups.

spore. A small reproductive body produced by some plants, fungi, bacteria, and protozoa.

sporotrichosis. An infectious disease caused by the fungus *Sporothrix schenckii*.

stachybotrys. A toxigenic black fungus (*Stachybotrys chartarum*) that grows in buildings, often in water-damaged areas.

staphylococci. Bacteria of the genus *Staphylococcus*.

sticky eye. *See* conjunctivitis.

strep throat. An acute sore throat caused by group A streptococci.

streptococci. Bacteria of the genus *Streptococcus*.

subacute sclerosing panencephalitis (SSPE). A progressive, usually fatal brain disorder occurring months to years after an attack of measles.

suppressor T cell. A T lymphocyte involved in the regulation of the immune system.

susceptible. Capable of contracting a given disease if exposed.

SV-40. Simian virus 40, a monkey virus that causes cancer in laboratory animals.

swamp fever. (1) Malaria. (2) Equine infectious anemia.

swimmer's itch. *See* schistosomiasis.

swine fever. *See* African swine fever; classical swine fever.

swine flu. *See* influenza.

swine vesicular disease (SVD). An infectious disease of swine, caused by a picornavirus.

swineherd's disease. *See* leptospirosis.

sylvatic plague. *See* plague.

synergistic effect. A situation in which the combined effect of two chemicals is greater than the sum of the effects of the individual chemicals if administered alone.

syphilis. A sexually transmitted disease caused by the spirochete *Treponema pallidum*.

T cell or **T lymphocyte**. Any of several types of small, antigen-specific lymphocyte that are involved in cellular immune reactions and antibody production.

taeniasis. Infestation with tapeworms, especially the beef tapeworm.

tapeworm. Any of a class of parasitic worms (Cestoda) found in humans and other vertebrates.

target organ. The site in the body where a given toxin causes its major effects.

tarichatoxin. A toxin produced by newts in the genus *Taricha*; chemically identical to tetrodotoxin.

teratogen. Any agent that causes defects in embryonic development.

tetanus. An acute infectious disease caused by a toxin produced by the anaerobic bacterium *Clostridium tetani*.

tetrodotoxin. A toxin produced by several species of pufferfish, ocean sunfishes, and porcupinefishes. *See* also maculotoxin; tarichatoxin.

three-day fever. *See* sandfly fever.

thrush. Oral candidiasis.

tick fever. Usually refers to Rocky Mountain spotted fever.

tickborne typhus fever. *See* Rocky Mountain spotted fever.

tinea. *See* ringworm.

tobamovirus. Tobacco mosaic virus.

togavirus. Any of a group of RNA viruses that cause diseases such as encephalitis and rubella.

tolerance. A state of decreased responsiveness to a toxic effect of a chemical, resulting from prior exposure.

TORCH infections. A group of infectious diseases that can cause birth defects if a pregnant woman contracts them; stands for toxoplasmosis, "other" (mainly varicella, Venezuelan equine encephalitis, mumps, coxsackievirus, parvovirus, and HIV), rubella, cytomegalovirus, and herpes.

toxic. Poisonous; having the properties or effects of a toxin.

toxic shock syndrome (TSS). A severe, invasive infection caused by *Staphylococcus aureus*, Group A streptococci, and other bacteria; has occurred with improper tampon use and as a complication of skin abscesses and nasal surgery.

toxicology. The study of the nature, effects, and detection of poisons in living organisms.

toxigenic. Producing a toxin or toxins.

toxin. A poison derived from a plant, animal, fungus, or microorganism.

toxocariasis. Infestation with the roundworm *Toxocara*.

toxoplasmosis. An infectious disease caused by the coccidian protozoan *Toxoplasma gondii*.

tracheal mite. A parasitic mite (*Acarapis woodi*) that infests honeybee colonies.

trachoma. An infectious eye disease caused by the bacterium *Chlamydia trachomatis*.

transmissible disease. *See* communicable disease.

transmissible spongiform encephalopathy (TSE). Any of a group of progressive neurological disorders including BSE in cattle, scrapie in sheep, and CJD in humans.

transmission (of an infectious agent). Any mechanism that exposes a susceptible host to an infectious agent.

trematode. Any of a group of parasitic flatworms.

trembles. An intoxication in cows that ingest the white snakeroot plant (*Eupatorium rugosum*).

trich. Slang term for trichomoniasis.

trichinellosis. *See* trichinosis.

trichinosis. A foodborne disease caused by the roundworm *Trichinella spiralis*.

trichomoniasis. A sexually transmitted disease caused by the protozoan *Trichomonas vaginalis*.

trichothecene. Any of a group of mycotoxins produced by molds such as *Fusarium*.

trypanosomiasis. An infectious disease caused by any of several protozoa in the genus *Trypanosoma*.

tuberculosis. A chronic infectious disease caused by *Mycobacterium tuberculosis* in humans and by *M. bovis* in livestock.

tularemia. An infectious disease caused by the bacterium *Francisella* (also called *Pasteurella*) *tularensis*.

type I allergic reaction. An allergic reaction caused by IgE antibodies (anaphylaxis or atopy).

type II allergic reaction. An allergic reaction caused by IgG and IgM antibodies.

type III allergic reaction. An immune complex disease.

type IV allergic reaction. A delayed-type (cell-mediated) allergic reaction.

typhoid fever. An infectious disease caused by the bacterium *Salmonella typhi*.

typhus fever. *See* endemic typhus; epidemic typhus.

ulcer. A persistent sore on the skin or a mucous membrane.

ulcer disease. An infection caused by the bacterium *Helicobacter pylori*, causing ulcers (sores) in the lining of the stomach or duodenum.

undulant fever or **undulating fever.** An infectious disease of livestock and humans, caused by the bacterium *Brucella abortus*.

urticaria. An allergic reaction with itching and raised edematous patches of skin or mucous membrane; hives.

urushiol. Any of several sensitizing chemicals found in the sap of poison ivy and related plants.

vaccination. The act of administering a vaccine.

vaccine. A preparation of killed, attenuated, or fully virulent microorganisms that is administered to produce or enhance immunity to a specific disease.

vaccinia. The poxvirus that causes cowpox.

valley fever. *See* coccidioidomycosis.

vancomycin. An antibiotic used against certain gram-positive bacteria.

varicella. *See* chickenpox.

variola. *See* smallpox.

variolation. An early form of smallpox vaccination.

varroa bee mite. A parasitic mite (*Varroa jacobsoni*) that infests honeybee colonies.

Glossary

vector. An insect or other invertebrate that transmits an infectious agent to a vertebrate host.

vehicleborne transmission. Transmission of an infectious agent to a susceptible host by way of a contaminated inanimate object, such as food, water, utensils, or clothing.

Venezuelan equine encephalitis. A form of encephalitis caused by a group A togavirus and transmitted by mosquitoes; may cause defects in a developing fetus.

venom. A poison that is secreted by certain animals and usually transmitted by biting or stinging.

venomous. Describes an animal that produces venom.

verruca. Warts.

vesicle. A small, fluid-filled blister on the skin.

vibrio. A bacterium of the genus *Vibrio*.

vibriosis. A disease caused by a vibrio, such as cholera.

violin spider. *See* recluse.

viper. Any of a family of snakes (Viperidae) that includes the Old World puff adders and vipers. Compare pit viper.

viral carditis. Inflammation of the myocardium or pericardium resulting from infection with any of a number of viruses.

viral meningitis. Meningitis caused by a virus (usually a picornavirus, arenavirus, or herpesvirus).

viral pneumonia. Pneumonia caused by a viral infection.

viremia. The presence of a virus in the bloodstream.

virion. A mature virus particle consisting of a nucleic acid core, a protein coat, and (in some cases) an outer lipid envelope.

viroid. A small circle of RNA that causes various plant diseases; replicated entirely by host cell enzymes and transmitted from plant to plant by insect vectors.

virulence. The ability of an agent to cause disease in a given host.

viruria. The presence of living viruses in the urine.

virus. An extremely small organism that can reproduce only as a parasite inside a living cell; classified as nonliving by some biologists.

visna. An infectious disease of sheep, caused by the maedi-visna retrovirus.

vivax malaria. *See* benign tertian malaria.

VRE. Vancomycin-resistant enterococci.

waterborne disease. A disease caused by an infectious agent that is present in water used for drinking or bathing.

weed. (1) Any plant that grows where it is not wanted. (2) A slang term for marijuana.

WER. Weekly Epidemiological Record, World Health Organization.

western equine encephalitis (WEE). A form of encephalitis caused by a group A togavirus and transmitted by mosquitoes.

West Nile encephalitis. A form of encephalitis caused by a group B togavirus and transmitted by mosquitoes.

whipworm. The nematode *Trichuris trichiura*.

white plague. *See* tuberculosis.

WHO. World Health Organization.

whooping cough. An infectious disease caused by the bacterium *Bordetella pertussis*.

wilt. Any of several plant diseases.

woolsorters' disease. *See* anthrax.

yaws. An infectious disease caused by the spirochete *Treponema pertenue*.

yellow fever. An infectious disease caused by a flavivirus and transmitted by mosquitoes.

yersiniosis. An infectious disease caused by bacteria in the genus *Yersinia*.

YLD. Years of life lived with disability.

YLL. Years of life lost.

zoonosis. An infection or infectious disease that is transmissible under natural conditions from vertebrate animals to human beings.

zoophobia. A pathological fear of animals.

Index

Index

Index

Index

Index

Index

Index

Index

About the Author

JOAN R. CALLAHAN is the award-winning author of numerous biological journal papers, environmental science documents, science and engineering books, and magazine articles. She received her doctorate in zoology from the University of Arizona and has worked as a consultant and researcher, most recently with a grant from the USGS Biological Resources Division. Her latest book is *Recent Advances and Issues in Environmental Science* (Oryx Press, 2000).